Mindfulness-Based Cognitive Therapy for Chronic Pain

Mindfulness-Based Cognitive Therapy for Chronic Pain

A Clinical Manual and Guide

Melissa A. Day

WILEY Blackwell

This edition first published 2017

Registered Office
John Wiley & Sons Ltd, The Atrium, Southern Gate, Chichester, West Sussex, PO19 8SQ, UK

Editorial Offices
350 Main Street, Malden, MA 02148-5020, USA
9600 Garsington Road, Oxford, OX4 2DQ, UK
The Atrium, Southern Gate, Chichester, West Sussex, PO19 8SQ, UK

For details of our global editorial offices, for customer services, and for information about how to apply for permission to reuse the copyright material in this book please see our website at www.wiley.com/wiley-blackwell.

Library of Congress Cataloging-in-Publication Data

Names: Day, Melissa A., author.
Title: Mindfulness-based cognitive therapy for chronic pain : a clinical manual and guide / Melissa A. Day.
Description: Chichester, West Sussex ; Malden, MA : John Wiley & Sons Inc., 2017. | Includes bibliographical references and index.
Identifiers: LCCN 2016051987| ISBN 9781119257615 (cloth) | ISBN 9781119257905 (paper) | ISBN 9781119257646 (epub) | ISBN 9781119257653 (pdf)
Subjects: LCSH: Chronic pain–Alternative treatment. | Mindfulness-based cognitive therapy.
Classification: LCC RB127 .D3934 2017 | DDC 616/.0472–dc23
LC record available at https://lccn.loc.gov/2016051987

A catalogue record for this book is available from the British Library.

Cover Design: Wiley
Cover Image: Laurie Prentice-Dunn

MIX
Paper from responsible sources
FSC® C013604
FSC
www.fsc.org

To all people living with unremitting pain and those who are working with them to alleviate their suffering.

Contents

Foreword

When I first heard about the proposal to develop a version of MBCT (Mindfulness-Based Cognitive Therapy) for patients living with chronic pain, I wondered whether acronyms had been confused, didn't they mean MBSR (Mindfulness-Based Stress Reduction)? Wasn't MBSR introduced to the world in the early 1980s through studies showing its impact on reducing chronic pain? Isn't chronic pain the "domain" of MBSR, whereas depression and anxiety are the "domain" of MBCT? These may have been quaint notions in the early days of the development and dissemination of MBSR and MBCT, but it is clear that they no longer apply. The participants who find their way into these interventions are often presenting with multiple diagnoses and, as has been amply demonstrated in the literature, pain and depression are often comorbid. We no longer have (if we ever did have) the conceptual luxury of segregating patients by diagnoses to treatments that address a singular problem. The answer instead, is to find the mechanisms that contribute to the perpetuation of symptoms and then find increasingly efficient and targeted ways of teaching patients how to address them.

This is exactly why Melissa Day's book outlining MBCT for chronic pain is so important. It represents a second generational format of the original MBCT framework that Mark Williams, John Teasdale, and I developed over 20 years ago. Marshaling psychological, neural, and social evidence, Day has identified internal and external drivers of the pain response and then modified the MBCT program to accommodate these elements. It actually reminds me of our own trajectory when we discussed how exactly to reconfigure the MBSR platform for patients who were recovering from a mood disorder.

This book will be embraced by clinicians who are interested in exploring Day's approach. Clear illustrations of how the central cognitive-behavioral therapy (CBT) and mindfulness components address pain amplification and maintenance are tied to specific sessions in which these elements are taught. In addition, the book is sensitive to and supports treatment integrity by emphasizing the importance of the therapist's own mindfulness practice, both as a way of knowing what is being taught "from the inside," but also to embody mindfulness more generally in ways that communicate grounding and presence, even if distressing experiences are present.

Finally, it is clear to see that this book is written with an intention toward service. The treatment manual outlines the eight-session structure and is supplemented by curricula for the therapist, handouts of class material, troubleshooting tips, and a workbook for clients—practically a one-stop shop for delivering the therapy. This book will serve as a model for others who may be looking to modify existing mindfulness-based interventions for increasingly complex patient groups. For right now, it already provides a valuable template for helping patients learn how to change their relationship to chronic pain in meaningful and significant ways.

Zindel V. Segal, PhD
The University of Toronto

Acknowledgments

In writing this book, and indeed in life, I have been fortunate to be supported by the most wonderful family, friends, and mentors. To my late grandparents, I am grateful to have been shown the embodiment of humility and compassion. To my parents and brother, for steadfastly being there for me with unwavering support. My friends, for the sense of humor and fun you bring into my life. And thank you to my mentors, Dr. Beverly Thorn, Dr. Mark Jensen and Dr. Dawn Ehde, for your generosity, patience, and confidence in me. Special thanks to Laurie Prentice-Dunn for allowing me to use an image of her beautifully made quilt as the cover image for the book, and to Lars Vester for his talented sketches, which are included in the text. Finally, I would like to thank Darren Reed at Wiley, for supporting me throughout the publishing process of this, my first book.

About the Companion Website

This book is accompanied by a companion website:

www.wiley.com/go/day/mindfulness_based_cognitive_therapy

The website includes:

- Appendices
- MP3 meditations
- Appendix A. Pre-Treatment Client Handouts
- Appendix B. Meditation Scripts
- Appendix C. MBCT for Chronic Pain Management: Daily Home Practice Record
- Appendix D. Example Program Completion Certificate
- Appendix E. Mindfulness-Based Cognitive Therapy Adherence Appropriateness and Quality Scale (MBCT-AAQS)
- Appendix F. The Brief 4-Session Clinical Manual
- Appendix G. Client Handouts for the 8-session Clinical Manual

Introduction

Pain is symbiotic with the human condition, a universal experience. When pain persists and becomes chronic however, it can be the cause of intense and sometimes even relentless suffering. Chronic pain affects hundreds of millions of individuals worldwide and changes the entire landscape of a person's everyday existence: one's sense of self, relationships, employment and financial situation, hobbies ... no aspect of experience is left untouched. All that is encompassed in people's thoughts, emotions and behavior, our entire phenomenal experience comes to fall within the landscape of ongoing pain. Chronic pain, by its very nature, is recalcitrant to traditional biomedical treatments consisting of medications and surgery alone. To address the pervasive landscape of chronic pain, psychological approaches—such as the Mindfulness-Based Cognitive Therapy (MBCT) approach we explore in this text—are incredibly beneficial across a range of pain types and target not just pain reduction, but also improved function, mood, quality of life and one's overall sense of well-being.

The majority of people living with persistent pain have seen an array of medical practitioners and most typically have a medical record bulging with various test results (some of which have led to various "conclusive" diagnoses along the way), have tried an armamentarium of pain medications, and many have had surgeries ultimately deemed "failures" as the pain persists and in some cases worsens. In the search to find some way to experience relief, most people living with persistent pain fall into the role of a passive recipient of biomedically driven healthcare. The approach described in this book, however, reverses that role, and places the person living with pain firmly and powerfully in the driver's seat: actively taking charge of managing their pain, suffering, and beyond that, their life. Thus, the MBCT for chronic pain approach is intended to be a complement, or in some cases an alternative to a traditional biomedical approach to pain. For most people, however, MBCT delivered as an integrated component within an interdisciplinary care team represents the ideal approach, and indeed, interdisciplinary treatment is considered the gold standard in chronic pain management (Ehde, Dillworth, & Turner, 2014).

There are a number of reasons as to *why* psychological approaches such as MBCT are effective for pain, although one primary, encompassing reason is that

Mindfulness-Based Cognitive Therapy for Chronic Pain: A Clinical Manual and Guide, First Edition. Melissa A. Day.

Companion website: www.wiley.com/go/day/mindfulness_based_cognitive_therapy

living with chronic pain is stressful and stress makes pain and suffering worse. If we target and improve stress management and coping skills, by default we also target the pain. Your client may say they are in pain but not stressed: well, psychological approaches such as MBCT can still help as they have been shown to enhance descending inhibition and modulation of pain, changing the way the brain processes pain itself. So if you are wondering who should be referred to such an approach as MBCT for chronic pain, the answer is anyone with chronic pain who wants to suffer less, and do more.

I see myself as both a scientist and a clinician, and initially I was hesitant in writing this book as I wanted to ensure that we first had a sufficiently large evidence base on MBCT for pain before facilitating the ready availability of its use. However, in the context of the relatively recent release of Segal, Williams, and Teasdale's excellent second edition of their MBCT for depression text, and the rapidly growing body of research over the past decade supporting its use for the treatment of an array of conditions, it is clear that MBCT is formed on a solid conceptual basis. Indeed, the widespread interest in mindfulness more broadly is growing at an exponential rate. In a recent review paper I wrote with my colleagues we reported that between 1990 and 2006 the number of published scientific articles on mindfulness went from fewer than 80 to over 600, and at the time we were writing that article there existed over 1,200 research articles in PubMed devoted to the topic (Day, Jensen, Ehde, & Thorn, 2014). We are now just at the beginning of witnessing the potential of MBCT for managing chronic pain, which is a particularly promising time.

My intention in writing this book is to provide a resource that is highly practical and of use to those of you who are clinicians (both experienced and in-training), researchers, or both, so that we can further our collective understanding and use of MBCT for chronic pain. Hence, this manual is intended to "bridge the gap" between researchers and clinicians, and I write the text from this perspective, as a true scientist practitioner. This book is not intended to spark a new and "trendy" revolution in therapy and research for chronic pain management. But primarily to provide a further treatment option for researchers to explore and for clinicians to use when it seems other available treatments aren't working or perhaps when they don't appeal to the client sitting in front of them. Just as we have multiple forms of antidepressant medication for depression in order to (hopefully) find the one class that best suits a given individual, so too do we need a range of psychological treatment options for chronic pain. MBCT represents another approach to pain management that may just reach that client whose pain is refractory to other treatment approaches.

My overarching aim is that in essence this book teaches the basics of *how to do*, or deliver, MBCT for chronic pain. And at base, in delivering MBCT and indeed any psychological approach for chronic pain, it is essential that the delivering clinician have a solid, in depth, core knowledge of pain, including pain theory, the neurophysiology of pain, the cognitive, emotional, behavioral, and societal correlates of living with chronic pain, as well as pain assessment and treatment. However, a recent pain psychology national needs assessment conducted in the USA identified that only 28% of graduate and postgraduate psychology training programs include at least 11 hr of training in pain instruction, and more than one-third of the psychologists/therapists surveyed reported little or no education in treating pain (Darnall et al., 2016). Hence, if you feel unprepared to treat individuals with chronic pain, do not fear, you are not alone! Thus, Part I of this book is intended to provide a working knowledge base of pain and pain psychology and I provide references to additional learning resources throughout the book. I then transition into describing how this knowledge has informed the development and continued evolution of psychosocial approaches for chronic pain—the foundation upon which MBCT for chronic pain is built. I conclude Part I by introducing and describing the MBCT theoretical model as developed and subsequently applied to chronic pain.

Part II opens by providing an overview of the MBCT approach, which includes a description of the steps needed to prepare and "be ready" to deliver your first MBCT for chronic pain program. I suggest opportunities for further training in pain psychology and more specifically in delivering MBCT, describe practical considerations to address prior to starting up your first program, and include recommendations for tracking client progress to optimize outcomes and prevent premature drop-out and treatment failure. Then in Chapters 5 through 12, I provide step-by-step, detailed guidance on delivering the eight-session MBCT for chronic pain treatment. Each session includes a therapist outline as well as client handouts (also available for download for ease of distribution to your clients), and built in to each of the sessions are troubleshooting tips, illustrative case scenarios, and clinical experiences, as well as basic supervision so that you can enhance your delivery of this approach. Part II concludes with a number of suggested ways you can implement and adapt the MBCT for chronic pain manual for optimal use in your own clinical practice and research setting, along with some caveats and considerations for retaining treatment integrity when doing so.

A large number of online supplementary materials are included to further your learning and knowledge of the techniques and treatment structure, and to foster seamless implementation of this program in to your clinical or research setting. Pre-treatment client handouts to foster positive and realistic client expectations coming into treatment, meditation scripts for each meditation delivered along with downloadable MP3 guided audio files, session-related client handouts and meditation practice log record forms, a therapist fidelity monitoring form as well as a four-session version of the manual are all available for free download at the companion webpage. Additionally, I conclude the text with a number of other recommended excellent resources for continued and advanced learning opportunities.

This text brings together the efforts of innovative thinkers, both in the broad psychotherapy and pain literatures, to describe this fresh approach to traditional cognitive therapy that does hold so much promise for chronic pain management. The feedback I have received over time from clinicians I have trained in MBCT for pain is a resounding "Ahh, this is what I have been missing in my cognitive-behavioral therapy work." The integration of mindfulness into traditional cognitive-behavioral therapy adds a dimension of depth that resonates, feels genuine, and provides a unique approach to shifting patients from unhelpful cognitive, emotional, and behavioral patterns into a way of being with their pain that allows them to adaptively live a life of meaning and value. I hope that in presenting this work—which truly rests on the shoulders of the groundbreaking work of many skilled scientist-practitioners in both the broad psychotherapy and pain literatures—that it will further our combined efforts to give people living with daily pain a way to live a meaningful life, with pain and all. May it be of benefit.

References

Darnall, B. D., Scheman, J., Davin, S., Burns, J. W., Murphy, J. L., Wilson, A. C., … Mackey, S. C. (2016). Pain psychology: A global needs assessment and national call to action. *Pain Medicine, 17,* 250–263.

Day, M. A., Jensen, M. P., Ehde, D. M., & Thorn, B. E. (2014). Towards a theoretical model for mindfulness-based pain management. *Journal of Pain, 15*(7), 691–703.

Ehde, D. M., Dillworth, T. M., & Turner, J. A. (2014). Cognitive behavioural therapy for indiviudals with chronic pain: Efficacy, innovations and directions for research. *American Psychologist, 69*(2), 153–166.

Part I

Chronic Pain

1

Defining Chronic Pain and its Territory

At some point in our lives nearly all of us have experienced pain. What I call "bare bones pain" is adaptive and is as essential to our everyday existence as being able to see, hear, touch, taste, and smell. Pain is our most profound teacher, claiming our attention, implanting itself in memory, readily recalled at a hint of danger. Rare individuals born with a congenital insensitivity to pain experience an abnormal amount of injuries and infections due to their inability to perceive and respond appropriately to painful stimuli and usually die young (Melzack & Wall, 1982). Most of the time when we experience pain, it naturally diminishes as the source (i.e., the injury in whatever form) heals. However, in some instances, pain persists beyond the normal or expected healing time, may arise with or without an identifiable "cause," is unamenable to traditional biomedical treatment options, and it becomes chronic. Along with the territory of chronic pain often comes depressed mood, stress, loss of gainful employment, relationship strain, and a host of other compounding circumstances—the pain is no longer "bare bones."

The International Association for the Study of Pain (IASP), the world's largest interdisciplinary forum devoted to science, clinical practice, and education in the field of pain defines pain as: "An unpleasant sensory and emotional experience associated with actual or potential tissue damage, or described in terms of such damage" (IASP Taxonomy, 1994, Part III, p. 3). Inclusion of the terms "unpleasant" and "emotional" in this definition clearly delineates psychology as integral in the experience of both acute and chronic pain. While there are a variety of taxonomies used to distinguish acute vs. chronic pain, the most common is a temporal profile. Depending on the type of pain and the various definitions, "chronic" is rather arbitrarily demarcated typically as pain experienced at least half of the days of the past 3 or 6 months (IASP Subcommittee on Taxonomy, 1986; NIH, 2011). For pain arising primarily from a specific injury, this 3- or 6-month time frame refers to the time that extends past the "normal" expected healing process from the initial injury (IASP Taxonomy, 1994); however, it often proves exceedingly difficult to determine the end of the healing process (Apkarian, Baliki, & Geha, 2009). Therefore, many have argued that such a taxonomy for classifying chronic pain is inadequate (Apkarian, Hashmi, & Baliki, 2011), and instead, some researchers have focused efforts on identifying brain maps and biomarkers for differentiating acute from chronic pain. However, one aspect from the various

Mindfulness-Based Cognitive Therapy for Chronic Pain: A Clinical Manual and Guide,
First Edition. Melissa A. Day.

Companion website: www.wiley.com/go/day/mindfulness_based_cognitive_therapy

definitions that is now widely agreed upon is that chronic pain is inherently biopsychosocial in nature as opposed to simply a biomedical phenomenon that can be explained purely in terms of the amount of tissue damage (which was the popular view held right up until the 20th century). In using the MBCT approach to treat pain, it is first helpful to hold a working understanding of such historical perspectives, as well as to be familiar with (and to be able to explain to patients) the current knowledge base of each aspect that makes up the experience of pain: the biological, psychological or human experience, and social factors. Keeping in mind, though, that although these shared features of the experience of pain are common, in reality our experience of pain is deeply personal.

A Historical Perspective of Pain

The Biopsychosocial Model: Pain ≠ Just Broken Bones and Tissue Damage

Traditionally pain has been understood from a biomedical perspective that has equated the amount of pain experienced to the amount of underlying tissue damage in a 1:1 relationship. The biomedical model originated from the 17th century with Descartes' mind–body dualism philosophy, and dominated illness and pain conceptualization for almost 300 years, right up until approximately mid-way through the last century. Pain was described purely in reductionistic, mechanistic, physical terms and the brain was considered to play a passive, receptive role of pain signals; psychosocial factors were considered essentially irrelevant. However, Beecher, who served as a physician in the US Army during the Second World War, provided one of the most famous early documented examples of evidence refuting the biomedical perspective (Beecher, 1946). Of the civilians and soldiers that Beecher treated who had experienced compound fractures, penetrating wounds to the abdomen, lost limbs or other intensely painful injuries, Beecher noticed that the majority of the soldiers (as many as 75%) reported no to moderate pain, and required far less pain medication than the civilians with comparable injuries. Beecher documented that the differentiating factor seemed to be the *meaning* that the civilians and soldiers were attributing to the injury. To the soldiers, this was their ticket home—they were evacuated and returned to the US for recuperation; to the civilians on the other hand, they were to leave the hospital to return to their war-torn homeland, and to likely a loss of wages due to an inability to return to work.

Other research began to accumulate supporting Beecher's observations. As one eloquent research example, Jensen and colleagues (Jensen et al., 1994) conducted a magnetic resonance imaging (MRI) study examining the lumbar spines of asymptomatic individuals (i.e., people with no pain, or history of pain) and found that only 36% had normal intervertebral discs at all levels, while the firm majority (64%) had bulges of at least one (and typically more) lumbar disc. In another study, Keefe and colleagues demonstrated that coping strategies were more predictive of self-reported osteoarthritic knee pain than X-ray evidence of the disease (Keefe et al., 1987). Other everyday examples of where the level of injury doesn't necessarily map on to the amount of pain experienced include when we see athletes playing through a game with a severe injury, maybe we hear on the news about a parent running through fire to rescue their child from a burning house, and yogis during deep meditation will not feel pain.

These observations and empirical findings, and a plethora of findings from other studies, called in to question the very foundation that the biomedical model was built upon, and clearly showed that "verifiable" tissue damage is a poor indicator of pain, and that the brain plays a dynamic, central role in pain processing and perception. Thus, mounting dissatisfaction with the biomedical models' account for illness and pain culminated in a tipping point when Engel (1977) formally challenged this prevailing conceptualization and proposed the integrated biopsychosocial model. The biopsychosocial model redefined illness (including but not specific to pain) as an entity not entirely subsumed under the biological sphere. Instead, manifest illness development, maintenance, and progression were viewed as the result of the convergence of a multitude of internal and external, biological, psychological, emotional, social, and behavioral influences. The shifted emphasis in Engel's approach—away from the purely physical realm—aligned perfectly with Melzack and Wall's (1965) "Gate Control Theory," and together these two models fueled a zeitgeist in the way pain was assessed and treated.

The Neuromatrix Model of Pain

The Gate Control Theory—now known as the Neuromatrix Model of Pain—is often delivered as an educational component of psychological pain treatments (including MBCT, as you shall see) to convey the rationale to clients as to why psychological treatments work for *real* pain, so it is worth spending some time here to go over it in detail. In essence, this revolutionary theory proposed by Melzack and Wall was the first to formally hypothesize that the brain plays an active, dynamic role in the interpretive processes of the sensory experience of pain (Melzack, 2001, 2005; Melzack & Wall, 1965, 1982). This theory is in stark contrast to the biomedical conceptualization, where the brain was considered a passive recipient of pain signals from a peripheral pain generator (i.e., the identified "source" of injury/pain). The Gate Control Theory represented, for the first time, a conceptualization of pain that took into account the unique and highly interconnected role of neurophysiological pathways, thoughts, emotions, and behavior in determining the experience we call "pain." The original theory described how descending (inhibitory or excitatory) signals from the brain were the stimulus that opened or closed a gating mechanism in the spinal column, and that this mechanism ultimately controlled the amount of pain signals that could reach the brain. Specifically, the theory proposed that if the "gates" are narrowed or closed (i.e., if descending inhibitory signals from the brain predominate), fewer pain signals are processed in the brain and less pain is experienced; however, if the gates are wide open (i.e., if descending excitatory signals from the brain predominate) more pain signals are processed in the brain and the felt experience of pain is amplified.

The Gate Control Theory and the subsequent Neuromatrix Model paved the way for an ensuing body of neuroimaging research. Through the use of technology such as functional MRI, studies have conclusively demonstrated that critical pain pathways travel through brain areas closely interconnected with cognitive and emotional activity (e.g., the thalamus, anterior cingulated cortex, and limbic system), and Melzack and Wall were the first to emphasize that this neuromatrix had the capacity to inhibit or enhance the sensory flow of painful stimuli. This important research on pain in the brain has demonstrated that psychological processes can actually shape the way painful stimuli are interpreted by the brain and thereby provides convincing evidence that psychological interventions for the treatment of chronic pain hold tremendous potential.

Models of Stress

As I touched on in the Introduction, living with daily pain as a persistent companion is typically stressful, and stress in turn makes pain worse. Thus, an integral component in many pain treatments is learning to manage stress more effectively. Stress has become a popular term that is a catchphrase for a multiplicity of situations, pressures, and experiences—what one person experiences as stress though, another person might see as the environment in which to thrive. The term "stress" historically has origins in the field of physics, where it describes the force that produces a strain to bend or break an object; however, the way we typically use the word "stress" today was first coined by Seyle in the 1950s (Selye, 1956). Seyle was a pioneer in advancing our understanding of the physiological processes involved when animals are injured or placed under unusual or extreme conditions and he popularized use of the word "stress" to describe the nonspecific response (in mind and body) to any (internal or external) pressure or demand (Selye, 1956, 1973). This nonspecific stress response has since been identified to initiate through the action of the hypothalamic–pituitary–adrenal (HPA) axis and includes cognitive, emotional, physiological (including hormonal and immunological) sequalae, and the inciting factor in triggering this response was termed by Seyle as a "stressor" (Brodal, 2010; McEwan, 2007; Selye, 1956, 1973).

Evolutionarily, back in the days of the caveman, the stress response and the associated rush of adrenaline and other physiological changes served an adaptive, critical life-preserving function for facing off against often larger, faster, more powerful predators (i.e., the classic example of the "saber tooth tiger") where the options were to freeze, run, fight, or, as a last resort, play dead (Bracha, 2004). Unfortunately, however, this maintained function of the primitive brain lacks sophisticated differentiation ability and it is comparatively far less adaptive in the developed world today where this network is responsible for triggering essentially the same physiological response when you are not able to get a good cup of coffee. Further, Seyle observed that when the stress response is prolonged or we are exposed to unresolved stressors, this can lead to what he called "diseases of adaptation" where the once adaptive system breaks down over long periods of heightened elevation, and disease or illness ensues. Research has since confirmed that chronic stress leads to wide-ranging negative effects for the body (i.e., increases in blood pressure, blood sugar dysregulation, greater abdominal fat, hormone imbalances, reduced neurological and immune function, chronic systemic inflammation, and reduced muscle strength) and has been linked to an enormous range of health conditions, including heart attack, stroke, respiratory disease, autoimmune conditions, depression, and chronic pain (Day, Eyer, & Thorn, 2013).

Sometimes not being able to get a good cup of coffee *is* enough to put us over the edge. As absurd as we know it is after the fact, in that moment, sometimes the smallest things can cause us to lose it. Taking this into account, a powerfully influential model in the evolution of biopsychosocial treatments for chronic pain was Lazarus and Folkman's (1984) Transactional Model of Stress. This model recognized that it is not always so much about the quality of the external stressor that matters, but equally important is the quality of the thought processes, judgments, or appraisals about what that stressor *means* to us at any given moment in time (Lazarus & Folkman, 1984). Lazarus and Folkman qualitatively differentiated among certain types of cognitions, considering them at varying levels, including immediate judgments in reaction to changes in the environment (termed primary appraisals, such as a threat, loss, or challenge), thought processes developed to guide choice of coping strategies (secondary appraisals), and more deeply held beliefs acquired over time. In Lazarus and Folkman's model, stress is the end result of something happening in the environment that is judged to tax or exceed our resources or ability to cope. Given that the very nature of living with chronic pain often becomes in and of itself a persistent stressor that "opens the gates" and makes the pain *worse*, it is no surprise that clinical pain researchers adopted Lazarus and Folkman's Transactional Model for refining the understanding and treatment of chronic pain, emphasizing that treatment can intervene at any of their proposed levels of cognition (Thorn, 2004).

Neurophysiological Underpinnings (*Bio*psychosocial)

Pain in the Brain

Extensive anatomical and electrophysiological data emerging from human and animal studies have converged to paint a comprehensive, reliable picture of the "biological" or neurological element of how pain is perceived and processed primarily in various regions of the brain (Jensen, 2010). Generally, pain perception (termed nociception) is conceptualized as a process that can be broken down into four (highly fluid and interconnected) elements: (1) *transduction*, the conversion of the painful stimuli detected by the pain receptors to an electrical message; (2) *transmission*, the process by which the electrical pain message is transmitted to the spinal column and brain; (3) *modulation*, the specific areas of the brain, including sensory, cognitive, and emotional processing areas, that are directly involved in descending signals that modulate the experience of pain; and (4) *perception*, the result of the "neuromatrix" of pain processing areas in the brain that process the pain signal, ultimately resulting in awareness of the experience of pain (Day, in press-b). Although some processing of pain signals does occur at the spinal cord level, the actual *experience* of pain is now widely understood to be the result of supraspinal (i.e., above the spine) neural activity.

Thus, at base, the specialized pain neuronal pathways stemming from the peripheral pain receptor to the cerebral cortex of the brain, termed the nociceptive system, comprises these four elements (Schnitzler & Ploner, 2000).

The first element, *transduction*, starts with pain receptors in the skin, muscles, and internal organs which are free nerve endings of neuronal cells that are called "nociceptors." Nociceptors are on the receiving end of pain-causing, noxious stimuli in the form of intense mechanical, thermal, electrical, or chemical stimulation. Nociceptors detect the noxious stimuli and convert the message to an electrical pain signal (transduction). This signal is transmitted to the axon, which are the thread-like fibers of the nerve cell. Two types of nerve fibers are involved in transmitting pain signals: (1) fast, myelinated axons for sharp, immediate pain; and (2) slow, nonmyelinated axons for chronic, dull, steady pain. At some point or another you may have accidently touched the stove or bumped the edge of the oven while removing a cake, and you likely recall an immediate sharp pain—this pain was transmitted by the fast, myelinated axons that are activated by strong physical pressure and temperature stimulation. This leads to a reflexive recoil of your hand away from the hot surface (the mechanism of which I will describe in more detail momentarily). Even after you ran your hand under cold water, you probably still felt a dull, more defuse type of pain in your hand afterwards—this is due to the slow, nonmyelinated fibers that are activated by the release of chemicals in the skin tissue when damaged. This slower pain serves a rehabilitative function in that it reminds us to protect the damaged body part. For either of these types of pain to elicit a behavioral (or cognitive/emotional) response however, the pain-related signal first needs to be carried along the axon to the spinal column (initial stage of *transmission*).

Once at the spinal column, the first level of pain processing occurs in neurons located in the dorsal horn (i.e., part of the gray matter towards the back of the spine), which respond specifically to the signals from the initial receiving nociceptors (Schnitzler & Ploner, 2000). The signal is transmitted across synapses from the nociceptor to the spine at the dorsal horn via an electrochemical process in which neurotransmitters are released and convey the message of the noxious stimuli. The axons of the neurons in the dorsal horn then cross the midline of the spine within one or two segments, and ascend to the brain via several partially independent pathways located within the spinothalamic tract. Neurons along this tract serve as relay stations conveying the noxious message and at all levels these ascending signals may be modulated by descending signals from the brain (this *modulation* process is described later in this section). However, for fast pain fiber types (the myelinated fibers), an "immediate" withdrawal from the pain stimulus is sometimes needed to minimize harm. Thus, in the example above where you might have accidently touched the side of the oven with your hand, rather than wait for the pain signal to be transmitted all the way to your brain, there is also a reflex mechanism processed at several synaptic links at the spinal column—termed the nociceptive flexion reflex pathway—which causes your hand to immediately recoil from the burning oven surface even prior to your brain processing the experience of pain (Purves et al., 2001).

The conscious *perception* of pain occurs when the pain signals are conveyed to various regions of the brain. If pain signals did not reach the brain, we would not be aware of the experience of pain. Importantly, one of the first brain regions the ascending fibers of the spinothalamic tract project to is the medulla oblongata and the reticular formation; processing here affects consciousness (with the severest of pain causing unconsciousness), and cardiovascular and respiratory responses to pain. Other ascending fibers of the spinothalamic tract project to the thalamus, which acts as a relay station disseminating and projecting the pain signals to various distributed areas of the cortex in an extensive central network of pain processing (Schnitzler & Ploner, 2000). Research has consistently shown that the brain regions most closely linked to pain are the primary somatosensory cortex (sensory–discriminative aspects of pain), secondary somatosensory cortex (recognition, learning, and memory of painful experiences), limbic system (emotional processing of pain), and the anterior cingulate cortex (allocation of attentional resources to pain and processing of pain unpleasantness and motivational–motor aspects of pain), insula (involved in processing information about one's physical condition, autonomic reactions, and potentially in affective aspects of pain-related learning and memory), and the prefrontal cortex (general executive functions such as planning of complex responses to pain) (Bantick et al., 2002; Jensen, 2010; Schnitzler & Ploner, 2000).

In parallel to the processes and regions associated with the experience of pain are areas of the brain that are directly involved in descending signals and in centrally *modulating* the experience of pain. Therefore, the perception of pain is also a function of the degree of modulation concurrently present. These are termed "descending" modulatory pathways as they stem from areas of the brain that sit above where ascending pain pathways project from the spinal column to the brain. Descending modulation circuitry is proposed to arise from multiple cortical and subcortical areas of the brain (including the hypothalamus, amygdala, and the rostral anterior cingulate cortex) that feed in to the periaqueductal gray region (PAG), and with outputs from the PAG to the medulla (specifically the nucleus raphe magnus and the nucleus reticularis gigantocellularis located within the rostral ventromedial medulla) (Ossipov, Dussor, & Porreca, 2010). Activation of the PAG projects to the medulla and then to neurons in the spinal or medullary dorsal horns, thereby activating an opioid sensitive circuit that reduces pain (Ossipov et al., 2010). Studies since the 1970s have shown that electrical stimulation of the PAG leads to analgesia. In one early study, Reynolds found that electrical stimulation of the PAG caused profound analgesia so powerful that a laparotomy surgery could be performed in a fully conscious rat without observable signs of distress (Reynolds, 1969).

To this day, activation of this opioid sensitive circuit underlies the action of the most widely used pain-relieving drugs used in humans, including opiates, cannabinoids, nonsteroidal anti-inflammatories (NSAIDs), and serotonin/norepinephrine reuptake blockers (Ossipov et al., 2010). These advances in understanding of the central modulation of pain have led to substantially more effective pain management over the past several decades, especially for *acute* pain management (Ossipov et al., 2010). However, for *chronic* pain, the long-term use of pain-relieving drugs is often associated with minimal pain relief and substantial negative side-effects, including possible addiction, tolerance effects, constipation, rebound pain, impaired cognition, and nausea (Ashburn & Staats, 1999; Trescot et al., 2008).

Not only are there differences in the pain medication treatment approaches most suitable for acute vs. chronic pain, but the brain itself and how pain is processed has been shown to change as a function of ongoing, persistent pain.

The Neuro-Signature of the Transition from Acute to Chronic Pain

Research is emerging to suggest that the way in which pain is processed by the brain changes as a function of pain duration, and critical differences between the brain in acute pain vs. chronic pain have been identified. In attempting to discover the explanatory pathway(s) underlying the transition from acute to chronic pain, researchers are hoping eventually to identify ways to interrupt this pathway and prevent pain chronicity from occurring. This line of research is particularly pertinent to pain resulting from some form of initial traumatic injury (as opposed to other degenerative conditions, such as arthritis, for example). However, given central sensitization (i.e., maladaptive neuroplasticity that heightens neurological pain processing and sensitivity) in chronic pain is also a factor underlying worsening outcomes for essentially all types of chronic pain, the findings of this research agenda may eventually hold widespread applicability (Apkarian et al., 2011; Woolf, 2011).

A promising line of laboratory-based research has attempted to gain insight into the transition from acute to chronic pain by comparing the brain activity of healthy individuals to those with chronic pain. One widely cited study implementing this approach utilized an experimental pain paradigm (specifically using a thermal pain stimulus) to examine the neurological response to the acute pain stimulus in the brains of healthy controls to those with a diagnosis of chronic low back pain (Baliki, Geha, Fields, & Apkarian, 2010). Results showed that brain activity was equivalent across these groups in areas of the brain associated with pain encoding and perception. Interestingly, however, activity in the bilateral nucleus accumbens (NAc)—an area of the brain responsible for both the encoding of the salience of the pain at stimulus onset (i.e., it signals *anticipation* of pain perception) and with the analgesia-related reward at stimulus offset—showed a disruption within the group of individuals with chronic low back pain. Specifically, this process was *reversed* in the individuals with chronic low back pain in that while healthy subjects were predicting a reward value at the cessation of the thermal pain causing stimulus, the NAc activity in the clinical sample showed they were *not* expecting reward at stimulus offset. Thus, the motivational value of analgesia was disrupted due to the presence of persistent pain. Further analysis showed that the reason for this disruption was a connective neural reorganization in the chronic pain group; in the healthy sample the NAc activity was mainly associated with the insula, whereas in the clinical sample the NAc was correlated with the medial prefrontal cortex (mPFC; a region that modulates emotional evaluations relative to the self). Moreover, the strength of this shift in connectivity in the clinical sample was in direct proportion to the amount of self-reported back pain intensity any given patient reported. Hence, both the chronicity as well as the intensity of the pain experienced were associated with brain reorganization (i.e., changes in areas of connectivity), notably within reward and motivational pathways in the context of chronic pain in this study.

In addition to chronic pain changing the way a pain stimulus is processed in specific pathways, research has also shown that living with persistent pain is associated with changes in brain processing in general, global (nonpain related) ways through disruption of critical homeostatic networks. In one seminal study comparing the brain activity of individuals with chronic low back pain to healthy controls while completing a minimally demanding visual attention task, no differences in performance or increases in brain activity were observed (Baliki, Geha, Apkarian, & Chialvo, 2008). However, marked differences in *decreased* activity were observed that correspond with a specific brain network, the default mode network, with the chronic pain group displaying reduced deactivation in several key areas of this region. This network represents the brain's activity in the resting state (i.e., in the absence of a subject doing anything) and a recent review of the literature reported this same reduced deactivation effect has been replicated across a number of chronic pain conditions (Apkarian et al., 2011). Research suggests that this disrupted default mode network becomes more pronounced as a function of chronic pain duration, with those individuals with a longer history of pain showing more disruption (Baliki et al., 2008). Importantly, in healthy individuals, the default mode network correlates negatively with activity in brain regions involved in attention and executive function, and an appropriate balance between these areas has been associated with memory function (Fornito, Harrison, Zalesky, & Simons, 2012). Thus, the findings of heightened default mode network activity in individuals with chronic pain may be a key reason why such individuals often report cognitive difficulties, such as trouble paying attention and declines in memory function.

Converging lines of research have demonstrated that chronic pain not only leads to changes in pain processing and associated connections, as well as general brain function (as described in the previous research on the default mode network) but there are also structural, anatomical brain changes that have been consistently observed in the presence of persistent, ongoing pain. Specifically, a loss in cortical regional gray matter volume has been found for a number of chronic pain conditions, including back pain (Schmidt-Wilcke et al., 2006), fibromyalgia (Luerding, Weigand, Bogdahn, & Schmidt-Wilcke, 2008), osteoarthritis of the knee (Rodriguez-Raecke, Niemeier, Ihle, Ruether, & May, 2009), and headache (Kim et al., 2008), among others. This loss in regional gray matter has been found to increase with longer duration of pain, higher intensity of pain, and as a function of the interaction between these factors (Apkarian et al., 2004; Geha et al., 2008; Kuchinad et al., 2007). Regional gray matter loss was also associated with cognitive declines in memory function in a sample of individuals with fibromyalgia pain (Luerding et al., 2008). Although the loss in gray matter volume may be an indicator of neuronal death, some research has found that these volume decreases are reversible when pain is relieved (Gwilym, Fillipini, Douaud, Carr, & Tracey, 2010; Obermann et al., 2009; Rodriguez-Raecke et al., 2009), suggesting that the observed structural changes in gray matter may more likely be caused by synaptic plasticity in these regions. The finding, however, that structural brain changes in the context of pain are reversible once adequate pain relief is achieved is certainly promising.

The exact timeline of the changes observed in the brain in acute vs. chronic pain has not been precisely identified, however, some research suggests that the neurological and psychological foundation for long-term pain is in place within hours of the initial injury (Carr & Goudas, 1999). Recent research is finding that the initial brain response to an inciting event (i.e., judgments of the intensity of the pain, quality, and meaning) potentially instigates a cascade of neurological changes that for some individuals sparks a gradual reorganization of the central nervous system, including structural changes, an increase in the number of pain receptors in the spinal cord, and a reduction in brain modulation processes (Apkarian, Baliki, & Farmer, 2013; Woolf & Salter, 2000). In one elegant study, the temporal causal relationship between injury, brain reorganization, and development of chronic pain (or recovery) was investigated by Apkarian and colleagues, who conducted brain imagining on individuals with subacute back pain, tracking them over a year to identify predictors of chronicity (Apkarian et al., 2013). Half of the sample went on to continue to experience the same magnitude of back pain 1 year later, and only these individuals (not those who recovered) showed a slow progression of gray matter density decreases. Findings showed that this loss of gray matter in the patients that went on to experience chronic pain was preceded by functional connectivity differences between the mPFC and NAc that were observable from the initial brain scans. This is consistent with the experimental research described above that identified this connectivity as a distinguishing feature of cortical reorganization in chronic pain (Baliki et al., 2010); what this study further demonstrated, however, was that the initial emotional response (as indicated by the mPFC-NAc disruption) represents a connectivity reorganization that ultimately may predict chronicity and also explain the structural changes observed as pain persists (Apkarian et al., 2013). Finally, this study also found that when an early pain medication treatment variable was included in the analyses along with the brain imaging data, results indicated that medication can play a protective role against pain chronification (Apkarian et al., 2013). The treatment parameter in isolation however, served no significant predictive function; the authors interpreted this finding as indicating that treatment outcome is contingent on the brain state. Although more research is needed to replicate and extend this finding, this research opens up exciting possibilities for the future in enhancing initial treatment that might prevent the transition from acute to chronic pain.

In sum, not all individuals who experience an acute injury go on to experience chronic pain; the correlates and predictors of who progresses to develop chronic pain and why this is the case are only beginning to be understood—we are at the tip of the iceberg. However, the evidence to date suggests that seemingly small differences in the initial brain state of the individual at the time of injury (and the period immediately following) can precipitate major differences in whether pain "heals" in the acute phase, or persists and becomes chronic. As discussed later in this chapter, the landscape for acute compared to chronic pain is vastly different not only at the level of neurological processing and cortical reorganization, but critically also in the cognitive, emotional, motivational, and behavioural response to pain. This, combined with our understanding of the theoretical models of the experience of pain, again provides a strong rationale for an interdisciplinary approach to chronic pain management that goes beyond pharmacopoeia.

The Human Experience (Bio*psycho*social)

The Emotional Impact of Chronic Pain

Chronic pain, for most people in most circumstances, is an aversive experience that typically elicits negative emotional and affective psychological responses. Thus, the bulk of the emotion research to date has focused on understanding the influence of negative emotions on pain and associated disability and rehabilitation. Due to their high comorbidity rates with chronic pain, particular attention has been devoted towards investigating the role of depression, anxiety, fear, and anger (Gatchel, Peng, Peters, Fuchs, & Turk, 2007). More recent research has shifted towards understanding the role of positive emotions and resiliency, which may serve a protective function and buffer the stress associated with chronic pain. Psychosocial treatments for chronic pain target both negative *and* positive emotions to mitigate the impact of chronic pain on emotional functioning.

Depression

Rates of comorbid depressive disorders within chronic pain populations have been found to be approximately 40–50%, although this is likely an underestimate as depression often goes undiagnosed (and untreated) (Banks & Kerns, 1996; Dersh, Gatchel, Mayer, Polatin, & Temple, 2006; Romano & Turner, 1985). Not only is depression a prevalent comorbidity for people with chronic pain, but the combination is deadly. Lifetime prevalence of suicidal ideation in these individuals is approximately 20% and rates of suicide attempts are estimated to be between 5% and 14%, which translates to risk of death by suicide being at least doubled in individuals with chronic pain (Tang & Crane, 2006). Further, in one study depression was found to uniquely predict the degree to which pain interferes with daily activities and overall life satisfaction, even while controlling for demographic and key psychological variables (Day & Thorn, 2010). Research has also identified that poorer outcomes are associated with the treatment of pain when comorbid depression goes untreated (Shmuely, Baumgarten, Rovner, & Berlin, 2001). For improvement of engagement in valued activities, quality of life, and for optimal pain treatment, it appears screening for and treating depression is critical.

Anxiety

Although epidemiological data on the rates of anxiety in pain populations are limited, anxiety and fear about pain is a common experience. One large-scale study conducted within a fibromyalgia sample reported that approximately 44–51% of individuals endorsed substantial anxiety symptoms (Wolfe et al., 1990). Anxiety may be especially common in individuals where a definitive diagnosis identifying the "cause" of the pain has not been possible, leaving these individuals "not knowing why" they have pain and therefore worrying about what certain symptoms "might mean." For example, someone who has persistent daily headaches might become anxious that these are caused by an undetected brain tumor, and they might become fearful about what the future will hold (note that this example also demonstrates the very close proximity between cognitive interpretations of symptoms, i.e., pain = brain tumor, and an associated anxiety response).

Many individuals fear the pain will become worse, and anxiety-related fear of pain, fear of movement (kinesiophobia), and fear of re-injury is particularly debilitating (Vlaeyen & Linton, 2000). Some research has found that fear-related factors more accurately predict functional limitations than even pain severity, duration, or other biomedical factors (Crombez, Vlaeyen, & Heuts, 1999; Vlaeyen, Kole-Snijders, Rotteveel, Ruesink, & Heuts, 1995). Critically, catastrophic cognitions are theorized to engender this fear, and this then subsequently leads to increased avoidance of engaging in activities (Vlaeyen & Linton, 2000). As we will see in the next section, behavioral avoidance of activity and more time "resting on the couch" is associated with heightened pain, more disability, and lower return to work rates, all of which not only add to the heightened suffering of the individual, but place a substantial increased economic burden on the medical system (Vlaeyen, Kole-Snijders, Boeren, & van Eek, 1995; Vlaeyen et al., 1995).

Anger

Another critical emotion to target in treatment is anger. Anger and associated blame towards self, significant other, healthcare providers, employers, insurance companies, the person who caused the accident... There are a whole host of reasons that a person living with chronic pain might have to feel angry (ranging from slight irritation or frustration, up to fury). One study within a multidisciplinary pain clinic identified that approximately 98% of patients at the time of their intake assessment reported feeling some degree of anger, and for most (74%) this anger was directed toward themselves (Okifuji, Turk, & Curran, 1999). Healthcare providers were identified by Okifuji and colleagues (1999) as the second most frequent target of patients' anger (62%), and research by Burns et al. found that this may lead to patients reporting a weaker working alliance with their clinicians (Burns, Higdon, Mullen, Lansky, & Mei Wei, 1999). Given that working alliance is a strong predictor of treatment outcome in its own right (Lambert, 1992), a disrupted alliance will likely substantially lessen the probability of treatment success. Indeed, research across a number of different pain types has found a consistent relation between anger and worse pain treatment outcomes, including higher pain intensity ratings, longer pain duration, increased analgesic medication intake, and higher impaired functioning (Gatchel et al., 2007; Greenwood, Thurston, Rumble, Waters, & Keefe, 2003; Trost, Vangronsveld, Linton, Quartana, & Sullivan, 2012). Finally, anger, anxiety, and depression are closely related, likely in reciprocal relationships (Trost et al., 2012), and often co-occur.

Resilience

Although the preponderance of pain literature has focused on the maladaptive role of negative emotions, the potential buffering, protective role of resiliency, and positive emotions/affect have more recently begun to receive an upsurge of empirical attention. There are two complementary theories that are the most widely cited which attempt to explain how positive emotion may improve pain and coping: Fredrickson's "Broaden and Build" theory (Fredrickson, 2001) and Zautra and colleagues' dynamic model of affect (Zautra, Smith, Affleck, & Tennen, 2001). The Broaden and Build theory proposes that people with more positive affect adapt more readily in the face of stress as they are able to broaden their outlook and build on their well-being that is already present, and in this way they are able to enhance their overall sense of well-being (Fredrickson, 2001). In support of this model, research suggests that positive emotions may foster recovery after pain flare-ups (Zautra et al., 2001), and one study found subjective happiness was associated with improved general health perception in individuals with low back pain (Takeyachi et al., 2003). In Zautra and colleagues' dynamic model of affect, they proposed a dynamic relationship between positive and negative affect such that during times of stress (e.g., when pain intensifies) the full range of affective experience collapses within a smaller, typically negative range. However, boosting affective complexity and the presence of positive emotions is hypothesized to be associated with decreased negative affective states, thereby functioning to preserve well-being during stressful times and build resilience (Zautra et al., 2001), and support for this hypothesis has been found (Davis, Thummala, & Zautra, 2014; Strand et al., 2006). Thus, both Fredrickson's notion of building on existing resources, and Zautra's theory of capitalizing on positive affect to dynamically counteract the negative affect associated with pain appear to be supported. One final potential protective factor worth mentioning is maintaining a sense of humor despite the pain. Humor and laughter are typically outward expressions of pleasant/positive emotions, and the use of humor has been shown to improve pain thresholds (Mahony, Burroughs, & Hieatt, 2001) and reduce pain intensity (Tse et al., 2010), and lead to the release of endorphins in the brain, a natural pain killer (Haig, 1988). Thus, appropriate use of humor in therapy might be a welcome addition for many reasons, including pain reduction!

The Behavioral Expression of Chronic Pain

The behavioral expression of chronic pain and the social ramifications of pain are difficult to distinguish, and although I describe them in separate sections here, as in all the other elements that coalesce in the experience of pain, they are closely interconnected. Spanning from the earliest investigations of the role of behavior in chronic pain adjustment, a key focus has been on understanding the influence of pain behaviors (Fordyce, 1976), which are functionally the communicative expression of pain. Pain behaviors can be verbal (e.g., statements such as, "I am hurting"), paraverbal (e.g., grunts, moans, sighs), and nonverbal (e.g., grimacing, wincing, resting, taking medication) (Fordyce, 1976; Sullivan, Adams, & Sullivan, 2004). Such behaviors may serve a protective, useful function in the short term when pain is acute by eliciting solicitous attention and responses, as well as assistance. However, when pain behavior engagement is maintained long term in the context of chronic pain, research has found that such behaviors predict reduced likelihood of return to work, higher compensation costs, and an increased number of lost work days, as well as increased self-reported disability (Prkachin, Schultz, & Hughes, 2007). Another study has found that decreases in guarding (i.e., protecting the site of pain by shielding the area to avoid it from being bumped etc.) and time spent resting were most strongly associated with improvement in self-reported disability during a multidisciplinary pain treatment (Jensen, Turner, & Romano, 2001). Along with individuals potentially lapsing into unhelpful patterns of specific pain behaviors, there are also broader more general patterns of avoidance behavior that are maladaptive in the context of chronic pain.

Avoidance Behavior

Compelling support for a disability model based on fear and maladaptive behavioral avoidance activity patterns—The Fear Avoidance Model—has been found in reviews of the literature, with fear conceptualized as underlying avoidance behavior, leading to disuse and disability (Asmundson, Norton, & Vlaeyen, 2004; Vlaeyen & Linton, 2000). The functional "opposite" of avoidance is behavioral engagement. Reviews of the literature have shown that appropriately paced engagement in valued activities despite the pain correlates with a range of positive outcomes, including less pain intensity, depression, pain-related anxiety, lower levels of physical and psychosocial disability, and improved globally rated daily activity and overall emotional well-being (McCracken & Samuel, 2007; McCracken & Vowles, 2006; Thompson & McCracken, 2011). Thus, reducing behavioral avoidance and enhancing engagement in valued activities are key treatment targets in the management of chronic pain.

Sleep

Although perhaps not precisely or neatly falling under the category of "behavioral" aspects of chronic pain, disturbances in sleep are a commonly reported problem. Epidemiological data indicate that as many as 53 to 88% of individuals with chronic pain also suffer from sleep disorders (Smith, Perlis, Smith, Giles, & Carmody, 2000; Tang, Wright, & Salkovskis, 2007; Wilson, Eriksson, D'Eon, Mikail, & Emery, 2002). Even when potentially confounding factors such as depression, anxiety, and other medical problems are controlled, people with chronic pain are at a significantly higher risk for developing insomnia compared to people without pain (Taylor et al., 2007). Conversely, over 40% of people with insomnia also report chronic pain (Ohayon, 2005); hence the relation between pain and sleep problems appears to be reciprocal (Smith & Haythornthwaite, 2004). Further demonstration of this reciprocal nature is found in research which has shown that effectively treating a comorbid sleep problem improves pain outcomes (Khalid, Roehrs, Hudgel, & Roth, 2011). Moreover, anxiety and depression symptoms are closely correlated with pain and disturbed sleep; and targeting improved mood in treatment may improve both pain and sleep outcomes (O'Brien et al., 2010; Schrimpf et al., 2015). On the other hand, sleep is one of the greatest homeostatic affect modulators, so improving sleep will also likely improve mood and pain (Palmer & Alfano, 2016). Pre-sleep cognitive arousal and pain catastrophizing may represent additional useful treatment targets for combined pain and sleep problems, as a recent study found these factors to be powerful cognitive predictors of disturbed sleep symptoms in a clinical pain population (Byers, Lichstein, & Thorn, 2015). These reciprocal relations show that although we are discussing the various aspects of the chronic pain experience in "isolated" sections here, these domains are closely interconnected and any one element has the capacity to initiate a domino effect, eliciting (either adaptive or maladaptive) change in all the other components.

Cognitive Factors and Chronic Pain

Unfortunately, many individuals with chronic pain who do not have an identified pathology or medical diagnosis for their pain are often directly or indirectly told by healthcare professionals that the pain is "all in their head." Well, although, as we saw in the earlier section, research has confirmed that pain *is* processed in the brain, our consideration of the role cognitive factors play in pain here in this section is not the same as saying that the pain is "not real." It is the *exceedingly* small minority of individuals who might engage in malingering. Clinically it is most helpful to communicate that the pain *is* real, *and* that the way we think about it influences how "wide the gates are" (i.e., to paraphrase the Gate Control Theory) and how much pain we feel. In support of this, a plethora of research has shown that cognitive factors play a key maintaining role in prolonging negative emotions, initiating unhelpful behavioral responses, and perpetuating poor pain-related outcomes (Thorn, 2004).

Attention

At base, pain is an overriding stimulus that demands attentional processes to pay heed and to selectively attend to the pain at the cost of other information in the environment (Crombez, Van Ryckeghem, Eccleston, & van Damme, 2013; Eccleston & Crombez, 1999). Ontogenetically and evolutionarily pain serves a survival functional, claiming attention, leading to a fear-based urge to escape, and behavioral interruption. Within the context of ongoing persistent pain, the intrinsic role of attention in urging escape becomes maladaptive as in chronic pain there *is* no escape and so the fear-based urge is maintained due to lack of goal fulfilment. In this context, many individuals living with persistent pain develop a *hypervigilant* attention to the emotionally laden pain stimulus, or as otherwise described, a cognitive attentional bias toward noticing painful stimuli. As attention is a limited resource that is required for a number of cognitive functions, and that pain places a toll on attentional resources, it is not surprising that many people with chronic pain report difficulty concentrating, making decisions, and an array of other executive function problems (Eccleston & Crombez, 1999). Moreover, attention is the foundational, initial cognitive factor underlying the primary appraisal processes theorized to play a key role in models of stress and coping.

Primary Appraisals

As discussed earlier, chronic pain and the wider landscape of what living with chronic pain entails are often stressful. So along with that, models of stress point to specific cognitions that maintain the stress response and exacerbate pain. Just to briefly recap, in the Transactional Model of Stress and coping framework (Lazarus & Folkman, 1984), the stress response is initiated (or not) on the basis of the *meaning* given to the contextual stimulus (the "stressor") once it has entered the field of awareness. Specifically, Lazarus and Folkman (1984) described three primary appraisal judgment categories about the meaning of a potentially stress-inducing stimulus (e.g., pain): (1) *threat*, which is the evaluation that pain represents a danger that outweighs one's ability to cope; (2) *loss/harm*, where pain is viewed as damaging, and/or as a loss of some form, for example, loss in the ability to work, engage in previously pleasurable activities etc.; or (3) *challenge*, where one perceives that he/she has the resources to cope with the pain. Of the three forms of primary appraisals, research has identified that threat appraisals are the most commonly reported within the context of chronic pain (Unruh & Richie, 1998). Threat appraisals and attentional processes are closely associated, and threat appraisals are theorized to be a key precipitating and maintaining factor in the development of hypervigilant attention to painful sensations (Crombez et al., 2013), leading to fear-avoidance beliefs that increase pain and disability, and negatively impact treatment and return to work rates (Pfingsten, Kroner-Herwig, Leibing, Kronshage, & Hildebrandt, 2000; Poiraudeau et al., 2006; Waddell, Newton, Henderson, Somerville, & Main, 1993). Further, beliefs that the feeling of hurt equals harm (i.e., pain equals damage) have been found to significantly predict physical dysfunction and poor adjustment to pain (Jensen et al., 1994). Loss appraisals in people with chronic pain have also been found to be frequently reported (Walker, Holloway, & Sofaer, 1999) and are theorized to lead to symptoms of depression, a sense of helplessness, and a reduction in adaptive coping behaviors (Thorn, 2004). Although research is limited on challenge appraisals in pain populations, one study found that only 14% of individuals appraised a recent painful experience as a challenge (Unruh & Richie, 1998).

Secondary Appraisals

Following closely on the heels of primary pain appraisals are ensuing secondary appraisals. Pain catastrophizing refers to an exaggerated negative mental set about actual or anticipated pain (Sullivan, Thorn, et al., 2001), and has variously been conceptualized as a primary appraisal, a secondary appraisal, and as a coping strategy (Thorn, 2004). Pain catastrophizing is by far the most researched and documented cognitive factor in the pain literature. A voluminous body of research has consistently demonstrated that it is a robust predictor of higher pain severity, disability, poorer social functioning, longer recovery times following surgery, greater healthcare utilization, and worse mood (e.g., depression and anxiety), above and beyond other factors such as disease severity, pain intensity, anxiety, and neuroticism (Day & Thorn, 2010; Drahovzal, Stewart, & Sullivan, 2006; Edwards, Cahalan, Mensing, Smith, & Haythornthwaite, 2011; Flor, Behle, & Birbaumer, 1993; Geisser, Robinson, Keefe, & Weiner, 1994; Keefe, Rumble, Scipio, Giordano, & Perri, 2004; Sullivan, Rodgers, & Kirsch, 2001; Sullivan, Thorn, et al., 2001). Pain catastrophizing is also theorized to be a primary precursor for exaggerated displays of pain behaviors, which serve a social communicative function in coping efforts to elicit solicitousness, empathy, and support from others in the environment (Sullivan, Thorn, et al., 2001). This theoretical framework has been called the Communal Coping Model of catastrophizing (Sullivan, Thorn, et al., 2001), and although available evidence is not entirely consistent with all its predictions (Sullivan, 2012; Tsui et al., 2012), a number of studies in both experimental and clinical samples has found support for many of its tenets (Giardino, Jensen, Turner, Ehde, & Cardenas, 2003; Holtzman & Delongis, 2007; Sullivan et al., 2004; Thibault et al., 2008; Tsui et al., 2012). Given the strong predictive role pain catastrophizing has been shown to play, over and above other factors, it represents a prime target for interventions aimed at improving pain coping, and in the next chapter I will describe specific interventions that have been designed to target this powerful predictor of the experience of pain (Thorn, 2004).

Adaptive Secondary Appraisals

As noted above in the emotion literature, in the past several decades there has been an upsurge in research devoted towards understanding the potential protective role of positive psychological factors. In the context of cognitions, beliefs related to pain management self-efficacy—the conviction one can cope with, and manage pain—is one form of secondary appraisal that a large body of research has identified to play a protective role in fostering adaptive physical and psychological adjustment to pain (Rudy, Lieber, Boston, Gourley, & Baysal, 2003). Furthermore, enhanced self-efficacy has been found to be a critical mechanism underlying improvements in pain, disability, depression, and adjustment following pain treatment (Altmaier, Russell, Kao, Lehmann, & Weinstein, 1993; Jensen et al., 2001; Keefe, Rumble, et al., 2004). However, some research suggests that perceived control over the *effects* of pain, rather than the sensation of pain per se, may be most important in regards to facilitating better adjustment and less disability (Tan, Jensen, Robinson-Whelen, Thornby, & Monga, 2002).

More recently, positive psychology-oriented research efforts have focused on identifying the potential protective role of mindfulness and pain acceptance, and particularly promising results have been found. Kabat-Zinn (1990) defines mindfulness as "...the awareness that emerges through paying attention on purpose, in the present moment, and non-judgmentally to the unfolding of experience, moment by moment" (p. 145). In one study by Schutze and colleagues (Schutze, Rees, Preece, & Schutze, 2010), higher levels of mindfulness predicted lower levels of pain, negative affect, pain catastrophizing, fear of pain, pain hypervigilance, and functional disability. Acceptance of pain, defined as the willingness to experience pain and to continue to engage in activities despite the pain (McCracken, Vowles, & Eccleston, 2004), has been shown to be associated with an array of better outcomes, including less pain, depression, anxiety, physical, and psychological disability (McCracken & Eccleston, 2003). Finally, a model of psychological flexibility (described in greater detail in the next chapter) has recently been proposed as an integrated model of several positive psychology constructs that may play a protective role in the context of pain. Preliminary support for individual aspects of this multifaceted (predominantly cognitively oriented) psychological flexibility model has been found, although more research is still needed to elucidate these factors in relation to the experience of pain specifically (Hann & McCracken, 2014; McCracken, Vowles, & Zhao-O'Brien, 2010; Sturgeon, 2014).

The Wider Ramifications of Chronic Pain (Biopsycho*social*)

How Big is the Problem and Who is at Risk?

At a nomothetic social level, chronic pain is a pervasive, major health concern, and has been referred to as a public healthcare crisis (Darnall et al., 2016; IOM, 2011) with worldwide point prevalence estimates ranging between 2% and over

55% (Blyth et al., 2001; Breivik, Collett, Ventafridda, Cohen, & Gallacher, 2006; Catala et al., 2002; Elliott, Smith, Penny, Smith, & Chambers 1999; Eriksen, Jensen, Sjøgren, Ekholm, & Rasmussen, 2003; Harstall & Ospina, 2003; Moulin, Clark, Speechley, & Morley-Forster, 2002; Neville, Peleg, Singer, Sherf, & Shvartzman, 2008; Sjøgren, Ekholm, Peuckmann, & Grønbæk, 2009; Verhaak, Kerssens, Dekker, Sorbi, & Bensing, 1998). In the United States, it is estimated that chronic pain affects 116 million adults, and prevalence is on the rise (IOM, 2011). This figure translates into pain affecting more Americans than diabetes, heart disease (including both coronary heart disease and stroke), and cancer combined (The American Academy of Pain Medicine, 2016). Low back pain is the most common source of chronic pain (28%), followed by severe headache or migraine pain (14%), and neck pain (14%) (National Centers for Health Statistics, 2013). Persistent pain is not always a primary condition, however, and is often a secondary condition that further complicates and impedes treatment for a vast spectrum of injuries and diseases, such as postoperative recovery and treatment of malignancy. However, all of these prevalence findings may be considered a vast *under*estimate as it is also well established that pain is both underdiagnosed and undertreated (IOM, 2011).

Risk for the development of chronic pain is not evenly proportionate across demographic groups: pain discriminates. Thus, compounding the pervasive underdiagnosis and undertreatment of pain is the well-documented existence of fundamental health, treatment, and ethnicity disparities across a broad range of samples, settings, and types of pain (Tait & Chibnall, 2005). Prior research in regards to such disparities indicates that a number of intervening factors potentially influence the relationship between healthcare access, treatment, and outcome (Day & Thorn, 2010). Age is one such intervening factor and although the relationship between age and increased risk for pain has not always been found to be linear, most population-based research consistently shows that chronic pain disproportionately affects older individuals (Bergman et al., 2001; Blyth et al., 2001; Ng, Tsui, & Chan, 2002). In an extensive review of the available research on gender differences in pain, Unruh found that women are more likely than men to experience a variety of recurrent pain conditions and women report pain of greater intensity, frequency, and duration than men (Unruh, 1996).

While the relationship between pain and race is complex, most of the research to date has focused on the comparison between African Americans and White Americans, and considerable evidence suggests that African Americans report greater pain intensity in acute clinical pain and in a variety of chronic pain conditions (Breitbart et al., 1996; Chibnall, Tait, Andreson, & Hadler, 2005; Selim et al., 2001). However, it has been suggested that individuals from minority racial groups may suffer from more severe symptoms before seeking treatment and that this is consequently an important point to consider when examining research conducted in clinical samples (McCracken, Matthews, Tang, & Cuba, 2001). Further, a disproportionate number of African Americans live in rural areas and represent a higher percentage of individuals classified as low socioeconomic status (SES), and evidence suggests that documented racial differences may be explained by these factors rather than biological differences associated with race per se (Day & Thorn, 2010; Kington & Smith, 1997; McIlvane, 2007; Williams & Collins, 1995). Taken together, the limited research on the experience of chronic pain in low SES and rural individuals suggests that annual income of less than US$25,000, no high school diploma, and rural residency are associated with a greater likelihood of having disabling chronic pain (Hoffman, Meier, & Council, 2002; Nguyen, Ugarte, Fuller, Haas, & Portnenoy, 2005; Portenoy, Ugarte, & Fuller, 2004). The overall impact is that people at the lowest end of the income gradient experience both intractable stressful circumstances and an impoverished lack of resources, which consequently combine to exacerbate their susceptibility to poor health and negative psychosocial indicants, and make them more vulnerable to experience chronic pain (Adler et al., 1994; Almeida, Neupert, Banks, & Serido, 2005).

Costs of Chronic Pain

Given the high prevalence rates of chronic pain it is not surprising that chronic pain is among the most common presenting complaints seen in medical practice, with some reports indicating pain accounts for more than 80% of physician visits (Gatchel, 2004). Low back pain has been reported as the second most frequent reason for visits to the physician (Hart, Deyo, & Cherkin, 1995), and headache pain alone accounts for 18 million physician visits per year in the United States (Schwartz, Stewart, Simon, & Lipton, 1998). Opioid analgesic medications are one of the most commonly prescribed treatments for chronic pain, but their misuse is now recognized as a healthcare crisis (IOM, 2011; NIH, 2011). The National Centers for Health Statistics, in their 2013 report, found a 300% increase in opioid analgesic consumption between 1999 and 2010, and death rates for poisoning involving opioid analgesics more than tripled between 2000 and 2010, resulting in over 16,000 opioid-involved overdose deaths in 2010 (National Centers for Health Statistics, 2013; NIH, 2011). Moreover, unrelieved pain is associated with longer hospital stays, increased rates of re-hospitalization, and often results in an inability of individuals to maintain health insurance (The American Academy of Pain Medicine, 2016), thereby further escalating the burden and cost chronic pain places on the healthcare system.

The direct and indirect economic costs of the widespread and debilitating nature of pain on society are astronomical. Most recent estimates in the United States reported that the total annual costs of pain ranged from $560 to $635 billion in 2010 constant dollars (Gaskin & Richard, 2012), an amount equivalent to approximately $2,000 annually for every person living in the US (IOM, 2011). Within this estimate, healthcare costs due to pain accounted for approximately $261 to $300 billion, and lost productivity costs (based on days of missed work, hours of work lost, and lower wages) due to pain ranged from $299 to $355 billion (Gaskin & Richard, 2012). Gaskin and Richard report these are conservative estimates as excluded from these figures are costs due to pain for nursing home residents, children, military personnel, and persons who are incarcerated (Gaskin & Richard, 2012). The costs of chronic pain are more than just financial, however, with chronic pain exacting a toll on every facet of life and functioning for the individual living in daily pain.

The Personal Social Cost

Focusing on just the macro-level societal and financial figures in isolation can detract from the human cost experienced at an everyday level for the individual and their friends, family, and loved ones living a life with chronic pain. The World Health Organization (WHO) reported findings from the IASP that one-third of people living with chronic pain are unable or less able to maintain an independent lifestyle due to the effects of the pain (WHO, 2004). Further, the WHO (2004) reported that approximately one-half to two-thirds of individuals with chronic pain are less able or unable to engage in physical exercise, enjoy normal sleep, attend to household chores, participate in social activities, drive a car, walk, or have sexual relations. Thus, the behavioral and social ramifications of pain are closely interconnected and extend across the entire spectrum of day-to-day living, from employment and level of independence, to the dynamic of interpersonal relationships, to what one can "do" in spare time or for hobbies.

A particular challenge for many individuals with worsening disability associated with chronic pain is that it negatively impacts one's ability to maintain gainful employment. Chronic pain has consistently been found to lead to higher rates of unemployment, which has a ripple on effect leading to downward socioeconomic drift (i.e., lower SES over time) and heightened associated stressors. Data collected within a primary care cohort study found that 13% of individuals with headache pain and 18% of individuals with back pain were unable to obtain or keep full-time employment over a 3-year period due to their pain (Stang, Von Korff, & Galer, 1998). Estimates from an Australian-based survey found that approximately 13% of those individuals who reported a chronic pain condition were unemployed, and over 17% were receiving disability benefit compensation (Blyth et al., 2001). Further, in this Australian-based study, higher levels of pain interference within those reporting chronic pain was associated with worse socioeconomic, health, and employment indicators (Blyth et al., 2001). Many people also change jobs due to pain (Magni, Caldieron, Rigatti-Luchini, & Merskey, 1990), which, depending on the type of change, may actually be beneficial. In a review of the literature, Teasell and Bombardier found that there is evidence to suggest that the availability of modified work or work autonomy is associated with less disability in people with chronic pain (Teasell & Bombardier, 2001). Thus, finding ways to enhance vocational rehabilitation in the context of chronic pain is critical.

Another co-occurring problem that often arises for individuals living with pain is that the pain (and its consequences) places a strain on relationships. Many individuals with chronic pain report pain to be an isolating experience and often feel their experience is not understood by family and friends. The WHO (2004) reported that one in four individuals living with chronic pain identify that relationships with a significant other, family, or friends are strained or broken due to the pain. Although the exact reasons for these deteriorations in relationships probably vary from person to person, it is likely that changes in what a person can or can't do any longer (i.e., possibly a companionable hike may have been a valued shared activity prior to the onset of pain and the loss of being able to do this together due to the pain may lead to strain), financial stress, and/or potentially comorbid depression and anger may play a role. Research has found that higher rates of outward expressions of anger and hostility directed toward a spouse may detrimentally impact the spouse's mood and over time, lead to more punishing, critical spousal responses to the individual living with chronic pain (Burns, Johnson, Mahoney, Devine, & Pawl, 1996). Moreover, a recent study implementing ecological momentary assessment to examine concurrent and lagged effects found that patient-perceived spouse criticism and hostility predicted increased patient pain intensity (Burns et al., 2013). Interestingly in this study, it was found that spouse observation of patient pain behaviors may be a precursor to the criticism and hostility perceived by the patient (Burns et al., 2013). Based on these findings, some pain treatment approaches, as we will cover in the next chapter, have included client partners within the therapy, with promising results emerging as a consequence (Keefe, Blumenthal, et al., 2014).

Summary

Pain in different contexts can entail a range of responses; consider, for example, the pain of child birth as compared to the pain of a compound fracture—contextual differences have a substantial influence on the experience. Contemporary models of chronic pain are firmly rooted within a biopsychosocial perspective, recognizing the critical synergistic role of biological, psychological, emotional, social, and behavioral contextual factors. However despite this, even today, the biomedical model is the most dominant model *implemented* in healthcare and in the treatment of chronic pain, one only has to look at the statistics on the number of medical visits, surgical procedures, and opioid prescriptions to see this is the case. Healthcare providers who are exposed to the biomedical model in training, but receive little in the way of chronic pain curriculum, still approach the problem of chronic pain via focusing on assessment to find the "physical" peripheral pain generator, and then establish treatment to remove this "cause" (Thorn & Walker, 2011). And in conditions where it is not possible to remove the cause (i.e., as in the case of arthritis and many other chronic pain conditions), palliative approaches are implemented in the form of analgesic pain medication. However, in chronic pain conditions, often a specific pain generator cannot be identified, and palliative approaches to management often entail serious adverse side effects (Trescot et al., 2008). Thus, while the biomedical model may work well for acute pain, in the instance of chronic pain, this approach reinforces a passive patient role, as the individual searches for a "cure" (that likely may not exist). For treatment to be effective, the *person* experiencing the pain must be considered in a completely holistic sense—including the neurophysiological aspect, as well as emotions, behavior, cognitions, and context. Effective chronic pain treatments target not simply "the pain" as an unwanted, separate, yet often defining part of self, but a radical shift in perspective toward living a valued life, with pain and all.

References

Adler, N. E., Boyce, T., Chesney, M. A., Cohen, S., Folkman, S., Kahn, R. L., & Syme, S. L. (1994). Socioeconomic status and health, the challenge of the gradient. *American Psychologist, 49*(1), 15–24.

Almeida, D. M., Neupert, S. D., Banks, S. R., & Serido, J. (2005). Do daily stress processes account for socioeconomic health disparities? *The Journals of Gerontology, 60*, 34–39.

Altmaier, E. M., Russell, D. W., Kao, C. F., Lehmann, T. R., & Weinstein, J. N. (1993). Role of self-efficacy in rehabilitation outcome among chronic low back pain patients. *Journal of Counseling Psychology, 40*(3), 335–339.

Apkarian, A. V., Baliki, M. N., & Farmer, M. A. (2013). Predicting transition to chronic pain. *Current Opinions in Neurology, 26*(4), 360–367.

Apkarian, A. V., Baliki, M. N., & Geha, P. Y. (2009). Towards a theory of chronic pain. *Progress in Neurobiology, 87*(2), 81–97.

Apkarian, A. V., Hashmi, J. A., & Baliki, M. N. (2011). Pain and the brain: Specificity and plasticity of the brain in clinical chronic pain. *Pain, 152*(3 Suppl), S49–S64.

Apkarian, A. V., Sosa, Y., Sonty, S., Levy, R. M., Harden, R. N., Parrish, T. B., & Gitelman, D. R. (2004). Chronic back pain is associated with decreased prefrontal and thalamic gray matter density. *The Journal of Neuroscience 24*(46), 10410–10415.

Ashburn, M. A., & Staats, P. S. (1999). Management of chronic pain. *The Lancet, 353*(9167), 1865–1869.

Asmundson, G. J., Norton, P., & Vlaeyen, J. W. (2004). Fear-avoidance models of chronic pain: An overview. In G. J. Asmundson, J. W. Vlaeyen, & G. Crombez (Eds.), *Understanding and treating fear of pain* (pp. 3–24). Oxford: Oxford University Press.

Baliki, M. N., Geha, P. Y., Apkarian, A. V., & Chialvo, D. R. (2008). Beyond feeling: Chronic pain hurts the brain, disrupting the default-mode network dynamics. *Journal of Neuroscience, 28*, 1398–1403.

Baliki, M. N., Geha, P. Y., Fields, H. L., & Apkarian, A. V. (2010). Predicting value of pain and analgesia: Nucleus accumbens response to noxious stimuli changes in the presence of chronic pain. *Neuron, 66*, 149–160.

Banks, S. M., & Kerns, R. D. (1996). Explaining high rates of depression in chronic pain: A diathesis-stress framework. *Psychological Bulletin, 119*, 95–110.

Bantick, S. J., Wise, R. G., Ploghaus, A., Clare, S., Smith, A. M., & Tracey, I. (2002). Imaging how attention modulates pain in humans using functional MRI. *Brain, 125*, 310–319.

Beecher, H. K. (1946). Pain in men wounded in battle. *Annals of Surgery, 123*(1), 96–105.

Bergman, S., Herrstrom, P., Hogstrom, K., Petersson, I. F., Svensson, B., & Jacobsson, L. T. (2001). Chronic musculoskeletal pain, prevalence rates, and sociodemographic associations in a Swedish population study. *Journal of Rheumatology, 28*(6), 1369–1377.

Blyth, F. M., March, L. M., Brnabic, A. J. M., Jorm, L. R., Williamson, M., & Cousins, M. J. (2001). Chronic pain in Australia: A prevalence study. *Pain, 89*, 127–134.

Bracha, H. S. (2004). Freeze, flight, fight, fright, faint: Adaptationist perspectives on the acute stress response spectrum. *CNS Spectrums, 9*(9), 679–685.

Breitbart, W., McDonald, M., Rosenfeld, B., Passik, S., Hewitt, D., Thaler, H., & Portenoy, R. (1996). Pain in ambulatory AIDS patients. *Pain, 68,* 315–321.

Breivik, H., Collett, B., Ventafridda, V., Cohen, R., & Gallacher, D. (2006). Survey of chronic pain in Europe: Prevalence, impact on daily life, and treatment. *European Journal of Pain, 10*(4), 287–333.

Brodal, P. (2010). *The central nervous system: Structure and function* (4th ed.). New York, NY: Oxford University Press.

Burns, J., Higdon, L., Mullen, J., Lansky, D., & Mei Wei, J. (1999). Relationships among patient hostility, anger expression, depression, and the working alliance in a work hardening program. *Annals of Behavioral Medicine, 21,* 77–82.

Burns, J. W., Johnson, B. J., Mahoney, N., Devine, J., & Pawl, R. (1996). Anger management style, hostility and spouse responses: Gender differences in predictors of adjustment among chronic pain patients. *Pain, 64,* 445–453.

Burns, J., Peterson, K. M., Smith, D. A., Keefe, F., Porter, L. S., Schuster, E., & Kinner, E. (2013). Temporal associations between spouse criticism/hostility and pain among patients with chronic pain: A within-couple daily diary study. *Pain, 154,* 2715–2721.

Byers, H. D., Lichstein, K. L., & Thorn, B. E. (2015). Cognitive processes in comorbid poor sleep and chronic pain. *Journal of Behavioral Medicine, 39,* 233–240.

Carr, D. B., & Goudas, L. C. (1999). Acute pain. *Lancet, 353,* 2051–2058.

Catala, E., Reig, E., Artes, M., Aliaga, L., Lopez, J. S., & Segu, J. L. (2002). Prevalence of pain in the Spanish population: Telephone survey in 5000 homes. *European Journal of Pain, 6,* 133–140.

Chibnall, J. T., Tait, R. C., Andreson, E. M., & Hadler, N. M. (2005). Race and socioeconomic differences in post-settlement outcomes for African American and Caucasian workers' compensation claimants with low back injuries. *Pain, 114,* 462–472.

Crombez, G., Van Ryckeghem, D. M. L., Eccleston, C., & van Damme, S. (2013). Attentional bias to pain-related information: A meta-analysis. *Pain, 154,* 497–510.

Crombez, G., Vlaeyen, J. W. S., & Heuts, P. (1999). Pain related fear is more disabling that pain itself: Evidence on the role of pain-related fear in chronic back pain disability. *Pain, 80,* 329–339.

Darnall, B. D., Scheman, J., Davin, S., Burns, J. W., Murphy, J. L., Wilson, A. C., … Mackey, S. C. (2016). Pain psychology: A global needs assessment and national call to action. *Pain Medicine, 17,* 250–263.

Davis, M. C., Thummala, K., & Zautra, A. J. (2014). Stress-related clinical pain and mood in women with chronic pain: Moderating effects of depression and positive mood induction. *Annals of Behavioral Medicine, 48,* 61–70.

Day, M. A. (2017). Pain and its optimal management. In J. Dorrian, E. Thorsteinsson, M. Di Benedetto, K. Lane-Krebs, M. Day, A. Hutchinson, K. Sherman., *Health Psychology in Australia* (pp. 261–281). Port Melbourne: Cambridge University Press.

Day, M. A., Eyer, J., & Thorn, B.E. (2013). Therapeutic relaxation. In S. G. Hofmann (Ed.), *The Wiley Handbook of Cognitive Behavioral Therapy: A Complete Reference Guide. Volume 1: CBT General Strategies* (Vol. *1*, pp. 157–180). Oxford: Wiley-Blackwell.

Day, M. A., & Thorn, B. E. (2010). The relationship of demographic and psychosocial variables to pain-related outcomes in a rural chronic pain population. *Pain, 151*(2), 467–474.

Dersh, J., Gatchel, R. J., Mayer, T. G., Polatin, P. B., & Temple, O. W. (2006). Prevalence of psychiatric disorders in patients in patients with chronic disabling occupational spinal disorders. *Spine, 31*, 1156–1162.

Drahovzal, D., Stewart, S., & Sullivan, M. (2006). Tendency to catastrophize somatic sensations: Pain catastrophizing and anxiety sensitivity in predicting headache. *Cognitive Behaviour Therapy, 35*(4), 226–235.

Eccleston, C., & Crombez, G. (1999). Pain demands attention: A cognitive-affective model of the interruptive function of pain. *Psychological Bulletin, 125*(3), 356–366.

Edwards, R. R., Cahalan, C., Mensing, G., Smith, M., & Haythornthwaite, J. A. (2011). Pain, catastrophizing, and depression in the rheumatic diseases. *Nature Reviews Rheumatology, 7*(4), 216–224.

Elliott, A. M., Smith, B. H., Penny, K. I., Smith, W. C., & Chambers, W.A. (1999). The epidemiology of chronic pain in the community. *Lancet, 354*, 1248–1252.

Engel, G. L. (1977). The need for a new medical model: A challenge for biomedicine. *Science, 196*(4286), 129–136.

Eriksen, J., Jensen, M. K., Sjøgren, P., Ekholm, O., & Rasmussen, N. K. (2003). Epidemiology of chronic non-malignant pain in Denmark. *Pain, 106*, 221–228.

Flor, H., Behle, D. J., & Birbaumer, N. (1993). Assessment of pain-related cognitions in chronic pain patients. *Behaviour Research and Therapy, 31*(1), 63–73.

Fordyce, W. E. (1976). *Behavioral methods for chronic pain and illness*. St. Louis, MO: Mosby.

Fornito, A., Harrison, B. J., Zalesky, A., & Simons, J. S. (2012). Competitive and cooperative dynamics of large-scale brain functional networks supporting recollection. *Proceedings of the National Academy of Sciences USA, 109*(31), 12788–12793.

Fredrickson, B. L. (2001). The role of positive emotions in positive psychology. The broaden-and-build theory of positive emotions. *American Psychologist, 56*(3), 218–226.

Gaskin, D. J., & Richard, P. (2012). The economic costs of pain in the United States. *The Journal of Pain, 13*(8), 715–724.

Gatchel, R. J. (2004). Comorbidity of chronic pain and mental health: The biopsychosocial perspective. *American Psychologist, 59*, 792–794.

Gatchel, R. J., Peng, Y. B., Peters, M. L., Fuchs, P. N., & Turk, D. C. (2007). The biopsychosocial approach to chronic pain: Scientific advances and future directions. *Psychological Bulletin, 133*(4), 581–624.

Geha, P. Y., Baliki, M. N., Harden, R. N., Bauer, W. R., Parrish, T. B., & Apkarian, A. V. (2008). The brain in chronic CRPS pain: Abnormal gray-white matter interactions in emotional and autonomic regions. *Neuron, 60*, 570–581.

Geisser, M. E., Robinson, M. E., Keefe, F. J., & Weiner, M. L. (1994). Catastrophizing, depression and the sensory, affective and evaluative aspects of chronic pain. *Pain, 59*(1), 79–83.

Giardino, N. D., Jensen, M., Turner, J. A., Ehde, D. M., & Cardenas, D. C. (2003). Social enviornment moderates the association between catastrophizing and pain among persons with spinal cord injury. *Pain, 106*, 19–25.

Greenwood, K. A., Thurston, R., Rumble, M., Waters, S. J., & Keefe, F. J. (2003). Anger and persistent pain: Current status and future directions. *Pain, 103,* 1–5.

Gwilym, S. E., Fillipini, N., Douaud, G., Carr, A. J., & Tracey, I. (2010). Thalamic atrophy associated with painful osteoarthritis of the hip is reversible after arthroplasty; a longitudinal voxel-based-morphometric study. *Arthritis and Rheumatology, 62,* 2930–2940.

Haig, R. A. (1988). *The anatomy of humor*. Springfield, IL: Charles C. Thomas.

Hann, K. E. J., & McCracken, L. M. (2014). A systematic review of randomized controlled trials of acceptance and commitment therapy for adults with chronic pain: Outcome domains, design quality, and efficacy. *Journal of Contextual Behavioral Science, 3*(4), 217–227.

Harstall, C., & Ospina, M. (2003). How prevalent is chronic pain? *Pain: Clinical Updates, 11,* 1–4.

Hart, L. G., Deyo, R. A., & Cherkin, D. C. (1995). Physician office visits for low back pain. *Spine, 20,* 11–19.

Hoffman, P., Meier, B., & Council, J. R. (2002). A comparison of chronic pain between an urban and rural population. *Journal of Community Health Nursing, 19,* 213–224.

Holtzman, S., & Delongis, A. (2007). One day at a time: The impact of daily satisfaction with spouse responses on pain, negative affect and catastrophizing among individuals with rheumatoid arthritis. *Pain, 131,* 202–213.

IASP Subcommittee on Taxonomy, C. o. c. p. (1986). Descriptions of chronic pain syndromes and definitions of pain terms. *Pain, 3,* S1–S226.

IASP Taxonomy, I. T. F. o. (1994). *Classification of chronic pain,* 2nd ed. Seattle, WA: IASP Press.

IOM. (2011). *Relieving pain in America: A blueprint for transforming prevention, care, education, and research.* Washington, DC: The National Academics Press.

Jensen, M. C., Brantzawadzki, M. N., Obuchowski, N., Modic, M. T., Malkasian, D., & Ross, J. S. (1994). Magnetic-resonance-imaging of the lumbar spine in people without back pain. *New England Journal of Medicine, 331*(2), 69–73.

Jensen, M., Turner, J. A., & Romano, J. M. (2001). Changes in beliefs, catastrophizing and coping are associated with improvement in multidisciplinary pain treatment. *Journal of Consulting and Clinical Psychology, 69,* 655–662.

Jensen, M. P. (2010). A neuropsychological model of pain: Research and clinical implications. *Journal of Pain, 11,* 2–12.

Kabat-Zinn, J. (1990). *Full catastrophe living: Using the wisdom of your body and mind to face stress, pain and illness.* New York, NY: Delacourt.

Keefe, F. J., Blumenthal, J., Baucom, D., Affleck, G., Waugh, R., Caldwell, D. S., … Lefebvre, J. (2004). Effects of spouse-assisted coping skills training and exercise training in patients with osteoarthritic knee pain: A randomized controlled study. *Pain, 110*(3), 539–549.

Keefe, F., Caldwell, D. S., Queen, K. T., Gil, K. M., Martinez, S., Crisson, J. E., … Nunley, J. (1987). Pain coping strategies in osteoarthritis patients. *Journal of Consulting and Clinical Psychology, 55,* 208–212.

Keefe, F. J., Rumble, M. E., Scipio, C. D., Giordano, L. A., & Perri, L. M. (2004). Psychological aspects of persistent pain: Current state of the science. *Journal of Pain, 5*(4), 195–211.

Khalid, I., Roehrs, T. A., Hudgel, D. W., & Roth, T. (2011). Continuous positive airway pressure in severe obstructive sleep apnea reduces pain sensitivity. *Sleep, 34*(12), 1687–1691.

Kim, J. H., Suh, S. I., Seol, H. Y., Oh, K., Seo, W. K., Yu, S. W., ... Koh, S. B. (2008). Regional grey matter changes in patients with migraine: A voxel-based morphometry study. *Cephalagia, 28*, 598–604.

Kington, R. S., & Smith, J. P. (1997). Socioeconomic status and racial and ethnic differences in functional status associated with chronic diseases. *American Journal of Public Health, 87*(5), 805–810.

Kuchinad, A., Schweinhardt, P., Seminowicz, D. A., Wood, P. B., Chizh, B. A., & Bushnell, M. C. (2007). Accelerated brain gray matter loss in fibromyalgia patients: premature aging of the brain? *The Journal of Neuroscience 27*(15), 4004–4007.

Lambert, M. J. (1992). Implications of outcome research for psychotherapy integration. In N. J. C. & M. R. Goldstein (Eds.), *Handbook of psychotherapy integration* (pp. 94–129). New York, NY: Basic Books.

Lazarus, R. S., & Folkman, S. (1984). *Stress, appraisal, and coping.* New York, NY: Springer.

Luerding, R., Weigand, T., Bogdahn, U., & Schmidt-Wilcke, T. (2008). Working memory performance is correlated with local brain morphology in the medial frontal and anterior cingulate cortex in fibromyalgia patients: Structural correlates of pain-cognition interaction. *Brain, 131*, 3222–3231.

Magni, G., Caldieron, C., Rigatti-Luchini, S., & Merskey, H. (1990). Chronic musculoskeletal pain and depressive symptoms in the general population. An analysis of the 1st National Health and Nutrition Examination Survey data. *Pain, 43*, 299–307.

Mahony, D. L., Burroughs, D. L., & Hieatt, A. C. (2001). The effects of laughter on discomfort thresholds: Does expectation become reality? *Journal of General Psychology, 128*(2), 217–226.

McCracken, L. M., & Eccleston, C. (2003). Coping or acceptance: What to do about chronic pain? *Pain, 105*, 197–204.

McCracken, L. M., Matthews, A. K., Tang, T. S., & Cuba, S. L. (2001). A comparison of blacks and whites seeking treatment for chronic pain. *The Clinical Journal of Pain, 17*, 249–255.

McCracken, L. M., & Samuel, V. M. (2007). The role of avoidance, pacing, and other activity patterns in chronic pain. *Pain, 130*, 119–125.

McCracken, L. M., & Vowles, K. E. (2006). Acceptance of chronic pain. *Current Pain and Headache Reports, 10*(2), 90–94.

McCracken, L. M., Vowles, K. E., & Eccleston, C. (2004). The Chronic Pain Acceptance Questionnaire. *Pain, 107*(1), 271–277.

McCracken, L. M., Vowles, K. E., & Zhao-O'Brien, J. (2010). Further development of an instrument to assess psychological flexibility in people with chronic pain. *Journal of Behavioural Medicine, 33*, 346–354.

McEwan, B. S. (2007). Physiology and neurobiology of stress and adaptation: Central role of the brain. *Physiological Reviews, 87*(3), 873–904.

McIlvane, J. M. (2007). Disentangling the effects of race and SES on arthritis-related symptoms, coping, and well-being in African American and White women. *Aging and Mental Health, 11*(5), 556–569.

Melzack, R. (2001). Pain and the neuromatrix in the brain. *Journal of Dental Education, 65,* 1378–1382.
Melzack, R. (2005). Evolution of the neuromatrix theory of pain. The Prithvi Raj Lecture: Presented at the third World Congress of World Institute of Pain, Barcelona 2004. *Pain Practice, 5,* 85–94.
Melzack, R., & Wall, P. D. (1965). Pain mechanisms: A new theory. *Science, 150*(699), 971–979.
Melzack, R., & Wall, P. D. (1982). *The challenge of pain.* New York, NY: Basic Books.
Moulin, D. E., Clark, A. J., Speechley, M., & Morley-Forster, P. K. (2002). Chronic pain in Canada-prevalence, treatment, impact and the role of opioid analgesia. *Pain Research and Management, 7,* 179–184.
National Centers for Health Statistics. (2013). Health, United States, with special features on prescription drugs. 37th. Retrieved from http://www.cdc.gov/nchs/data/hus/hus13.pdf
Neville, A., Peleg, R., Singer, Y., Sherf, M., & Shvartzman, P. (2008). Chronic pain: A population-based study. *Israel Medical Association Journal, 10,* 676–680.
Ng, K. F., Tsui, S. L., & Chan, W. S. (2002). Prevalence of common chronic pain in Hong Kong adults. *The Clinical Journal of Pain, 18,* 275–281.
Nguyen, M., Ugarte, C., Fuller, I., Haas, G., & Portnenoy, R. (2005). Access to care for chronic pain: Racial and ethnic differences. *The Journal of Pain, 6,* 301–314.
NIH. (2011). *Interagency pain research coordinating committee: National Pain Strategy.* Retrieved from https://iprcc.nih.gov/docs/DraftHHSNationalPainStrategy.pdf
Obermann, M., Nebel, K., Schumann, C., Holle, D., Gizewski, E. R., Maschke, M., ... Katsarava, Z. (2009). Grey matter changes related to chronic posttraumatic headache. *Neurology, 73,* 978–983.
O'Brien, E. M., Waxenberg, L. B., Atchison, J. W., Gremillion, H. A., Staud, R. M., McCrae, C. S., & Robinson, M. E. (2010). Negative mood mediates the effect of poor sleep on pain among chronic pain patients. *Clinical Journal of Pain, 26*(4), 310–319.
Ohayon, M. M. (2005). Relationship between chronic painful physical condition and insomnia. *Journal of Psychiatric Research, 39,* 151–159.
Okifuji, A., Turk, D. C., & Curran, S. L. (1999). Anger in chronic pain: Investigations of anger targets and intensity. *Journal of Psychosomatic Research, 47,* 1–12.
Ossipov, M. H., Dussor, G. O., & Porreca, F. (2010). Central modulation of pain. *The Journal of Clinical Investigation, 120*(11), 3779–3787.
Palmer, C. A., & Alfano, C. A. (2016). Sleep and emotion regulation: An organizing, integrative review. *Sleep Medicine Reviews* DOI: 10.1016/j.smrv.2015.12.006
Pfingsten, M., Kroner-Herwig, B., Leibing, E., Kronshage, U., & Hildebrandt, J. (2000). Validation of the German version of the Fear-Avoidance Beliefs Questionnaire (FABQ). *European Journal of Pain, 4,* 259–266.
Poiraudeau, S., Rannou, F., Baron, G., Le Henanff, A., Coudeyre, E., Rozenberg, S., ... Ravaud, P. (2006). Fear-avoidance beliefs about back pain in patients with subacute low back pain. *Pain, 124,* 305–311.
Portenoy, R., Ugarte, C., & Fuller, I. (2004). Population-based survey of pain in the United States: Differences among White, African American, and Hispanic subjects. *The Journal of Pain, 5,* 317–328.

Prkachin, K. M., Schultz, I. Z., & Hughes, E. (2007). Pain behavior and the development of pain-related disability: The importance of guarding. *Clinical Journal of Pain, 23,* 270–277.

Purves, D., Augustine, G. J., Fitzpatrick, D., Katz, L. C., LaMantia, A., McNamara, J. O., & Williams, S. M. (2001). *Neuroscience* (2nd ed.). Sunderland, MA: Sinauer Associates.

Reynolds, D. V. (1969). Surgery in the rat during electrical analgesia induced by focal brain stimulation. *Science, 164*(13), 1099–1109.

Rodriguez-Raecke, R., Niemeier, A., Ihle, K., Ruether, W., & May, A. (2009). Brain grey matter decrease in chronic pain is the consequence and not the cause of pain. *Journal of Neuroscience, 29,* 13746–13750.

Romano, J., & Turner, J. A. (1985). Chronic pain and depression: Does the evidence support a relationship? *Psychological Bulletin, 97,* 18–34.

Rudy, T. E., Lieber, S. J., Boston, J. R., Gourley, L. M., & Baysal, E. (2003). Psychosocial predictors of physical performance in disabled individuals with chronic pain. *Clinical Journal of Pain, 19,* 18–30.

Schmidt-Wilcke, T., Leinisch, E., Ganssbauer, S., Draganski, B., Bogdahn, U., Altmeppen, J., & May, A. (2006). Affective components and intensity of pain correlate with structural differences in gray matter in chronic back pain patients. *Pain, 125*(1–2), 89–97.

Schnitzler, A., & Ploner, M. (2000). Neurophysiology and functional neuroanatomy of pain perception. *Journal of Clinical Neurophysiology, 17*(6), 592–603.

Schrimpf, M., Liegl, G., Boeckle, M., Leitner, A., Geisler, P., & Pieh, C. (2015). The effect of sleep deprivation on pain perception in health subjects: A meta-analysis. *Sleep Medicine, 16,* 1313–1320.

Schutze, R., Rees, C., Preece, M., & Schutze, M. (2010). Low mindfulness predicts pain catastrophizing in a fear-avoidance model of chronic pain. *Pain, 148,* 120–127.

Schwartz, B. S., Stewart, W. F., Simon, D., & Lipton, R. B. (1998). Epidemiology of tension-type headache. *Journal of the American Medical Association, 279*(5), 381–383.

Selim, A. J., Fincke, G., Ren, X. S., Deyo, R. A., Lee, A., Skinner, K., & Kazis, L. (2001). Racial differences in the use of lumbar spine radiographs: Results from the Veterans Health Study. *Spine (Phila Pa 1976), 26*(12), 1364–1369.

Selye, H. (1956). *The stress of life.* New York, NY: McGraw-Hill.

Selye, H. (1973). The evolution of the stress concept. *American Scientist, 61,* 692–699.

Shmuely, Y., Baumgarten, M., Rovner, B., & Berlin, J. (2001). Predictors of improvement in health-related quality of life among elderly patients with depression. *International Pyschogeriatrics, 13,* 63–73.

Sjøgren, P., Ekholm, O., Peuckmann, V., & Grønbæk, M. (2009). Epidemiology of chronic pain in Denmark: An update. *European Journal of Pain, 13,* 287–292.

Smith, M. T., & Haythornthwaite, J. A. (2004). How do sleep disturbance and chronic pain inter-relate? Insights from the longitudinal and cognitive-behavioral clinical trials literature. *Sleep Medicine Reviews, 8*(2), 119–132.

Smith, M. T., Perlis, M. L., Smith, M. S., Giles, D. E., & Carmody, T. P. (2000). Sleep quality and presleep arousal in chronic pain. *Journal of Behavioral Medicine, 23*(1), 1–13.

Stang, P., Von Korff, M., & Galer, B. S. (1998). Reduced labor force participation among primary care patients with headache. *Journal of General Internal Medicine, 13,* 296–302.

Strand, E. B., Zautra, A. J., Thoresen, M., Ødegard, S., Uhlig, T., & Finset, A. (2006). Positive affect as a factor of resilience in the pain-negative affect relationship in patients with rheumatoid arthritis. *Journal of Psychosomatic Research, 60,* 477–484.

Sturgeon, J. A. (2014). Psychological therapies for the management of chronic pain. *Psychology Research and Behavior Management, 7,* 115–124.

Sullivan, M. J. L. (2012). The communal coping model of pain catastrophizing: Clinical and research implications. *Canadian Psychology, 53*(1), 32–41.

Sullivan, M. J. L., Adams, H., Sullivan, M. E. (2004). Communicative dimensions of pain catastrophizing: Social cueing effects on pain behaviour and coping. *Pain, 107,* 220–226.

Sullivan, M. J., Rodgers, W. M., & Kirsch, I. (2001). Catastrophizing, depression and expectancies for pain and emotional distress. *Pain, 91*(1–2), 147–154.

Sullivan, M. J., Thorn, B., Haythornthwaite, J. A., Keefe, F., Martin, M., Bradley, L. A., & Lefebvre, J. C. (2001). Theoretical perspectives on the relation between catastrophizing and pain. *Clinical Journal of Pain, 17*(1), 52–64.

Tait, R. C., & Chibnall, J. T. (2005). Racial and ethnic disparities in the evaluation and treatment of pain: psychological perspectives. *Professional Psychology: Research and Practice, 36*(6), 595–601.

Takeyachi, Y., Konno, S., Otani, K., Yamauchi, K., Takahashi, I., Suzukamo, Y., & Kikuchi, S. (2003). Correlation of low back pain with functional status, general health perception, social participation, subjective happiness and patient satisfaction. *Spine, 28*(13), 1461–1467.

Tan, G., Jensen, M. P., Robinson-Whelen, S., Thornby, J. I., & Monga, T. (2002). Measuring control appraisals in chronic pain. *Journal of Pain, 3*(5), 385–393.

Tang, N. K. Y., & Crane, C. (2006). Suicidality in chronic pain: A review of the prevalence, risk factors and psychological links. *Psychological Medicine, 36*(5), 575–586.

Tang, N. K., Wright, K. J., & Salkovskis, P. M. (2007). Prevalence and correlates of clinical insomnia co-occurring with chronic back pain. *Journal of Sleep Research, 16,* 85–95.

Taylor, D. J., Mallory, L. J., Lichstein, K. L., Durrence, H. H., Riedel, B. W., & Bush, A. J. (2007). Comorbidity of chronic insomnia with medical problems. *Sleep, 30,* 213–218.

Teasell, R. W., & Bombardier, C. (2001). Employment-related factors in chronic pain and chronic pain disability. *Clinical Journal of Pain, 17*(4), S39–S45.

The American Academy of Pain Medicine. (2016). AAPM facts and figures on pain. Retrieved from http://www.painmed.org/PatientCenter/Facts_on_Pain.aspx

Thibault, P., Loisel, P., Durand, M. J., & Sullivan, M. J. L. (2008). Psychological predictors of pain expression and activity intolerance in chronic pain patients. *Pain, 139,* 47–54.

Thompson, M., & McCracken, L. M. (2011). Acceptance and related processes in adjustment to chronic pain. *Current Pain and Headache Reports, 15*(2), 144–151.

Thorn, B. E. (2004). *Cognitive therapy for chronic pain: A step-by-step guide.* New York, NY: Guilford Press.

Thorn, B. E., & Walker, B. B. (2011). Chronic pain: Closing the gap between evidence and practice. In H. S. Friedman (Ed.), *The Oxford handbook of health psychology*. New York, NY: Oxford University Press, 375–393.

Trescot, A. M., Glaser, S. E., Hansen, H., Benyamin, R., Patel, S., & Manchikanti, L. (2008). Effectiveness of opioids in the treatment of chronic non-cancer pain. *Pain Physician, 11*(2 Suppl), S181–S200.

Trost, Z., Vangronsveld, K., Linton, S. J., Quartana, P. J., & Sullivan, M. J. L. (2012). Cognitive dimensions of anger in chronic pain. *Pain, 153*, 515–517.

Tse, M., Lo, A., Cheng, T., Chan, E., Chan, A., & Chung, H. (2010). Humor therapy: Relieving chronic pain and enhancing happiness for older adults. *Journal of Aging Research, 2010*, 1–9.

Tsui, P., Day, M. A., Thorn, B. E., Rubin, N., Alexander, C., & Jones, R. (2012). The communal coping model of catastrophizing: Patient-health provider interactions. *Pain Medicine, 13*, 66–79.

Unruh, A. M. (1996). Gender variations in clinical pain experience. *Pain, 65*, 123–167.

Unruh, A. M., & Richie, J. A. (1998). Development of the pain appraisal inventory: Psychometric properties. *Pain, 65*, 105–110.

Verhaak, P. F. M., Kerssens, J. J., Dekker, J., Sorbi, M. J., & Bensing, J. M. (1998). Prevalence of chronic benign pain disorder among adults: A review of the literature. *Pain, 77*, 231–239.

Vlaeyen, J. W., Kole-Snijders, A. M., Boeren, R. G., & van Eek, H. (1995). Fear of movement/(re)injury in chronic low back pain and its relation to behavioral performance. *Pain, 62*, 363–372.

Vlaeyen, J. W. S., Kole-Snijders, A., Rotteveel, A., Ruesink, R., & Heuts, P. (1995). The role of fear of movement/(re)injury in pain disability. *Journal of Occupational Rehabilitation, 5*, 235–252.

Vlaeyen, J. W. S., & Linton, S. J. (2000). Fear-avoidance and its consequences in chronic musculoskeletal pain: A state of the art review. *Pain, 85*, 317–332.

Waddell, G., Newton, M., Henderson, I., Somerville, D., & Main, C. J. (1993). A Fear Avoidance Beliefs Questionnaire (FABQ) and the role of fear-avoidance beliefs in chronic low back pain and disability. *Pain, 52*, 157–168.

Walker, J., Holloway, I., & Sofaer, B. (1999). In the system: The lived experience of chronic back pain from the perspectives of those seeking help from pain clinics. *Pain, 80*, 621–628.

Williams, D. R., & Collins, C. (1995). US socioeconomic and racial differences in health: Patterns and explanations. *Annual Review Sociology, 21*, 349–386.

Wilson, K. G., Eriksson, M. Y., D'Eon, J. L., Mikail, S. F., & Emery, P. C. (2002). Major depression and insomnia in chronic pain. *Clinical Journal of Pain, 18*, 77–83.

Wolfe, F., Smythe, H. A., Yunus, M. B., Bennett, R. M., Bombardier, C., Goldenberg, D. L. ... Sheon, R. P. (1990). The American College of Rheumatology 1990 criteria for the classification of fibromyalgia: Report of the Multicenter Criteria Committee. *Arthritis and Rheumatology, 33*, 160–172.

Woolf, C. J. (2011). Central sensitization: Implications for the diagnosis and treatment of pain. *Pain, 152*(3), S2–15.

Woolf, C. J., & Salter, M. W. (2000). Neuronal plasticity: Increasing the gain in pain. *Science, 288*, 1765–1768.

World Health Organization (2004). World Health Organization supports global effort to relieve chronic pain. Retrieved from http://www.who.int/mediacentre/news/releases/2004/pr70/en/

Zautra, A. J., Smith, B., Affleck, G., & Tennen, H. (2001). Examinations of chronic pain and affect relationships: Applications of a dynamic model of affect. *Journal of Consulting and Clinical Psychology, 69*, 786–795.

2

Psychosocial Chronic Pain Management: Current State of the Theory and Evidence

We now know with greater conviction than ever before that pain, and particularly chronic pain, is clearly much more intimately linked to supraspinal cortical activity and processes than peripheral activity (Apkarian et al., 2009; Jensen, 2010). Brain imaging research shows that psychological processes shape the way pain is interpreted and contribute to central sensitization and the chronification of pain; this provides convincing evidence that treatments based on psychological principles for pain are viable, ideally suited approaches that hold tremendous potential. Psychological approaches to chronic pain have been in continuous development since the 1960s, and research shows that they are at least as efficacious as medically based treatments such as surgery and medication management (Eccleston, Palermo, Williams, Lewandowski, & Morley, 2009; Morley & Williams, 2015). Further, while many of the available biomedical approaches entail potentially serious side-effects (Trescot et al., 2008), the side-effect profile of psychological treatments for pain is typically positive in that we often see the alarmingly high rates of comorbid emotional problems (e.g., depression, anxiety), unhelpful cognitions, and the behavioral and social ramifications associated with chronic pain also improve. In this section we will explore the rich theoretical, clinical, and empirical tradition of the application of psychological treatments for chronic pain management, which will provide clarity for later understanding the contextual theory upon which MBCT for chronic pain is founded.

Behavioral Approaches

Theory

Wilbert E. Fordyce, the founding father of multidisciplinary pain treatment, was the first to apply psychological principles to the management of pain (Fordyce, 1976). Fordyce theorized that the application of behavioral technology stemming from Skinner's (1953) operant conditioning principles had the capacity to shape and enhance adaptive coping responses in the context of daily persistent pain. Skinner detailed how operants—which are intentional actions or behaviors that produce an effect on the surrounding environment—increase in frequency and

Mindfulness-Based Cognitive Therapy for Chronic Pain: A Clinical Manual and Guide, First Edition. Melissa A. Day.

Companion website: www.wiley.com/go/day/mindfulness_based_cognitive_therapy

are repeated when reinforced, and are reduced or extinguished when not reinforced. Based on this, Fordyce hypothesized that certain interpersonal and social consequences of chronic pain (or more precisely, consequences of the outward behaviors of the person *in* chronic pain) create powerful environmental contingencies that function to operantly condition increased maladaptive pain behaviors (e.g., pain contingent resting, grimacing, guarding) and reduced adaptive behaviors (e.g., paced activity, social interaction).

For example, a partner may respond to the patient rubbing his/her back while vacuuming by jumping in, providing a solicitous response, and by further attending to the pain behavior by offering to take over the vacuuming. Unwittingly (for both the partner *and* often also the patient), this may actually serve to reinforce (and sustain) the maladaptive pain behavior, leading to increased pain contingent resting. Alternatively, a partner who responds with encouragement of normal activity appropriately paced throughout the day would reinforce the patient continuing to engage normal role function. Fordyce recognized the importance of such environmental context and associated learning theory, and he hypothesized that these operant conditioning processes played a central role in predicting disability and function over time.

Techniques and Application

Through Fordyce's pioneering work, Behavioral Therapy (BT) became the first psychological approach that was applied to the management of pain (Fordyce, 1976). In practice, Fordyce's model programs were based on the premise of first analyzing a client's pain behavior tendencies and their function within specific contexts. Next, contingency management and reinforcement principles were applied that were specifically designed to target the shaping of an increase in adaptive well behavior, and a decrease in maladaptive pain behavior. Within this model, Fordyce recognized the importance of appropriate quota-based reactivation and pacing. Specifically, some individuals become fearful of the pain and "underdo," and for these individuals a quota-based reactivation plan with the goal of systematically increasing their baseline activity capacity by a goal (quota) of approximately 5% each day (while not allowing pain to guide behavior) would be recommended. On the other hand, some individuals fall in to patterns of "overdoing" at times where their pain feels better only to then "pay the penalty later." Fordyce described this pattern as repeated "boom and bust" behaviors, which over time increases the risk for pain flare-ups and results in muscle atrophy associated with the usually increasingly longer periods of the inactivity phase; hence, pacing skills would be recommended to these individuals to develop a more consistent, regular pattern of behavioral activity, which was again not guided by levels of pain (i.e., whether it is a "good day" or "bad day"). More modern BT approaches have expanded the repertoire of techniques taught to include a variety of relaxation approaches, behavioral activation, assertiveness training, expressive writing, and a host of other behavioral skills training activities.

An additional, more recently developed behaviorally focused application of learning theory has emerged from Vlaeyen's fear-avoidance model (FAM), which incorporates graded in vivo exposure-based techniques explicitly designed to target fear of pain. Within this approach, fear of pain is considered a classically conditioned response to catastrophizing about ongoing pain, leading to safety-seeking behavioral patterns of avoidance and escape which, over the long term, ultimately leads to more rest time, deconditioning of muscles, and heightened disability (Vlaeyen & Linton, 2000). Based on this, the primary treatment targets are to reduce fear of pain and avoidance behavior through the application of graded exposure techniques, where clients learn that engagement in feared/avoided behaviors does not lead to serious consequences (Leeuw et al., 2007; Vlaeyen, de Jong, Geilen, Heuts, & van Breukelen, 2001). Psychoeducation on the fear-avoidance model is also typically included in these programs, along with application of reinforcement principles to encourage confronting feared activities and engaging in enjoyable, pleasurable activities (Woods & Asmundson, 2008).

Evidence and Limitations

Fordyce's behavioral principles are a key component of many currently investigated treatment approaches. A large body of research has documented the efficacy of behavioral approaches for a variety of chronic pain conditions in improving functioning and adjustment to chronic pain in the short and long term (Henschke et al., 2010; Keefe & Lefebvre, 1999; Ostelo et al., 2005). Reviews of the literature have reported that BT is particularly effective for headache pain (Andrasik, 2003, 2007) and low back pain (Henschke et al., 2010), however other approaches that include cognitive therapy components (described below) appear to be equally as effective (Henschke et al., 2010; Thorn et al., 2007). A behavioral treatment based on behavioral activation (Martell, Dimidjian, & Herman-Dunn, 2010) applied to chronic fibromyalgia pain was also found to be efficacious, resulting in improvement across a variety of pain-related functioning, emotional, and medical outcomes (Lundervold, Talley, & Buermann, 2008). A building body of research supports the efficacy of the more recently developed exposure-based approaches, with results showing improved pain, fear of pain, catastrophizing, disability, and return to work rates (Linton et al., 2008; Staal et al., 2006; Sullivan, Adams, Rhodenizer, & Stanish, 2006; Vlaeyen, de Jong, Geilen, Heuts, & van Breukelen, 2002; Woods & Asmundson, 2008). However, comparatively, research on average suggests that the efficacy of this approach is equal to that based on operant graded activity principles (as in Fordyce's model) (Henschke et al., 2010; Leeuw et al., 2007).

One lasting legacy of Fordyce's work is his emphasis on the social context. As described in the previous chapter, a large body of research has documented the significant role a partner's response to pain behaviors plays in predicting whether those pain behaviors are maintained (and perpetuate negative pain outcomes) or are extinguished (Flor & Turk, 2011; Romano, Jensen, Turner, Good, & Hops, 2000). Research has found that treatment programs that include a client's support system (i.e., partner, family members) lead to increased adaptive coping efforts and a tendency toward decreased pain intensity (Keefe, Blumenthal, et al., 2004; Keefe et al., 1996; Keefe & Somers, 2010). However, little is known about the comparative efficacy of these programs relative to a treatment approach that does not include the client's support system.

Although strict BT is rarely still implemented, behavioral principles remain highly influential in present conceptualizations of the experience of chronic pain, and current widely used interventions draw heavily from, and build upon, the foundation laid by Fordyce's seminal work. While efficacious, the main criticism of BT approaches is that they may not be an adequate stand alone. For example, Linton and colleagues found in their study that many patients had additional issues beyond just fear of pain (i.e., maladaptive cognitive beliefs, family issues, workplace changes) that needed to be acknowledged and targeted (Linton et al., 2008). Recognition of this limitation of the strictly behavioral approach sparked the "cognitive revolution" in the 1970s when clinicians across multiple fields began to emphasize the importance of therapeutically targeting maladaptive cognitions within behavioral interventions (Beck, 1979; Foreyt & Rathjen, 1978; Meichenbaum, 1977). In the early 1980s, pain researchers began integrating cognitive therapy and behavioral approaches such that these issues, along with maladaptive behaviors, could concurrently be addressed.

Cognitive-Behavioral Therapy

Theory

The cognitive-behavioral perspective has arguably been the most influential of the biopsychosocial models of chronic pain in terms of the breadth and depth of the research stemming from its theoretical tenets, and its broad international clinical application. The emergence of cognitive-behavioral therapy (CBT) for pain represented a paradigm shift (Kerns, Turk, Holzman, & Rudy, 1986; Turk, Meichenbaum, & Genest, 1983; Turner, 1982; Turner & Clancy, 1988), broadening the focus of biopsychosocial treatment beyond the behavioral patterns that were the cornerstone of Fordyce's model programs, to include an integrated focus on targeting maladaptive thoughts, beliefs, and perceptions. Further, the evolving CBT approach includes an expanded repertoire of BT techniques that are designed to theoretically target the aforementioned learning theory principles applied by Fordyce, Keefe, Vlaeyen, and others.

Theoretically, the rationale for the integration of the cognitive element with BT learning theory principles in CBT was to explicitly target change in not just maladaptive behaviors (as in BT), but also change in maladaptive cognitive content (i.e., *what* an individual thinks about pain). So along with the aforementioned BT theory, there are also three levels of cognitions simultaneously theoretically targeted by CBT for pain, which stem from Aaron Beck's original cognitive therapy (CT) theory (Beck, 1979). The first is the level of automatic thoughts, which may be thought of as the running stream of mental commentary happening just below the surface of consciousness that we are not typically aware of until we bring attention to it (pain catastrophizing is conceptualized at this level). The second level is intermediate beliefs, which theoretically give rise to automatic thoughts, and typically center around the rules or "should beliefs" we hold about how ourselves, others, and the world should be, ought to be or must be. The third, most deep seated level is core beliefs, which are deeply held beliefs about ourselves (often developed in childhood) around themes typically about our lovability, worth, and competency, and which theoretically give rise to intermediate beliefs and subsequent patterns of automatic thoughts. We all have these automatic thoughts, intermediate and core beliefs, they are a large part of what we base our identity around, and they help us to navigate our world. However, during times of prolonged stress (such as in the context of chronic pain), negative or unhelpful thoughts and beliefs tend to rise to the surface and predominate, and patterns of thinking can become overly strict, rigid, or harsh, which is theorized in time to lead to worse pain outcomes.

Returning back to the Transactional Model of Stress (Lazarus & Folkman, 1984), recall that the root of stress is not the outer "stressful" circumstance per se. Rather, it is the underlying cognitive pathways (e.g., primary loss appraisals that might map on to the core belief "I am worthless," and ensuing secondary appraisals mapping onto automatic thoughts such as, "There is nothing I can do") that translate the initial stimulus and response into "unmanageable" and "threatening" (Thorn, 2004). From this perspective, chronic pain and other situations are considered stressful if the individual judges or appraises the stimulus as taxing and as exceeding one's coping resources, which then subsequently leads to initiation of the stress response. In the context of chronic pain, this is particularly damaging as if these stress-inciting judgments and thoughts predominate over time, then the stress response remains persistently "switched on," leading to chronically elevated blood pressure, damaging levels of stress hormones such as cortisol, weakened immune system functioning, and worsening pain outcomes (Kabat-Zinn, 1990, 2013). Thus, in CBT the aim is to take an antecedent-oriented pain management approach to intervene at the level of the maladaptive thoughts, beliefs, and behaviors arising in the context of chronic pain and related stress *before* they cascade and potentially trigger a downward spiral of negative emotions, symptoms, and behaviors that feed into each other in a vicious cycle, culminating in worsening pain and stress over time (Hofmann & Asmundson, 2008).

Techniques and Application

Although there is no "standard" CBT protocol, a critical component of CBT for chronic pain is promoting a more positive and realistic reappraisal of situations initially judged as overwhelming and stressful, and to activate adaptive behavioral responses. To this end, one of the central cognitive techniques taught in most CBT-based interventions is cognitive restructuring (although other techniques are also applied), which aims to target the quality and content of thoughts. In essence, cognitive restructuring entails first enhancing a client's awareness of automatic thoughts, intermediate and core beliefs (with beliefs targeted later in treatment than automatic thoughts), such that patients are taught to recognize "red flags" in their thinking patterns (Thorn, 2004). For example, words such as "always," "never," "should" suggest the possibility for rigid or overly negative thinking, and thought patterns such as "Fortune Telling" (i.e., catastrophizing about the future) and "Mind Reading" (i.e., "My doctor thinks my pain is not real") and others can be identified as unhelpful frequent fliers. Once these thoughts are noted in awareness, patients are then taught to weigh the evidence for and against the thought/belief to determine its level of truth (and helpfulness)—much like a judge in a court room. Once the evidence is collected, the overly rigid or maladaptive thought is challenged and restructured (with the help of Socratic dialogue), to develop more realistic, helpful, and adaptive alternative thoughts/beliefs, which can also be placed on coping cards to remind patients of their more adaptive thoughts throughout the day. Further, the cognitive restructuring skill set is mastered via completion of thought records and column technique worksheets completed by clients as take-home activities between sessions. In this way, thoughts and beliefs come to be viewed as simply ideas that can be challenged and changed, and are not fact. Over time, this process of repeatedly identifying and examining the validity of negative and unhelpful thoughts allows patients to distance themselves from the thoughts, thereby engendering a decentered, more generalized change in worldview.

A variety of behavioral techniques are also taught—sometimes prior to the cognitive component of the program, sometimes following, and sometimes integrated into the same session, depending on any number of reasons and factors—to enhance stress management and increase well behaviors. Behavioral techniques often used in CBT for pain programs include relaxation, biofeedback, assertiveness training, expressive writing (or another form of emotional expression), setting and working towards behavioral goals (such as increasing pleasurable or rewarding activities), behavioral activation, and guidance on activity pacing (Ehde et al., 2014; Turner & Romano, 2001). The behavioral techniques taught in session are assigned for further at-home practice between sessions; for example, an audio recording of a guided relaxation is often provided for patients' use.

Evidence and Limitations

The initial empirical investigations of CBT for a variety of heterogeneous chronic pain conditions by leaders in the field such as Turk, Turner, Kerns, and others demonstrated the tremendous potential of this approach (Kerns et al., 1986; Turner, 1982; Turner & Clancy, 1988). Three decades later, CBT has become the first-line psychosocial treatment for chronic pain (Ehde et al., 2014), with the efficacy of this approach documented by a proliferation of RCTs, as well as in meta-analyses and systematic reviews. Although there is strong evidence for this approach in nonadult populations, most of the research to date has been conducted within adult populations with chronic back pain, headache, orofacial pain, or arthritis related pain, and to a lesser degree across an array of other pain conditions, including cancer-related pain (Ehde et al., 2014). In terms of specific outcomes following CBT for chronic pain, a large body of research has shown this approach leads to short- and long-term improvement in pain intensity, interference in daily activities due to pain, mood, physical function, and disability, as well as pain catastrophizing and a variety of other outcomes (Aggarwal et al., 2011; Andrasik, 2007; Eccleston et al., 2009; Ehde et al., 2014; Hoffman, Papas, Chatkoff, & Kerns, 2007; Williams, Eccleston, & Morley, 2012). However, a recent systematic review of psychological approaches specifically for neuropathic pain found there was limited evidence to suggest CBT is effective in this population (Eccleston, Hearn, & Williams, 2015).

Research has found that the cognitive process of pain catastrophizing precedes and is a robust predictor of poor pain-related outcomes (Quartana, Campbell, & Edwards, 2009), and based on this body of research and the cognitive theory perspective underlying many CBT for pain programs, pain catastrophizing has become a focus mechanism variable targeted by modern CBT for pain approaches. A number of studies have found that treatment-related reductions in pain catastrophizing during CBT correlates with improvement in pain-related outcomes (Jensen et al., 2001; Turner, Holtzman, & Mancl, 2007). Further, research by Thorn and colleagues found that tailoring CBT specifically toward the reduction of catastrophizing is particularly effective for headache pain, with treatment-related reductions in pain catastrophizing correlating with improvement in several treatment outcome variables (Thorn et al., 2007). Other cognitive variables that have been found to correlate with improved outcomes during CBT include self-efficacy (Holroyd, Labus, & Carlson, 2009; Thorn et al., 2007; Turner et al., 2007), perceived pain control (Jensen et al., 2001; Spinhoven et al., 2004; Turner et al., 2007), pain helplessness (Burns, Johnson, Mahoney, Devine, & Pawl, 1998), and other pain-related beliefs (Jensen et al., 2001). Two other studies investigating a CBT-oriented interdisciplinary treatment program for chronic pain used lagged and cross-lagged analyses and found that early-treatment reductions in pain catastrophizing predicted late-treatment improvements in pain-related outcomes, but not vice versa (Burns, Glenn, Bruehl, Harden, & Lofland, 2003; Burns, Kubilus, Bruehl, Harden, & Lofland, 2003). However, a more recent sophisticated, nuanced design found that CBT may be beneficial not only due to change in cognitive variables, but via widespread adaptive changes across a number of theory specific and nonspecific coping skills (Burns et al., 2015). Indeed, a recent study identified that pain acceptance (which is a treatment target theoretically specific to acceptance-based treatments) was correlated with improvement in pain outcomes during a CBT-based multidisciplinary pain program (Akerblom, Perrin, Fischer, & McCracken, 2015), and another study showed mindfulness improved during CBT and this was associated with improved pain outcomes (Cassidy, Atherton, Robertson, Walsh, & Gillett, 2012).

The evidence base for CBT as a first-line treatment approach in managing a wide variety of chronic pain conditions is expansive and growing, however a limitation of this broad literature is that comparatively little is known about the mechanisms of CBT for pain. Recent research efforts have focused on advancing our understanding of how this approach engenders beneficial outcomes and for whom this approach is most suited so that the CBT treatment package can be streamlined and optimized (Day, Ehde, & Jensen, 2015; Jensen, 2011; Thorn & Burns, 2011). The research to date suggests that change in pain catastrophizing and pain beliefs may be critical for improvement in pain-related outcomes to occur during CBT, although other mechanisms likely exert an effect. Despite the great advancements in pain treatment that have been made with the application of CBT, effect sizes are on average modest, and not everyone who engages in a CBT program achieves clinically meaningful benefit (Eccleston et al., 2009).

Thus, the more recently developed treatment approaches based on acceptance and mindfulness principles afford promising potential and provide additional alternative treatment options for individuals living with persistent pain.

First, a Brief Note on the Difference Between Acceptance- and Mindfulness-Based Approaches

Acceptance and Commitment Therapy (ACT; and other acceptance approaches) are sometimes included under the umbrella of mindfulness approaches as to some extent they do include a selection of mindfulness enhancing elements; and vice versa, mindfulness-based interventions (MBIs) are sometimes included under the umbrella of acceptance-based treatments as MBIs also include an emphasis on cultivating acceptance (Veehof, Oskam, Schreurs, & Bohlmeijer, 2011). Indeed, one of the most common questions I am asked at workshops and during presentations is: "How are mindfulness approaches different from ACT?" Although there are some similarities, the key difference lies in the theory underlying acceptance-based interventions vs. MBIs, which is fundamentally unique across the two approaches; the two also typically involve unique procedural elements (Day, Jensen, et al., 2014). Therefore, to avoid confusion in the field, our research group (Day, Jensen, et al., 2014; Day, Thorn, & Burns, 2012) as well as other prominent research groups (Chiesa & Serretti, 2010; Veehof, Trompetter, Bohlmeijer, & Schreurs, 2016) have recommended that these two theoretically and procedurally different treatment approaches be considered distinct interventions and semantic separation of the descriptive labels for the treatments maintained. Hence, here acceptance-oriented interventions are described in a section as separate from MBIs.

Acceptance-Oriented Approaches

Theory

Similar to the BT model described earlier, acceptance-based interventions such as ACT have roots in learning theory and basic behavioral processes (Hayes, 2004; McCracken, MacKichan, & Eccleston, 2007; McCracken & Vowles, 2014). Unique to ACT however, is its core theoretical basis in processes of language and cognition from within the perspective of Relational Frame Theory (RFT) (Hayes, 2004), as well as a theoretical emphasis on psychological flexibility (McCracken & Morley, 2014). While a more detailed account of RFT is available elsewhere (Hayes, 2004; Hayes, Luoma, Bond, Masuda, & Lillis, 2006), a parsimonious take on the model is to consider that the central tenet of this theory is its emphasis on associative learning principles.

Briefly, RFT emphasizes the importance of stimulus relations (i.e., relations that are learned without direct training) and language-based representations (i.e., a verbal label or descriptor) that are elicited automatically. This model recognizes that once an association has been made between a phenomenal experience and a language-based representation of that experience, it cannot be unlearned. For example, once one experiences a noxious stimulus and labels this experience "pain," the verbal label "pain" then encapsulates the association with the felt sensation of the noxious insult, and this association cannot be *removed* from memory and is henceforth elicited automatically in certain contexts. Although learned associations cannot be *un*learned, theoretically the relational network of associations connected to a label such as "pain" can be *broadened* with the learning of new associations—in either a helpful or unhelpful way! To elucidate, when pain becomes chronic and *coping is maladaptive*, associations with the noxious stimuli may be broadened to rigid representations (e.g., "hurt," "harm," "damage," "avoid"), to various emotions with a negative valence (e.g., fear, anxiety, sadness), catastrophic thoughts (e.g., "this pain is ruining my life"), and perhaps to avoidance behavior. The behavioral function of these associations or links (rather than the symptoms of the pain per se) become theoretical treatment targets in ACT for chronic pain, as does the development of new, *adaptive coping* associations that can broaden and build and then positively influence the impact of contextual cues on thoughts, emotions, and behavior, leading to improved pain outcomes.

There are six continuum-based theoretical processes in ACT that are harnessed as a means to broaden associative responses in different contexts, which are subsumed within the psychological (in)flexibility model (Hayes, Strosahl, & Wilsons, 2012) which has more recently been applied to pain (McCracken & Morley, 2014). On the psychological flexibility end of the continuum (reflecting adaptive pain coping), these processes reflect behavior that is "open, aware, and active" whereas the other end of the continuum represents psychological *in*flexibility (reflecting maladaptive pain coping) and constitutes a model of suffering and unhelpful behavioral responses (McCracken & Morley, 2014). Specifically, these six processes of flexibility vs. *in*flexibility (or rigidity), respectively, are: (1) acceptance vs. experiential avoidance; (2) cognitive defusion vs. cognitive fusion; (3) flexible present-focused attention vs. past or future-oriented preoccupation; (4) self-as-observer vs. inability to take a perspective separate from thoughts and feelings; (5) values vs. lack of value clarity or failure to pursue values; and (6) committed action vs. rigid behavioral persistence, inaction, or impulsive avoidance. McCracken and Morley provide an excellent detailed definition and account of these six processes in the context of chronic pain (McCracken & Morley, 2014). In sum, based on the theory underlying the ACT model, the form, frequency, and appearance of thoughts or emotions in and of themselves is not problematic, rather the focus is on their function in context. Therapeutically the focus is therefore to apply various techniques to move that functioning in a healthier direction, towards the processes embodied in psychological flexibility.

Techniques and Application

Hayes (the developer of ACT) emphasized that the techniques delivered within this framework need to target increasing psychological flexibility, and engendering either change or persistence in behavior in such a way that behavior serves valued ends (Hayes, 2004). To accomplish this, Hayes suggests that many traditional behavior therapy change and activation methods can be delivered and assigned as homework within the ACT framework (e.g., exposure, scheduling in more valued activities that bring a sense of pleasure or mastery), and that all delivered techniques and homework assignments should be linked to short-, medium-, and long-term behavioral change goals. The emphasis on the behavior–goal linkage in ACT for chronic pain is so that the client moves towards living a life that is progressively more consistent with what is valued, despite the pain. Along with this, ACT works with values assessment and clarification, and differential reinforcement to shape behavior towards increasing behavioral activity that is aligned with valued domains. Formal mindfulness meditation has not traditionally been included in ACT, however bringing mindfulness into everyday activities is sometimes included and other techniques to enhance defusion (which is an aspect of mindfulness) are taught. An example of such a defusion technique in ACT would be to repeat a thought over and over again out loud, until it becomes a meaningless sound.

The use of various metaphors is also a cornerstone technique in the delivery of ACT for activating the six psychological flexibility processes. For example, a popular ACT metaphor developed by Hayes and colleagues that encapsulates the full psychological flexibility model is the "Passengers-on-the-Bus" metaphor (Hayes, Strosahl, & Wilson, 1999). However, there are literally hundreds of metaphors that have been used in the ACT framework to tap into the various psychological flexibility processes, and for some clients this approach has been found to be highly beneficial.

Evidence and Limitations

Acceptance-based interventions such as ACT (Hayes, 2004) and Contextual Cognitive-Behavioral Therapy (McCracken et al., 2007) are increasingly being successfully applied to chronic pain and evidence for their efficacy is rapidly building. Research investigating the efficacy of ACT for a variety of chronic pain conditions has found significant positive outcomes associated with this approach including improved physical performance and quality of life, fewer sick days, and reduced pain intensity, disability, medical utilization, daytime rest, distress, depression, and pain-related anxiety (Dahl, Wilson, Luciano, & Hayes, 2005; McCracken et al., 2007; McCracken & Vowles, 2008, 2014; Veehof et al., 2016; Vowles, McCracken, & O'Brien, 2011; Vowles, Witkiewitz, Sowden, & Ashworth, 2014; Wetherell et al., 2011). The most consistent reported benefits of ACT applied to chronic pain include improved physical and social functioning and a reduction in pain-related medical visits, with these benefits reported to be maintained up to 3 years following treatment (McCracken & Vowles, 2014). Overall, the accumulated evidence for the effectiveness of ACT for chronic pain has been recognized as constituting the strongest possible evidence grading of the American Psychological Association (APA, 1998).

Most of the research examining ACT for chronic pain has focused on establishing the efficacy of this approach, although studies examining treatment processes are emerging. Two studies have found that increased pain acceptance during treatment was significantly correlated with improved disability, and symptoms of anxiety and depression at post-treatment (McCracken, Vowles, &

Eccleston, 2005; Vowles & McCracken, 2008). Further, maintenance of these pain-related improvements at 3 months post-treatment was correlated with pre- to post-treatment improvement in pain acceptance, general acceptance, mindfulness, and values-based action (McCracken & Gutierrez-Martınez, 2011). A recent diary study showed that reduction in efforts to control pain and increased engagement in activities during ACT was reliably associated with reduced disability at 3-month follow-up (Vowles, Kink, & Cohen, 2014). To the best of my knowledge, only three other studies to date have implemented formal tests of mediation in the context of ACT for chronic pain and found evidence for aspects of psychological flexibility as the underlying process associated with treatment-related improvement (Vowles et al., 2014; Wicksell, Olsson, & Hayes, 2010, 2011).

Increasing evidence is supporting the efficacy of acceptance-based approaches for chronic pain, and preliminary support is accumulating to suggest ACT may exert beneficial effects for the reasons specified by theory. Hayes (Hayes et al., 2006), the developer of ACT considers this approach "third wave" CBT and it is certainly a promising intervention, of benefit to many people. However, others have questioned whether ACT (and mindfulness-based approaches) is "new wave or old hat" (Hofmann & Asmundson, 2008). Specifically, a criticism of ACT in the literature is that the key theorized mechanisms of ACT (as well as the techniques referred to as "ACT-based") closely resemble CBT concepts (Hofmann & Asmundson, 2008). Although RFT seems unique to ACT, the cornerstone mechanism of psychological flexibility appears to share substantial conceptual overlap with other approaches. For example, defusion and self-as-an-observer closely resemble models of mindfulness (described below) as well as the aspect of observing thoughts to weigh their evidence and apply restructuring in CBT, and committed behavioral action is a major focus of BT (Day & Thorn, 2014). Additionally, while ACT has traditionally *not* included formal mindfulness meditation as a technique (which is at the core of MBIs), more recently in clinical practice some practitioners have been including formal seated mindfulness meditations within ACT. It will be interesting in the future, if formal mindfulness meditation does become a more typical component in ACT, to see what this inclusion would mean in terms of the functional therapeutic distinction between what is one approach vs. another (i.e., what is ACT vs. BT vs. MBIs). And along with that, what approach does accumulating empirical evidence for "ACT" actually support?

Mindfulness-Based Interventions

In this section I will focus on mindfulness-based approaches *other* than MBCT, to lay the foundation for then discussing MBCT in depth in the next chapter.

Theory

Mindfulness shares conceptual kinship with a number of philosophical and psychological traditions (Brown, Ryan, & Creswell, 2007); however, the term "mindfulness" is most systematically articulated within Eastern Buddhist philosophy where it is a central pathway within a traditional spiritual system developed to alleviate human suffering (Hanh, 1976). Mindfulness as defined within the majority of Buddhist traditions (termed "sati" in Pali, "smrti" in Sanskrit, and "tren-ba" in Tibetan) commonly denotes presence of mind. However, in the past several decades, the principles and practices associated with mindfulness have been integrated into Western psychology and healthcare, and along with this has come a concurrent development of numerous conceptual, secularized definitions and applied mindfulness theory (Bishop, 2002; Shapiro & Carlson, 2009; Shapiro, Carlson, Astin, & Freedman, 2006).

Perhaps the most widely cited definition of mindfulness in the scientific community is the definition I provided earlier in Chapter 1, proffered by Jon Kabat-Zinn, the founder of mindfulness-based approaches within the Western medical (allopathic) community. Stemming from Kabat-Zinn's definition, Shapiro and colleagues proposed that the quality of mindfulness is cultivated via three theoretical pathways: (1) a clear intention as to why one practices meditation; (2) an attentional focus on one's moment-to-moment experiences; and (3) an attitude one brings to attention characterized by acceptance, kindness, openness, curiosity, patience, equanimity, non-striving, and non-evaluation (Shapiro et al., 2006). Shapiro and Carlson (2009) later provided a further theoretical delineation by operationally defining mindfulness as both a *construct/outcome*, and as a *practice* (i.e., meditation). The debate about how to best operationalize and theoretically define mindfulness as a construct continues, and Carmody (2009) as well as Brown and colleagues (2007) offer a more in depth exploration of the various viewpoints.

Mindfulness as a practice for the management of a variety of conditions, including but not limited to pain, is typically taught within integrated programs such as Mindfulness-Based Stress Reduction (MBSR) (Kabat-Zinn 1990, 2013). MBSR and other meditative therapies (e.g., Mindfulness Oriented Recovery Enhancement; Garland, 2016; Garland et al., 2014) emphasize the practice of mindfulness meditation as a means to systematically train the mind to intentionally observe the full range of inner experiences—including thoughts, emotions, and bodily sensations (including but not limited to pain)—on a moment-to-moment basis with a non-judgmental, open, and accepting attitude, such that they are perceived as transient experiences with natural variation. Any experience, regardless of its affective valence—whether it be pleasant, unpleasant, or neutral—is observed with equanimity (Desbordes et al., 2015). Theoretically, this "observing" quality of attention (i.e., to see oneself as having a thought vs. being identified with the thought) decoupled from emotion is harnessed in meditation to accelerate the shift towards relating *to* thoughts (as objects of awareness), rather than *from* thoughts (as necessarily reflecting reality) (Kabat-Zinn, 2013; Segal, Williams, & Teasdale, 2013). Within this perspective, whether the inherent characteristics of the thought, emotion, or sensation itself changes or does not change is secondary; the focus is on harnessing the qualities of mindfulness through meditation to change one's *relationship* to these experiences: to observe them as transient experiences that are nonrepresentative of the self, and are not *the* truth.

Until recently, there was a notable gap in the literature as there existed no explicit theoretical rationale for applying mindfulness principles specifically to chronic pain. My colleagues and I sought to begin to fill this gap by proposing an initial evidence-based theoretical model of MBIs for pain management that integrated mindfulness and pain theory, and relevant empirical findings (Day, Jensen, et al., 2014). I will come back to this model in more detail in Chapter 3. However, at base, this model recognizes the use of mindfulness meditation as the core practice of MBIs to train the mind to intentionally cultivate each of the qualities of mindfulness discussed above. Building on this, we theorized that meditation may be likened to a form of exposure, and therefore has parallels with exposure-focused approaches for pain based on the FAM (Vlaeyen & Linton, 2000). Further, the yoga component of MBSR (described below) may contribute to reduced fear of movement and fear of pain/re-injury, which are factors that are frequently associated with disability and that are emphasized in the FAM (Vlaeyen & Linton, 2000). The emphasis on the intentional values clarification component in MBIs and the cultivation of acceptance and cognitive, emotional and behavioral flexibility shares conceptual kinship with ACT-based philosophy. And the central emphasis on reducing identification with thoughts, emotions, and physical sensations (i.e., reperceiving) in MBIs is similarly a shared mechanism of CBT and ACT for chronic pain. In the next chapter I will discuss further the unique and shared theoretical kinship between MBIs and other pain treatments, to explicate how and for whom mindfulness-based approaches are most likely to be of benefit.

Techniques and Application

MBSR and other meditative therapies typically consist of four to eight sessions (an extended meditation retreat is sometimes included) and are delivered in a fundamentally secular manner typically within a group setting (Kabat-Zinn, 1990, 2013). In MBSR, a didactic component conveying psychoeducation on the psychology and physiology of the stress response is typically included, along with information on how mindfulness may be applied to more effectively respond to pain and stress. The MBSR protocol includes a series of formal and informal mindfulness meditation practices. To illustrate the mindfulness meditation training technique, a basic breath-focused sitting meditation is described hereafter:

> The client settles into a dignified sitting posture, and anchors the attention on the movements of the breath; aware as the breath enters the body, aware as the breath leaves the body, and aware of the pauses in between. Inevitably the mind will at times wander from the breath, and the moment of awareness that the mind has wandered and is no longer on the breath is mindfulness itself. The training is simply to notice when a thought, emotion, or sensation arises and calls for attention, to acknowledge it, to non-judgmentally label it—"thinking" or "sadness"—and then, with kindness and gentleness, to usher the attention back to resuming awareness of the movements of the breath. Each time the mind wanders, this same, compassionate response is applied. The breath is harnessed as an anchor to the present moment, always available to return to.

As can be seen in this seated meditation description, distraction in any number of forms (e.g., thoughts, memories, painful sensations, emotions, daydreaming…) is not seen as any particular "failing" and is not to be taken as an indication that one is a "bad meditator"—indeed it is no problem at all—it *is* the mindfulness practice itself. Distraction of any kind is viewed as an opportunity to notice the tendencies of the mind and then to train in stabilizing the mind by calmly and nonjudgmentally returning awareness to the focus of attention. The premise is not necessarily to gain deep insight (although this may happen over time), but simply to nonjudgmentally notice what arises in the field of awareness without reacting with attachment or aversion.

In MBSR, generally the Body Scan is the first formal meditation technique taught, followed by a variety of seated meditations, mindful walking, and mindful hatha yoga. Such techniques incorporate similar procedures to the breath-focused sitting meditation described above, and encourage the same nonjudgmental and accepting attitudes; the primary difference between the meditation techniques is the object of focus to sustain attention. Yoga, for example, involves tuning into the sensations and signals of the body as gentle movements are done, with moment-to-moment awareness, to slowly move the body into various configurations or postures. Guided audio files of the techniques taught in session are provided for between-session practice, and clients are instructed to practice meditation for 45 min per day. Furthermore, clients are encouraged to infuse mindful awareness into everyday tasks (such as when eating, washing the dishes etc.) to cultivate mindfulness into everyday activities.

Evidence and Limitations

A rapidly growing body of research is supporting the efficacy of mindfulness-based approaches for a range of clinical populations, including chronic pain. Reviews of the effectiveness of MBIs applied to heterogeneous health conditions have consistently found clinically and statistically significant gains from pre- to post-treatment on standardized measures of physical health and psychological well-being (Bohlmeijer, Prenger, Taal, & Cuijpers, 2010; Fjorback, Arendt, Ornbol, Fink, & Walach, 2011; Grossman, Niemann, Schmidt, & Walach, 2004; Keng, Smoski, & Robins, 2011; Schmidt et al., 2011). Although still preliminary, an increasing number of clinical trials have examined the effectiveness of MBIs specifically for the management of chronic pain, and to date most of these studies have compared MBSR to standard medical care. Beneficial outcomes have been reported in these trials with respect to improved pain intensity, disability, pain coping, pain interference, quality of life, depression, anxiety, and measures of affect immediately post-treatment and also at follow-up (Fjorback et al., 2011; Grossman et al., 2004; Keng et al., 2011; Veehof et al., 2016). The published effect sizes for pain intensity in these studies are typically between $d = 0.27$ (i.e., a small effect) and $d = 0.73$ (i.e., a medium–large effect) (Fjorback et al., 2011; Grossman et al., 2004; Keng et al., 2011; Veehof et al., 2016), which is comparable to the range of effect sizes seen with CBT and other psychosocial interventions for chronic pain (Morley, 2011). One recent study by Davis and colleagues (Davis, Zautra, Wolf, Tennen, & Yeung, 2015) that implemented daily diary methodology within a rheumatoid arthritis sample found that a mindfulness-based approach was significantly *more* effective than both CBT and pain education for improving pain catastrophizing, morning disability, fatigue, and stress-related anxious affect. In one of the largest RCTs conducted to date investigating MBSR vs. CBT vs. usual care in chronic low back pain, it was found that MBSR was as effective as CBT (both of which were significantly better than the control) for improving back pain and associated functional limitations, with benefit maintained at long-term follow-up (Cherkin et al., 2016). Taken together, these efficacy findings suggest that CBT, acceptance and mindfulness-based approaches are appropriate for delivery in mainstream healthcare for chronic pain.

Preliminary mechanism research suggests that there are a number of potential pathways through which MBIs may engender the observed improvements in pain outcomes (Day, Jensen, et al., 2014). Brain state research using fMRI and electroencephalography (EEG) technology with healthy individuals and long-term meditators has found state- and trait-related brain changes with meditation in cortical structures that may modulate pain via enhancement of the frontal attentional control systems, reduced evaluative/emotional responses, improved emotion regulation (i.e., as evidenced by increased positive affect and decreased negative affect), increased approach-oriented coping, and reduced arousal (Brown & Jones, 2010; Cahn & Polich, 2006; Chiesa & Serretti, 2010; Fell, Axmacher, & Haupt, 2010; Grant, Courtemanche, Duerden, Duncan, & Rainville, 2010; Grant, Courtemanche, & Rainville, 2011; Holzel et al., 2011; Zeidan, Grant, Brown, McHaffie, & Coghill, 2012). Further, consistent with theory, measures of mindfulness have been found to correlate with treatment gains during MBSR for irritable bowel syndrome (Garland et al., 2012) and fibromyalgia (Schmidt et al., 2011). However, in a secondary analysis of the RCT described above that compared MBSR vs. CBT vs. usual care, Turner and colleagues compared the mechanisms of MBSR to CBT and found that not only did both active treatments exert similar effects as reported in the original trial, but that long term (i.e., at 52 weeks) they seem to do so through the *same* mechanism pathways—change in mindfulness, acceptance, self-efficacy, and pain catastrophizing—suggesting mindfulness may not be a mechanism unique to MBIs, nor change in pain-related cognitions a mechanism specific to CBT (Turner et al., 2016).

Finally, some evidence has found that the amount of meditation practice engaged in (i.e., the dose of meditation) corresponded to treatment-related increases in mindfulness, which in turn led to symptom reduction and improved well-being (Carmody & Baer, 2008). Another recent study in a fibromyalgia sample found that the reported number of times per week that meditation was practiced at 2-months follow-up significantly predicted reductions in pain and fibromyalgia symptom severity, but not perceived stress, fatigue, physical function, or cortisol (Cash et al., 2015). However, meditation dose–treatment response findings are not consistent and more research in this area is needed to identify the optimal dose for a given individual (Carmody & Baer, 2009; Davis, 2015).

The clinical and empirical interest in MBSR and other meditative therapies for chronic pain management has grown exponentially in recent years, and based on this, it is expected that the current preliminary evidence supporting the use of MBIs in this context will continue to build. It is not clear based on the current empirical literature whether the theoretical focus of MBSR on targeting cognitive processes without a concurrent explicit emphasis on the cognitive content targeted by CBT may constrain the potential benefit of this approach for chronic pain; current evidence suggests both of these approaches exert similar effects. The recent research by Cherkin, Turner, and colleagues represents the current state-of-the-art evidence on MBSR. Further well-controlled trials examining the efficacy and mechanisms of MBIs compared to other active psychosocial treatments such as CBT and ACT are needed to confirm the beneficial effects found, and to identify the potential unique and shared mediators of MBIs and other psychosocial treatments for pain.

Summary

The development, adaption, and application of psychosocial treatments for chronic pain has evolved and advanced substantially in the past half century. Spanning from the earliest models of behavioral therapy, to the integration of cognitive therapy principles, and most recently, to the successful application of acceptance and mindfulness-based approaches, researchers and clinicians have made tremendous gains in working towards refining and optimizing treatments in efforts to find tailored approaches to the problem of intractable pain. Recognizing this advancement and the abundance of supporting evidence, leading international pain organizations are now beginning to endorse and recommend cognitive and behavioral psychological approaches alongside pharmacotherapy as the first-line treatment approach for headache (Penzien, Rains, & Andrasik, 2002). Based on the accumulating evidence, one would expect that other organizations representing various other forms of chronic pain will closely follow suit. Although I have focused in this chapter on the most widely used approaches for chronic pain, there are also other approaches which have been found to be tremendously beneficial, in particular self-hypnosis (Jensen, 2011). An important shared denominator across all of these psychosocial approaches is that they give patients *skills they can use*, which is empowering for the individual with chronic pain as it allows them to step out of a passive patient role and become an active participant in the management of their pain. This empowers clients to live a meaningful life despite the "full catastrophe" (as Jon Kabat-Zinn so aptly refers to it; 1990, 2013) that chronic pain—and indeed life more broadly—entails.

References

Aggarwal, V. R., Lovell, K., Peters, S., Javidi, H., Joughin, A., & Goldthorpe, J. (2011). Psychosocial interventions for the management of chronic orofacial pain. *Cochrane Database of Systematic Reviews, 11*, 1–57.

Akerblom, S., Perrin, S., Fischer, M. R., & McCracken, L. (2015). The mediating role of acceptance in multidisciplinary cognitive-behavioral therapy for chronic pain. *The Journal of Pain, 16*, 606–615.

Andrasik, F. (2003). Behavioral treatment approaches to chronic headache. *Neurological Sciences, 24,* S80–S85.
Andrasik, F. (2007). What does the evidence show? Efficacy of behavioural treatments for recurrent headaches in adults. *Neurological Sciences, 28,* S70–S77.
APA. (1998). Acceptance and commitment therapy for chronic pain. Retrieved from http://www.div12.org/psychological-treatments/disorders/chronic-or-persistent-pain/acceptance-and-commitment-therapy-for-chronic-pain/
Apkarian, A. V., Baliki, M. N., & Geha, P. Y. (2009). Towards a theory of chronic pain. *Progress in Neurobiology, 87*(2), 81–97.
Beck, A. T. (1979). *Cognitive therapy of depression.* New York, NY: Guilford Press.
Bishop, S. R. (2002). What do we really know about mindfulness-based stress reduction? *Psychosomatic Medicine, 64,* 71–83.
Bohlmeijer, E., Prenger, R., Taal, E., & Cuijpers, P. (2010). The effects of mindfulness-based stress reduction therapy on mental health of adults with a chronic medical disease: A meta-analysis. *Journal of Psychosomatic Research, 68,* 539–544.
Brown, C. A., & Jones, A. K. (2010). Meditation experience predicts less negative appraisal of pain: Electrophysiological evidence for the involvement of anticipatory neural responses. *Pain, 150*(3), 428–438.
Brown, K. W., Ryan, R. M., & Creswell, J. D. (2007). Mindfulness: Theoretical foundations and evidence for salutary effects. *Psychological Inquiry, 1,* 211–237.
Burns, J. W., Glenn, B., Bruehl, S., Harden, R. N., & Lofland, K. (2003). Cognitive factors influence outcome following multidisciplinary chronic pain treatment: A replication and extension of a cross-lagged panel analysis. *Behaviour Research and Therapy, 41*(10), 1163–1182.
Burns, J. W., Johnson, B. J., Mahoney, N., Devine, J., & Pawl, R. (1998). Cognitive and physical capacity process variables predict long-term outcome after treatment of chronic pain. *Journal of Consulting and Clinical Psychology, 66,* 434–439.
Burns, J. W., Kubilus, A., Bruehl, S., Harden, R. N., & Lofland, K. (2003). Do changes in cognitive factors influence outcome following multidisciplinary treatment for chronic pain? A cross-lagged panel analysis. *Journal of Consulting and Clinical Psychology, 71*(1), 81–91.
Burns, J., Nielson, W. R., Jensen, M. P., Heapy, A., Czlapinski, R., & Kerns, R. D. (2015). Does change occur for the reasons we think it does? A test of specific therapeutic operations during cognitive-behavioral treatment of chronic pain. *Clinical Journal of Pain, 31,* 603–611.
Cahn, B. R., & Polich, J. (2006). Meditation states and traits: EEG, ERP, and neuroimaging studies. *Psychological Bulletin, 132,* 180–211.
Carmody, J. (2009). Evolving conceptions of mindfulness in clinical settings. *Journal of Cognitive Psychotherapy: An International Quarterly, 23*(3), 270–280.
Carmody, J., & Baer, R. A. (2008). Relationships between mindfulness practice and levels of mindfulness, medical and psychological symptoms and well-being in a mindfulness-based stress reduction program. *Journal of Behavioral Medicine, 31*(1), 23–33.
Carmody, J., & Baer, R. A. (2009). How long does a mindfulness-based stress reduction program need to be? A review of class contact hours and effect sizes for psychological distress. *Journal of Clinical Psychology, 65*(6), 627–638.

Cash, E., Salmon, P., Weissbecker, I., Rebholz, W. N., Bayley-Veloso, R., Zimmaro, L. A., ... Sephton, S. E. (2015). Mindfulness meditation alleviates fibromyalgia symptoms in women: Results of a randomized clinical trial. *Annals of Behavioral Medicine, 49*, 319–330.

Cassidy, E. L., Atherton, R. J., Robertson, N., Walsh, D. A., & Gillett, R. (2012). Mindfulness, functioning and catastrophizing after multidisciplinary pain management for chronic low back pain. *Pain, 152*(3), 644–650.

Cherkin, D. C., Sherman, K. J., Balderson, B. H., Cook, A. J., Anderson, M. L., Hawkes, R. J., ... Turner, J. A. (2016). Effect of mindfulness-based stress reduction vs cognitive behavioral therapy or usual care on back pain and functional limitations in adults with chronic low back pain: A randomized controlled trial. *Journal of the American Medical Association, 315*(12), 1240–1249.

Chiesa, A., & Serretti, A. (2010). A systematic review of neurobiological and clinical features of mindfulness meditations. *Psychological Medicine, 40*(8), 1239–1252.

Dahl, J. C., Wilson, K. G., Luciano, C., & Hayes, S. C. (2005). *Acceptance and commitment therapy for chronic pain*. Reno, NV: Context Press.

Davis, M. (2015). Mindfully considering treatment of fibromyalgia: A comment on Cash et al. *Annals of Behavioral Medicine, 49*, 299–300.

Davis, M. C., Zautra, A. J., Wolf, L. D., Tennen, H., & Yeung, E. W. (2015). Mindfulness and cognitive-behavioral interventions for chronic pain: Differential effects on daily pain reactivity and stress reactivity. *Journal of Consulting and Clinical Psychology, 83*(1), 24–35.

Day, M. A., Ehde, D. M., & Jensen, M. P. (2015). Psychosocial pain management moderation: The limit, activate and enhance model. *The Journal of Pain, 16*(10), 947–960.

Day, M. A., Jensen, M. P., Ehde, D. M., & Thorn, B. E. (2014). Towards a theoretical model for mindfulness-based pain management. *Journal of Pain, 15*(7), 691–703.

Day, M. A., & Thorn, B. E. (2014). Using theoretical models to clarify shared and unique mechanisms in psychosocial pain treatments: A commentary on McCracken and Morley's theoretical paper. *The Journal of Pain, 15*(3), 237–238.

Day, M. A., Thorn, B. E., & Burns, J. (2012). The continuing evolution of biopsychosocial interventions for chronic pain. *Journal of Cognitive Psychotherapy: An International Quarterly, 26*(2), 114–129.

Desbordes, G., Gard, T., Hoge, E. A., Hölzel, B. K., Kerr, C., Lazar, S. W., Olendzki, A., & Vago, D.R. (2015). Moving beyond mindfulness: Defining equanimity as an outcome measure in meditation and contemplative research. *Mindfulness, 6*(2), 356–372.

Eccleston, C., Hearn, L., & Williams, A. C. (2015). Psychological therapies for the management of chronic neuropathic pain in adults. *Cochrane Database of Systematic Reviews, 29*(10), 1–32.

Eccleston, C., Palermo, T. M., Williams, A. C., Lewandowski, A., & Morley, S. (2009). Psychological therapies for the management of chronic and recurrent pain in children and adolescents. *Cochrane Database of Systematic Reviews*(2), CD003968.

Ehde, D. M., Dillworth, T. M., & Turner, J. A. (2014). Cognitive behavioural therapy for indiviudals with chronic pain: Efficacy, innovations and directions for research. *American Psychologist, 69*(2), 153–166.

Fell, J., Axmacher, N., & Haupt, S. (2010). From alpha to gamma: Electrophysiological correlates of meditation-related states of consciousness. *Medical Hypotheses, 75*(2), 218–224.

Fjorback, L. O., Arendt, M., Ornbol, E., Fink, P., & Walach, H. (2011). Mindfulness-based stress reduction and mindfulness-based cognitive therapy: A systematic review of randomized controlled trials. *Acta Psychiatry Scandinavia, 124*(2), 102–119.

Flor, H., & Turk, D. C. (2011). *Chronic pain: An integrated biobehavioral perspective.* Seattle, WA: IASP Press.

Fordyce, W. E. (1976). *Behavioral methods for chronic pain and illness.* St. Louis, MO: Mosby.

Foreyt, J. P., & Rathjen, D. P. (1978). *Cognitive-behavior therapy: Research and application.* New York, NY: Plenum.

Garland, E. L. (2016). Restructuring reward processing with mindfulness-oriented recovery enhancement: Novel therapeutic mechanisms to remediate hedonic dysregulation in addiction, stress, and pain. *Annals of the New York Academy of Sciences, 1373*, 25–37.

Garland, E. L., Gaylord, S. A., Palsson, O., Faurot, K., Mann, J. D., & Whitehead, W. E. (2012). Therapeutic mechanisms of a mindfulness-based treatment for IBS: Effects on visceral sensitivity, catastrophizing, and affective processing of pain sensations. *Journal of Behavioral Medicine, 35*(6), 591–602.

Garland, E. L., Manusov, E. G., Froeliger, B., Kelly, A., Williams, J. M., & Howard, M. O. (2014). Mindfulness-oriented recovery enhancement for chronic pain and prescription opioid misuse: Results from an early-stage randomized controlled trial. *Journal of Consulting and Clinical Psychology, 82*(3), 448–459.

Grant, J. A., Courtemanche, J., Duerden, E. G., Duncan, G. H., & Rainville, P. (2010). Cortical thickness and pain sensitivity in zen meditators. *Emotion, 10*(1), 43–53.

Grant, J. A., Courtemanche, J., & Rainville, P. (2011). A non-elaborative mental stance and decoupling of executive and pain-related cortices predicts low pain sensitivity in Zen meditators. *Pain, 152*(1), 150–156.

Grossman, P., Niemann, L., Schmidt, S., & Walach, H. (2004). Mindfulness-based stress reduction and health benefits. A meta-analysis. *Journal of Psychosomatic Research, 57*, 35–43.

Hanh, T. N. (1976). *The miracle of mindfulness: A manual for meditation.* Boston, MA: Beacon.

Hayes, S. C. (2004). Acceptance and Commitment Therapy, Relational Frame Theory, and the third wave of behavioral and cognitive therapies. *Behavior Therapy, 35*, 639–664.

Hayes, S. C., Luoma, J. B., Bond, F. W., Masuda, A., & Lillis, J. (2006). Acceptance and commitment therapy: Model, processes, and outcomes. *Behavior Research and Therapy, 44*, 1–25.

Hayes, S. C., Strosahl, K. D., & Wilson, K. G. (1999). *Acceptance and commitment therapy: An experiential approach to behavior change.* New York, NY: Guilford Press.

Hayes, S. C., Strosahl, K. D., & Wilsons, K. G. (2012). *Acceptance and Commitment Therapy: The process and practice of mindful change* (2nd ed.). New York, NY: Guilford Press.

Henschke, N., Ostelo, H., van Tulder, M. W., Vlaeyen, J. W., Morley, S., Assendelft, W. J. J., & Main, C. J. (2010). Behavioural treatment for chronic low-back pain. *Cochrane Database of Systematic Reviews, 7*, 1–125.

Hoffman, B. M., Papas, R. K., Chatkoff, D. K., & Kerns, R. D. (2007). Meta-analysis of psychological interventions for chronic low back pain. *Health Psychology, 26*(1), 1–9.

Hofmann, S. G., & Asmundson, G. J. G. (2008). Acceptance and mindfulness-based therapy: New wave or old hat? *Clinical Psychology Review, 28*, 1–16.

Holroyd, K. A., Labus, J. S., & Carlson, B. (2009). Moderation and mediation in the psychological and drug treatment of chronic tension-type headache: The role of disorder severity and psychiatric comorbidity. *Pain, 143*, 213–222.

Holzel, B. K., Carmody, J., Vangel, M., Congleton, C., Yerramsetti, S. M., Gard, T., & Lazar, S. W. (2011). Mindfulness practice leads to increases in regional brain gray matter density. *Psychiatry Research, 191*(1), 36–43.

Jensen, M., Turner, J. A., & Romano, J. M. (2001). Changes in beliefs, catastrophizing and coping are associated with improvement in multidisciplinary pain treatment *Journal of Consulting and Clinical Psychology, 69*, 655–662.

Jensen, M. P. (2010). A neuropsychological model of pain: Research and clinical implications. *Journal of Pain, 11*, 2–12.

Jensen, M. P. (2011). *Hypnosis for chronic pain management: Therapist guide*. Oxford: Oxford University Press.

Kabat-Zinn, J. (1990). *Full catastrophe living: Using the wisdom of your body and mind to face stress, pain and illness*. New York, NY: Delacourt.

Kabat-Zinn, J. (2013). *Full catastrophe living (revised edition): Using the wisdom of your body and mind to face stress, pain, and illness*. New York, NY: Bantam Books.

Keefe, F. J., Blumenthal, J., Baucom, D., Affleck, G., Waugh, R., Caldwell, D. S., ... Lefebvre, J. C. (2004). Effects of spouse-assisted coping skills training and exercise training in patients with osteoarthritic knee pain: A randomized controlled study. *Pain, 110*, 539–549.

Keefe, F. J., Caldwell, D. S., Baucom, D., Salley, A., Robinson, E., Timmons, K., ... Helms, M. (1996). Spouse-assisted coping skills training in the management of osteoarthritic knee pain. *Arthritis Care Research, 9*(4), 279–291.

Keefe, F. J., & Lefebvre, J. C. (1999). Behavior therapy. In R. Melzack & P. D. Wall (Eds.), *Textbook of pain* (pp. 1445–1461). London: Churchill Livingstone.

Keefe, F. J., & Somers, T. J. (2010). Psychological approaches to understanding and treating arthritis pain. *Nature Reviews Rheumatology, 6*, 210–216.

Keng, S. L., Smoski, M. J., & Robins, C. J. (2011). Effects of mindfulness on psychological health: A review of empirical studies. *Clinical Psychology Review, 31*(6), 1041–1056.

Kerns, R. D., Turk, D. C., Holzman, A. D., & Rudy, T. E. (1986). Comparison of cognitive-behavioral and behavioral approaches to the outpatient treatment of chronic pain. *Clinical Journal of Pain, 1*, 195–203.

Lazarus, R. S., & Folkman, S. (1984). *Stress, appraisal, and coping*. New York, NY: Springer.

Leeuw, M., Goossens, M. E., Linton, S. J., Crombez, G., Boersma, K., & Vlaeyen, J. W. (2007). The fear-avoidance model of musculoskeletal pain: Current state of scientific evidence. *Journal of Behavioral Medicine, 30*, 77–94.

Linton, S. J., Boersma, K., Jansson, M., Overmeer, T., Lindblom, K., & Vlaeyen, J. W. (2008). A randomized controlled trial of exposure in vivo for patients with spinal pain reporting fear of work-related activities. *European Journal of Pain, 12*(6), 722–730.

Lundervold, D. A., Talley, C., & Buermann, M. (2008). Effect of behavioral activation treatment on chronic fibromyalgia pain: Replication and extension. *International Journal of Behavioral Consultation and Therapy, 4*(2), 146–157.

Martell, C. R., Dimidjian, S., & Herman-Dunn, R. (2010). *Behavioral activation for depression: A clinician's guide*. New York, NY: Guilford.

McCracken, L. M., & Gutierrez-Martınez, O. (2011). Processes of change in psychological flexibility in an interdisciplinary group-based treatment for chronic pain based on acceptance and commitment therapy. *Behavioural Research and Therapy, 49*, 267–274.

McCracken, L. M., MacKichan, F., & Eccleston, C. (2007). Contextual cognitive-behavioral therapy for severely disabled chronic pain sufferers: Effectiveness and clinically significant change. *European Journal of Pain, 11*(3), 314–322.

McCracken, L. M., & Morley, S. (2014). The psychological flexibility model: A basis for integration and progress in psychological approaches to chronic pain management. *The Journal of Pain, 15*(3), 221–234.

McCracken, L. M., & Vowles, K. E. (2008). A prospective analysis of acceptance of pain and values-based action in patients with chronic pain. *Health Psychology, 27*(2), 215–220.

McCracken, L. M., & Vowles, K. E. (2014). Acceptance and Commitment Therapy and mindfulness for chronic pain: Model, process, and progress. *American Psychologist, 69*(2), 178–187.

McCracken, L. M., Vowles, K. E., & Eccleston, C. (2005). Acceptance based treatment for persons with complex longstanding chronic pain: A preliminary analysis of treatment outcome in comparison to a waiting phase. *Behavior Research and Therapy, 43*, 1335–1346.

Meichenbaum, D. H. (1977). *Cognitive-behavioral modification: An integrative approach*. New York, NY: Plenum.

Morley, S. (2011). Efficacy and effectiveness of cognitive behaviour therapy for chronic pain: Progress and some challenges. *Pain, 152*(3 Suppl), S99–106.

Morley, S., & Williams, A. (2015). New developments in the psychological management of chronic pain. *The Canadian Journal of Psychiatry, 60*(4), 168–175.

Ostelo, R. W., van Tulder, M. W., Vlaeyen, J. W., Linton, S. J., Morley, S. J., & Assendelft, W. J. (2005). Behavioural treatment for chronic low-back pain. *Cochrane Database of Systematic Reviews, 1*, CD002014.

Penzien, D. B., Rains, J. C., & Andrasik, F. (2002). Behavioral management of recurrent headache: Three decades of experience and empiricism. *Applied Psychophysiology and Biofeedback, 27*(2), 163–181.

Quartana, P. J., Campbell, C. M., & Edwards, R. R. (2009). Pain catastrophizing: A critical review. *Expert Reviews in Neurotherapeutics, 9*(5), 745–758.

Romano, J. M., Jensen, M. P., Turner, J. A., Good, A. B., & Hops, H. (2000). Chronic pain patient-partner interactions: Further support for a behavioral model of chronic pain. *Behavior Therapy, 31*(3), 415–440.

Schmidt, S., Grossman, P., Schwarzer, B., Jena, S., Naumann, J., & Walach, H. (2011). Treating fibromyalgia with mindfulness-based stress reduction: Results from a 3-armed randomized controlled trial. *Pain, 152*(2), 361–369.

Segal, Z. V., Williams, J. M. G., & Teasdale, J. D. (2013). *Mindfulness-based cognitive therapy for depression*. New York, NY: Guilford.

Shapiro, S. L., & Carlson, L. E. (2009). *The art and science of mindfulness: Integrating mindfulness into psychology and the helping professions*. Washington, DC: American Psychological Association.

Shapiro, S. L., Carlson, L. E., Astin, J. A., & Freedman, B. (2006). Mechanisms of mindfulness. *Journal of Clinical Psychology, 62*, 373–386.

Skinner, B. F. (1953). *Science and Human Behavior*. New York, NY: The Free Press, The Macmillan Company.

Spinhoven, P., Kuile, M., Kole-Snijders, A. M. J., Mansfeld, M. H., Ouden, D., & Vlaeyen, J. W. S. (2004). Catastrophizing and internal pain control as mediators of outcome in the multidisciplinary treatment of chronic low back pain. *European Journal of Pain, 8*, 211–219.

Staal, J. B., Hlobil, H., Köke, A. J., Twisk, J. W., Smid, T., & van Mechelen, W. (2006). Graded activity for workers with low back pain: Who benefits most and how does it work. *Arthritis and Rheumatism, 59*, 642–649.

Sullivan, M., Adams, A., Rhodenizer, T., & Stanish, W. (2006). A psychosocial risk factor targeted intervention for the prevention of chronic pain and disability following whiplash injury. *Physical Therapy, 86*, 8–18.

Thorn, B. E. (2004). *Cognitive therapy for chronic pain: A step-by-step guide*. New York, NY: Guilford Press.

Thorn, B. E., & Burns, J. W. (2011). Common and specific treatment mechanisms in psychosocial pain interventions: The need for a new research agenda. *Pain, 152*(4), 705–706.

Thorn, B. E., Pence, L. B., Ward, L. C., Kilgo, G., Clements, K. L., Cross, T. H., ... Tsui, P. W. (2007). A randomized clinical trial of targeted cognitive behavioral treatments to reduce catastrophizing in chronic headache sufferers. *The Journal of Pain, 8*(12), 938–949.

Trescot, A. M., Glaser, S. E., Hansen, H., Benyamin, R., Patel, S., & Manchikanti, L. (2008). Effectiveness of opioids in the treatment of chronic non-cancer pain. *Pain Physician, 11*(2 Suppl), S181–S200.

Turk, D. C., Meichenbaum, D., & Genest, M. (1983). *Pain and behavioral medicine: A cognitive-behavioral perspective*. New York, NY: Guilford Press.

Turner, J. A. (1982). Comparison of group progressive-relaxation training and cognitive-behavioral group therapy for chronic low back pain. *Journal of Consulting and Clinical Psychology, 50*(5), 757–765.

Turner, J. A., Anderson, M. L., Balderson, B. H., Cook, A. J., Sherman, K. J., & Cherkin, D. C. (2016). Mindfulness-based stress reduction and cognitive-behavioral therapy for chronic low back pain: Similar effects on mindfulness, catastrophizing, self-efficacy, and acceptance in a randomized controlled trial. *Pain* DOI: 10.1097/j.pain.0000000000000635

Turner, J. A., & Clancy, S. (1988). Comparison of operant behavioral and cognitive-behavioral group treatment for chronic low back pain. *Journal of Consulting and Clinical Psychology, 56*, 261–266.

Turner, J. A., Holtzman, S., & Mancl, L. (2007). Mediators, moderators, and predictors of therapeutic change in cognitive-behavioral therapy for chronic pain. *Pain, 127,* 276–286.

Turner, J. A., & Romano, J. M. (2001). Cognitive-behavioral therapy for chronic pain. In J. D. Loeser & J. J. Bonica (Eds.), *Bonica's management of pain* (3rd ed., pp. 1751–1758). Philadelphia, PA: Lippincott Williams & Wilkins.

Veehof, M. M., Oskam, M. J., Schreurs, K. M., & Bohlmeijer, E. T. (2011). Acceptance-based interventions for the treatment of chronic pain: A systematic review and meta-analysis. *Pain, 152*(3), 533–542.

Veehof, M. M., Trompetter, H. R., Bohlmeijer, E. T., & Schreurs, K. M. G. (2016). Acceptance- and mindfulness-based interventions for the treatment of chronic pain: A meta-analytic review. *Cognitive Behaviour Therapy, 45*(1), 5–31.

Vlaeyen, J. W., de Jong, J., Geilen, M., Heuts, P. H., & van Breukelen, G. (2001). Graded exposure in vivo in the treatment of pain-related fear: A replicated single-case experimental design in four patients with chronic low back pain. *Behaviour Research and Therapy, 39*(2), 151–166.

Vlaeyen, J. W., de Jong, J., Geilen, M., Heuts, P. H., & van Breukelen, G. (2002). The treatment of fear of movement/(re)injury in chronic low back pain: Further evidence on the effectiveness of exposure in vivo. *Clinical Journal of Pain, 18*(4), 251–261.

Vlaeyen, J. W. S., & Linton, S. J. (2000). Fear-avoidance and its consequences in chronic musculoskeletal pain: A state of the art review. *Pain, 85,* 317–332.

Vowles, K. E., Kink, B., & Cohen, L. (2014). Acceptance and commitment therapy for chronic pain: A diary study of treatment process in relation to reliable change in disability. *Journal of Contextual Behavioral Science, 3,* 74–80.

Vowles, K. E., & McCracken, L. M. (2008). Acceptance and values-based action in chronic pain: A study of treatment effectiveness and process. *Journal of Consulting and Clinical Psychology, 76*(3), 397–407.

Vowles, K. E., McCracken, L. M., & O'Brien, J. Z. (2011). Acceptance and values-based action in chronic pain: A three-year follow-up analysis of treatment effectiveness and process. *Behaviour Research and Therapy, 49*(11), 748–755.

Vowles, K. E., Witkiewitz, K., Sowden, G., & Ashworth, J. (2014). Acceptance and commitment therapy for chronic pain: evidence of mediation and clinically significant change following an abbreviated interdisciplinary program of rehabilitation. *Journal of Pain, 15*(1), 101–113.

Wetherell, J. L., Afari, N., Rutledge, T., Sorrell, J. T., Stoddard, J. A., Petkus, A. J., ... Atkinson, J. H. (2011). A randomized, controlled trial of acceptance and commitment therapy and cognitive-behavioral therapy for chronic pain. *Pain, 152*(9), 2098–2107.

Wicksell, R. K., Olsson, G. L., & Hayes, A. F. (2010). Psychological flexibility as a mediator of improvement in acceptance and commitment therapy for patients with chronic pain following whiplash. *European Journal of Pain, 14,* 1059. e1051–1059.e1011.

Wicksell, R. K., Olsson, G. L., & Hayes, S. C. (2011). Mediators of change in acceptance and commitment therapy for pediatric chronic pain. *Pain, 152,* 2792–2801.

Williams, A. C., Eccleston, C., & Morley, S. (2012). Psychological therapies for the management of chronic pain (excluding headache) in adults. *Cochrane Database of Systematic Reviews, 11*, CD007407.

Woods, M. P., & Asmundson, G. J. (2008). Evaluating the efficacy of graded in vivo exposure for the treatment of fear in patients with chronic back pain: A randomized controlled clinical trial. *Pain, 136*, 271–280.

Zeidan, F., Grant, J. A., Brown, C. A., McHaffie, J. G., & Coghill, R. C. (2012). Mindfulness meditation-related pain relief: Evidence for unique brain mechanisms in the regulation of pain. *Neuroscience Letters, 520*(2), 165–173.

3

The Development of MBCT for Chronic Pain

An innovative psychological approach developed around the turn of the 21st century saw the recalibration of traditional cognitive therapy to include mindfulness-based principles to form the approach called Mindfulness-Based Cognitive Therapy (MBCT; Segal, Williams, & Teasdale, 2002). Originally developed by Dr. Zindel Segal, Dr. Mark Williams, and Dr. John Teasdale to target relapse prevention in depression, MBCT is based on a rich theoretical tradition that incorporates empirically supported psychological principles from mindfulness, cognitive, and behavioral backgrounds. The approach has now been widely applied to a diverse range of populations and conditions with great success, and evidence is continuing to build exponentially.

In the realm of chronic pain, although CBT is considered the so-called first-line psychosocial treatment approach, we know that not everyone obtains clinically meaningful benefit from CBT, and moreover the approach is not universally appealing (for both clinicians and patients alike!). Thus, I followed with great interest the development and advancement of MBCT over the years, and in February 2009, Dr. Beverly Thorn and I decided to attend a 5-day intensive group retreat led by Dr. Zindel Segal and Dr. Steven Hickman at the Joshua Tree retreat center in California, learning about the intricacies of the theory, principles, and practice of MBCT. Following this immersive experience, combined with my own personal experience of practicing meditation since my teenage years, I was convinced that this approach held great potential for the advancement of chronic pain treatment, and that it might represent a viable alternative to CBT.

On the plane ride back from the retreat, Beverly Thorn and I started writing the grant that would eventually fund the first clinical trial of MBCT specifically for chronic pain. As a first step to adapting the MBCT approach for pain however, we needed a theoretical rationale as to why this approach maps onto the complex problem of chronic pain, and why we expected it to hold tremendous capacity for alleviating pain and suffering. So first, let me start by describing an overview of the original model developed by Segal, Williams, and Teasdale (for a detailed account of their model, the interested reader is directed to both their original as well as the second edition of their text as excellent resources), and retrace my steps to begin placing the original MBCT model within pain theory.

Mindfulness-Based Cognitive Therapy for Chronic Pain: A Clinical Manual and Guide,
First Edition. Melissa A. Day.

Companion website: www.wiley.com/go/day/mindfulness_based_cognitive_therapy

Adapting MBCT Theory for Pain

The Initial MBCT Theoretical Framework for Depressive Relapse Prevention

When I first read Segal, Williams, and Teasdale's (2002) original edition of their MBCT approach, I found myself drawn to the middle way MBCT represented in terms of its seamless integration of solid cognitive and behavioral therapy principles with the approach of Jon Kabat-Zinn's MBSR. Segal, Williams, and Teasdale's MBCT framework masterfully weaved together core components of the CBT and MBSR broad theoretical models to place an explicit emphasis upon cognitions, while concurrently explicitly targeting emotions and bodily sensations. Still holding central the idea that automatic thought processes are a key component to coping, combined with the training in nonjudgmental, kind attention to the present moment through meditation, it seemed that an adapted version of the innovative MBCT treatment package was ideally designed to explicitly address pain catastrophizing, hypervigilant attentional pain bias, stress, and emotional regulation—all of which have been demonstrated to robustly predict pain-related outcomes and coping.

In their development of the MBCT approach, a central premise hypothesized by Segal, Williams, and Teasdale (2002) was that while the explicit focus of CBT is upon changing unhelpful, negative automatic thoughts, they proposed that changing the thoughts per se may not be necessary. Rather, they proposed that the sustained, long-term improvements demonstrated with CBT may actually stem from an implicit shift in the patient's relationship to their thoughts, such that thoughts are regarded simply as mental events, not as the truth and not as some reflection of one's identity. This decentralized perspective on thoughts is described by Teasdale as "meta-cognitive insight" (Teasdale, 1999), although a variety of other terms are also variously applied, such as reperceiving (Shapiro & Carlson, 2009), decentering (Russel & Barrett, 1999), cognitive defusion (Hayes et al., 1999), distancing (Carmody, Baer, Lykins, & Olendzki, 2009), and deautomatization (Deikman, 1982).

Through their early experiences in attending MBSR courses, Segal and colleagues observed that the mindfulness meditation technique that is at the core of MBSR effectively targeted this underlying shift in relationship to thoughts (that is engendered implicitly in CBT), to make it the direct, explicit focus of the treatment itself. Hence, while CBT and MBSR differ fundamentally in their treatment rationale, it was theorized that they share a common pathway for treatment success that is critical for improved outcome: facilitation of a shift in the patients' relationship to their thoughts, while the experience itself may remain (changed or unchanged). Moreover, they noticed that in the delivery of MBSR, this decentered perspective was expanded to include not only targeting thoughts, but also in relating to emotions and bodily sensations. Further, in MBSR, there was an additional emphasis bought to bear with decentering: the attitude one brings in relating to thoughts, feelings, and sensations, which is characterized by a nonjudgmental acceptance, kindness, and self-compassion.

In order for this shift toward a mindful, open, decentered perspective to be sustained in the MBCT treatment context, Segal, Williams, and Teasdale built upon cognitive and learning theory (in the specific context of depression, relapse, and emotional reactivity models) and theorized that accumulated experiential learning at a deep level in mind and body in *being* in this mode of mind is needed. They proposed that this deep-level learning could be facilitated by integrating CBT oriented exercises with training in mindfulness to accelerate enhancement of awareness of patterns of changes in thought, emotion, and body when automatically reacting (and running on automatic pilot or when the mind is in "doing mode") vs. these patterns when intentionally responding (when the mind is in the present moment, in "being mode"). Thus, the cognitive therapy aspect was theorized to enhance this capacity for discerning awareness of the present mode of mind, while synchronously the fully integrated mindfulness practices were theorized to provide experiential training in learning how to intentionally switch mental gears from doing mode to being mode. Together, this enhanced awareness and training of the mind was theorized to open up the opportunity to *choose* how to respond (in a way to reduce suffering), rather than just simply running off of well-worn automatic habits of mind, emotion, and body (which only add to suffering). In essence this approach thereby targets a shift in the entire nature of how we typically relate to experience. The question was, though, how did this theory fit specifically within the context of models of pain, and how might it be adapted to best meet the unique, complex demands that living a life in daily pain entails?

Integrating the MBCT Framework with Pain Theory: Early Ideas

The challenge was to clearly articulate *why* MBCT should be effective for pain specifically, and *how* it might be expected to be different from other extant pain treatment approaches—in essence, to develop an MBCT for chronic pain theoretical model. Armed with an appropriate theoretical model, we could then move forward with adapting the MBCT protocol. In approaching this challenge, we first sought to understand fully what was already known on the topic of mindfulness for pain. In reviewing the literature at the time, it was clear that there was already a rapidly growing body of research investigating MBIs for pain (most typically, MBSR); seminal in the field was Kabat-Zinn's extensive work on MBSR applied broadly to coping with stress, pain, and illness. Further, various mindfulness theoretical models had been proposed in the broad psychotherapy literature, and in addition to this, we also felt it was necessary to study and consider the traditional Eastern Buddhist texts on suffering from which Westernized concepts emerged.

Surprisingly, I came to realize that at this point in time, there was no unified, testable scientific theory however that provided an explicit rationale for applying MBIs specifically to pain. This was the gap in the literature I referred to in the previous chapter when I touched on introducing our recently proposed theoretical model of MBIs for pain that was intended to be a starting point in filling this gap (Day, Jensen, et al., 2014). However, backtracking in time to when I first realized this gap, it meant we had to reset our starting point in adapting the MBCT approach for pain—it was no longer just a matter of adjusting extant mindfulness for pain theory and integrating well-established cognitive and behavioral therapy for pain principles, rather the MBCT model for pain needed more extensive development from the ground up.

As a fresh starting point, one excellent article published at that time by Hoffman and Asmundson from the broad psychotherapy literature particularly stood out and caught my attention. The title of the article posed the question: "Acceptance and mindfulness-based therapy: New wave or old hat?" (Hofmann & Asmundson, 2008). In this article, Hoffman and Asmundson argued that acceptance and mindfulness-based treatments share a great deal of common ground with CBT, and that all of these approaches (despite acknowledged differences in their philosophical foundations) may best be conceptualized in the larger context of the emotion regulation literature.

Specifically, in the broad psychotherapy context, Hoffman and Asmundson conceptualized CBT as primarily an "antecedent-focused" approach, and MBIs and ACT as "response-focused" emotional regulation approaches. Mapping this model onto the theory of CBT for pain discussed in the previous chapter: Theoretically CBT for pain is goal oriented and a key focus is on stress management and changing maladaptive, negative, or otherwise unhelpful automatic thoughts about pain to make them more realistic and positive—in essence to address these *antecedent* thoughts before they cascade and lead to worsening mood, pain, and function. From the perspective of Hoffman and Asmundson's framework, given that pain catastrophizing has been shown to precede and predict poor pain-related outcomes, it represents a critical, "antecedent-focused" mechanism of CBT.

On the other hand, Hoffman and Asmundson considered mindfulness and acceptance interventions (as delivered in the psychotherapy context for psychological disorders, such as depression) "response-focused" treatments as the core techniques of these approaches target unhelpful emotional *responses*. Applying this to build a theoretical model of MBIs for pain then: Theoretically in MBSR for pain, meditation is taught as the core technique to train the cultivation of moment-to-moment awareness in response to *all* thoughts, emotions, and bodily sensations (including but not limited to pain) as they arise with a "response-focused" attitude of nonstriving and with an emphasis upon cultivation of nonjudgmental awareness and acceptance of pain. Hence, the processes of mindfulness and acceptance might well be conceptualized as key "response-focused" mechanisms in MBIs for pain.

With Hoffman and Asmundson's conceptualization in mind, it seemed possible that a viable model of MBCT for pain was that this approach, with its combination of CBT and MBSR principles and techniques, theoretically targeted *both* antecedent- and response-focused coping and therefore might have the capacity to extend and build upon the effects observed when these treatments are applied in isolation. Further, given the MBCT model places an explicit emphasis upon cognitions, but also directly addresses emotions and bodily sensations, it seemed that an adapted version of the MBCT theoretical premises made specific to pain had the capacity to target each of the key biopsychosocial elements that interconnect in the experience we call "pain." This seemed a plausible rationale and at that time provided a missing theoretical link specifying why MBCT should be effective for chronic pain. With this model, Beverly Thorn and I had the final missing piece for our grant proposal for the Anthony Marchionne Foundation that we started writing on the plane trip back from Joshua Tree, and then later that year for the National Headache Foundation. It is never predictable, but as fate would have it, both of these grant proposals were successful, and provided the resources we needed to begin testing and refining the theory, and to begin to obtain empirical data speaking to the feasibility, acceptability, and efficacy of the adapted MBCT for chronic pain protocol.

Evolving Theoretical Underpinning of MBCT for Chronic Pain

Despite both of our first MBCT for chronic pain grants being successful, as things went along and as I bounced ideas around with my primary collaborators—Dr. Beverly Thorn, Dr. Mark Jensen, Dr. Dawn Ehde, and Dr. Chuck Ward—I found myself becoming less and less convinced that the antecedent- and response-focused distinction was altogether useful for the purposes that we had been using it for. Our discussions kept returning to the fact that CBT for pain truly is *not* only about antecedent-focused stress management, but also includes response-focused techniques, and vice versa with MBSR. Moreover, in coping with chronic pain, what can truly be designated as coming before (i.e., the antecedent) and what as after (i.e., the response)? When does one response end and another begin? It was a theory exceptionally difficult to test, to prove or to disprove and therefore not entirely useful. For the theory of MBCT for pain to be of practical and scientific use, it needed more specificity and testability.

Around the time that we were in the midst of running our first funded pilot research and the initial MBCT for chronic pain trial, Mark Jensen proposed an overarching theoretical model describing the mechanisms of how *all* psychosocial pain treatments exert beneficial effects (Jensen, 2011). This was a model that shifted my way of thinking. Although broad and inclusive just as Hoffman and Asmundson's theory was, Mark Jensen's model included more specificity, and also made nuanced predictions about the mechanisms of various psychosocial pain treatments. In the original model, treatments were hypothesized to be of benefit by influencing one or more of five elements: (1) cognitive content (i.e., *what* people think about the pain, the contents of consciousness); (2) cognitive process (i.e., *how* people think about the pain); (3) behavior; (4) brain states; and (5) the environment/social variables. In our next revised version of this model, we proposed an additional sixth element; (6) emotion and affect (Day, Jensen, et al., 2014). The figure below illustrates the revised organizational framework.

This highly interconnected organizational framework provided the structure for the development of a more precise theoretical model for MBCT than our initial attempt. Using this structure, combined with consideration of the vast empirical understanding of the multidimensional experience of pain, the original MBCT theory, as well as an updated review of the building evidence base of MBIs for pain, we had what we needed to build an explicit, evidence-based, testable theory of MBCT for chronic pain. Central to building this theory was to identify the domains of functioning targeted specifically by MBCT for pain, and to contrast this to the shared targeted domains that are influenced, but nonspecifically, by MBCT as well as a number of other approaches.

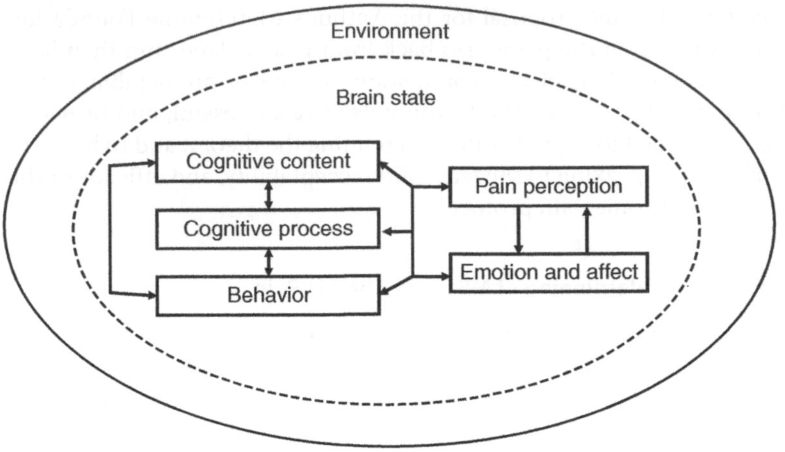

The revised organizational framework. Reprinted from *Journal of Pain*, *15*(7), Day, M.A., Jensen, M.P., Ehde, D.E., and Thorn, B.E. "Toward a theoretical model for mindfulness-based pain management" Copyright (2014), with permission from Elsevier.

Our initial model, using Hoffman and Asmundson's approach, theorized that MBCT engendered improvement primarily via targeting both antecedent and response-focused mechanisms, respectively the core targets of CBT and MBSR. In Mark Jensen's framework however, what was theorized is that CBT and MBSR respectively primarily target cognitive content (i.e., cognitive restructuring to target the content of catastrophic thoughts) and cognitive process (i.e., meditation to enhance mindfulness). Thus, similar to our earlier integration attempt, here we viewed the MBCT for chronic pain protocol as building upon both the CBT and MBSR frameworks to directly incorporate key techniques from these approaches (Kabat-Zinn, 1990; Thorn, 2004) that explicitly target both pain-related cognitive content *and* cognitive process. Unlike our earlier antecedent and response-focused model however, this model was testable with available psychometrically sound assessment instruments.

Consistent with our evolving ideas on how MBCT for pain might engender benefit, our review of the literature (Day, Jensen, et al., 2014) identified that MBCT does instigate change in both cognitive processes specific to MBIs (i.e., mindfulness, which has also been shown to potentially moderate MBI outcomes) as well as nonspecific processes shared by MBIs and other psychosocial treatments (i.e., pain catastrophizing, pain acceptance[1]) (Day, Jensen, et al., 2014; Garland et al., 2012; Shapiro, Brown, Thoresen, & Plante, 2011). Moreover, MBCT has also been shown to lead to changes in cognitive content variables also similarly targeted by other cognitive and behavioral approaches (e.g., pain management self-efficacy beliefs) (Day, Jensen, et al., 2014). Thus, there appeared tentative support for the primary role that *both* cognitive content and cognitive process play in MBCT for pain. An additional cognitive mechanism emerging in our review, although not specific to MBCT or indeed MBIs more broadly, is stimulating positive, realistic expectations that treatment will be of benefit (Goossens, Vlaeyen, Hidding, Kole-Snijders, & Evers, 2005; Peerdeman et al.,

2016; Smeets et al., 2008). Expanding beyond the cognitive domain, we also sought to identify the other mechanisms that might be at work in MBCT operating broadly within the brain state sphere—behaviors and emotions/affect—as well as the contextual environmental sphere.

In terms of behavioral mechanisms, the practice of mindfulness meditation is the most overt form of behavioral change associated specifically with MBIs, including but not limited to MBCT. Despite the standard meditation dose recommendations of 45 min per day initialized in MBSR and carried forward into the original MBCT for depression relapse approach, we identified in our review that there is currently limited evidence that has examined dose–response relations to determine empirically what dose is ideal for a given individual (Day, Jensen, et al., 2014). In our pilot MBCT research (which will be discussed in more detail later in this chapter), we found that the average length of practice recorded by participants in their daily meditation diaries was 25 min; however, for those completing treatment, the average dose was 40 min (Day, Thorn, et al., 2014). The one significant factor we identified that was associated with the amount of at-home practice was therapist rated client engagement: those participants who were observed by the therapist to be more engaged during session practiced significantly more outside of session (Day, Halpin, & Thorn, 2016). Interestingly, our review of the brain imaging research related to MBIs hinted at further behavioral mechanisms: approach-oriented coping (and associated decreased avoidance, which is consistent with mindfulness theory) and increased task persistence (Cahn & Polich, 2006; Chiesa & Serretti, 2010).

Consistent with Hoffman and Asmundson's (2008) assertion that emotional regulation is a core emphasis in mindfulness interventions, converging evidence from brain imaging and self-report data show increased positive affect and decreased negative affect following MBIs (Cahn & Polich, 2006; Chiesa & Serretti, 2010). As described in Chapter 1, neuroimaging studies have demonstrated that similar areas of the brain are activated in processing negative emotions as in processing pain (e.g., the amygdala, anterior cingulate cortex and insula), and support for the Gate Control Theory or Neuromatrix Model shows that ramping down activity in these areas improves pain. Based on this, the observed changes in increased positive affect and decreased negative affect following MBIs might represent key mechanisms underlying pain relief associated with MBIs. Historically, affect and emotional variables have typically been conceptualized as secondary outcomes in pain research; however, based on the evidence, it is just as plausible that treatment-related changes in these variables during MBCT may actually play a causative mechanism role in improving pain.

Further findings from brain imaging research suggest that other select changes in brain state seem to be associated with MBIs, including but not specific to MBCT. To date, most of this research has been conducted with healthy individuals and/or long-term meditators, however the results have shown mindfulness meditation is associated with increased cortical thickness (within the hippocampus, brain stem, posterior and anterior insula, midcingulate cortex, and parietal and prefrontal cortices), enhanced frontal attentional control systems, as well as an observed effect of a decoupling of sensory-discriminative networks from cognitive-evaluative brain networks (i.e., indicative of a decentered perspective)

(Day, Jensen, et al., 2014; Jensen, Day, & Miró, 2014). The degree to which MBCT might target these brain state changes in comparison to other MBIs is not known at this time. In an exciting line of recent research however, Mark Jensen and colleagues have found preliminary evidence that baseline brain state may moderate MBI outcomes (Jensen et al., 2014). Specifically, they found that lower levels of slow oscillations (8–13 Hz, or alpha; as assessed by EEG) prior to treatment was associated with greater pain reduction in the mindfulness meditation condition only; this same effect was not observed in any of the other conditions (hypnosis, neurofeedback, active or sham transcranial direct current stimulation). Although additional trials with larger samples are needed to see if this finding replicates, it suggests that individuals with fewer alpha brainwaves at pre-treatment (i.e., which is our brain wave pattern when we are in a state of physical and mental relaxation while still aware of what is happening in our moment-to-moment experience) might be ideally suited to MBCT, as this approach is theoretically designed to help "overactive" brain states and to foster mindfulness.

In addition to these theoretically "internal" mechanisms of MBCT for pain, there are a variety of shared, nonspecific "external" environmental/social contextual mechanisms that are as critical in this psychosocial treatment approach as in many others. Although I did not mention this in Chapter 2, a powerful influence on outcomes across all psychological treatments is exerted by common factors, such as group cohesion and therapist alliance. MBCT for chronic pain is most often delivered in a group setting (although as I will discuss in Chapter 13, the approach can also easily be adapted to be delivered in individual therapy), and for many patients an important part of being involved in a group delivered treatment is that they learn that they are not alone and that their experiences are commonly shared by others also living with chronic pain (Day, Thorn, & Kapoor, 2011). Some evidence even suggests that group factors such as social learning and cohesion can become agents of change in and of themselves (Yalom & Leszcz, 2005). Further, preliminary research in nonpain populations has found that mindfulness meditation might facilitate improved social relationships and support, which consequently might be associated with improved treatment outcomes.

Arguably the most robust environmental mechanism in MBCT (as in other psychosocial pain treatments) is the importance of a strong therapeutic alliance. A massive body of research has repeatedly affirmed the critical role of alliance in influencing outcome across a range of studies, research groups, settings, and population types. Necessary but perhaps not sufficient, the therapeutic alliance has been described as the foundation upon which all other effects and therapeutic processes build. Therapeutic alliance is particularly important in MBCT given that patient–therapist collaboration is central to at least two core elements that we will discuss in more detail shortly: (1) the therapist-initiated guided inquiry into the participants' moment-to-moment experience with meditation in a curious, open, and warm manner; and (2) therapeutically leading mindfulness meditation practices while co-participating such that collaboration is maintained during the meditation practice (Felder, Dimidjian, & Segal, 2012).

The figure below illustrates pictorially the full theoretical model emerging from our review which I have described in this section. This model is based on

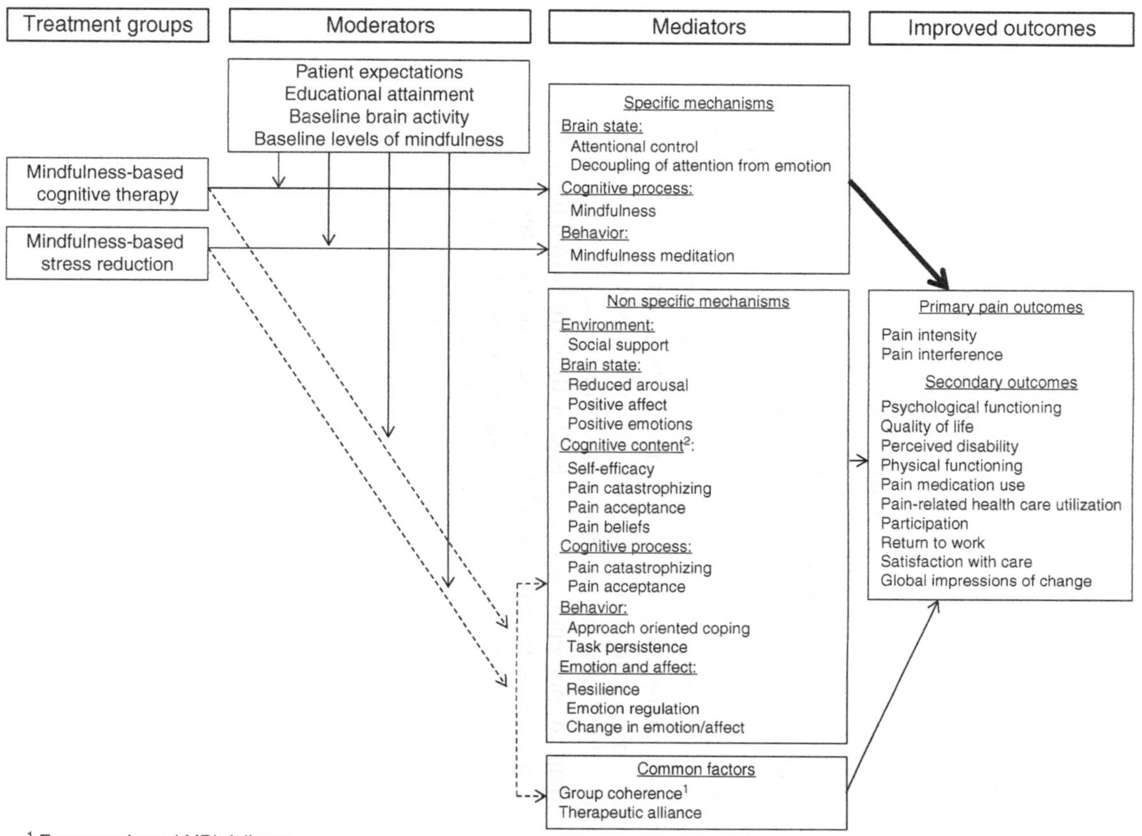

[1] For group-based MBI delivery

[2] This may be a more potent mechanism for MBCT compared to MBSR, given MBCT integrates key cognitive therapy principles

The full theoretical model emerging from the review. Reprinted from *Journal of Pain*, *15*(7), Day, M.A., Jensen, M.P., Ehde, D.E., and Thorn, B.E. "Toward a theoretical model for mindfulness-based pain management" Copyright (2014), with permission from Elsevier.

the currently available evidence, and given there is limited research that has investigated MBCT for pain specifically, this model is currently generalized to include MBSR. However, as I have described, there is already some evidence consistent with MBCT theory that suggests the integrated CBT component in this protocol might lead to stronger effects on cognitive content than MBSR. This model and the theory of MBCT will continue to evolve and be refined as more evidence accumulates.

Adapting the MBCT for Chronic Pain Treatment Structure

Tailoring the Approach to Pain

In developing the first edition of the manualized protocol described in Part II, a key focus was to stay as close as possible to the originally described MBCT approach (Segal, Williams, & Teasdale, 2002), while tailoring it and adapting it specifically to map on to our theoretical model to meet the individual needs and challenges of individuals living with chronic pain (Kabat-Zinn, 1990; Thorn, 2004). The MBCT for pain approach, as in the original protocol, maintains one of the strengths of CBT protocols in that cognitive exercises are included that train the mind to be more aware, more often, of cognitions, emotions, behaviors, and pain, and the links between them. Unlike in CBT however, the CBT-oriented exercises in the MBCT protocol are not aimed toward *changing* any of these aspects of moment-to-moment experience. Rather they are geared toward simply heightening awareness, thereby providing an entry point to stepping *out* of automatic pilot and doing mode, and *into* being mode. Similar to the original MBCT protocol, the first half of treatment is focused on enhancing awareness of our habitual patterns, and this awareness is built upon in the second half of treatment to enhance skillful, wise responding (i.e., choosing to intentionally *respond* rather than *react*—this is what is meant by "skillful" here).

The CBT Component

Throughout the MBCT for pain approach, you will see that each of the cognitively oriented exercises from the original protocol have been adapted to be specific and relevant to chronic pain. If I were to distill that down however, in essence, the psychoeducation and CBT-oriented exercises included in the adapted MBCT for chronic pain protocol are designed to assist in developing awareness of the following: (1) stressful and pleasant experiences, and their connection to cognitions, behaviors, emotions, pain, and physiological changes; (2) patterns of negative automatic thinking, with a specific emphasis on patterns of pain-related automatic thoughts such as pain catastrophizing, ruminating about the pain, and an absorptive focus on the pain; (3) the idea that "thoughts are not fact"; (4) nourishing activities and depleting activities (and how to increase the former, and decrease the latter to foster better self-care); and (5) awareness of red flags that might precipitate pain and stress flare-ups (e.g., overdoing, underdoing, allowing pain to guide behavior etc.).

More specifically, in terms of key pain-related CBT-oriented content that is included within the MBCT for pain protocol, in Session 1, psychoeducation and an interactive discussion on the Gate Control Theory is presented. This is adapted from the approach we developed in one of Beverly Thorn's trials on CBT for pain (Kuhajda, Thorn, Gaskins, Day, & Cabbil, 2011; Thorn et al., 2011), and the qualitative feedback we received from patients was that inclusion of this component at the outset of the program sent the clear message that (1) yes, we believe your pain is real; and that (2) psychological approaches such as the one we are teaching here work to improve real pain, and change the way pain is processed in the brain (Day et al., 2011). Thus, inclusion of the Gate Control Theory in the first MBCT session provides patients with an easy-to-understand, scientific reason as to why this approach should be of benefit for pain, fostering positive expectations and buy-in.

A further traditional CBT for pain exercise is included in Session 2, where a key theme of the session is on increasing awareness of how stress increases pain, and how a large part of our stress is influenced by the ways in which we think about our experiences. This is a critical component early on in CBT approaches for chronic pain, which is why this aspect is emphasized early in the MBCT for pain protocol. Thus, integrating the notions advocated in Beverly Thorn's *Cognitive Therapy for Chronic Pain* (Thorn, 2004), this session has been adapted to include psychoeducation on key concepts of the Stress–Pain–Appraisal model illustrating the importance of stepping out of "automatic pilot" and increasing our awareness of our thoughts, judgments, and appraisals, and their connection with stress, pain, emotions, and behaviors. The final CBT-oriented exercise delivered in this session has roots in behavioral activation and is the "Pleasant Experiences Diary" (termed the "Pleasant Events Calendar" in the original protocol), which functions to further illustrate the connection between how our judgments of events (i.e., as "pleasant") powerfully influence pain, emotions, and how we think. Moreover, while stress and pain "put the blinders on" for many people in that they often lose sight of anything *but* the pain, this exercise (which is assigned as a take-home activity) increases awareness of those experiences in life that may bring a sense of pleasure—if we notice them.

In Session 3 further practice to enhance assimilation of the concepts of the Stress–Pain–Appraisal model is provided by the "Stressful Experiences Diary," which is assigned for homework the week following this session and was called the "Unpleasant Events Calendar" in Segal, Williams, and Teasdale's original version. The new label here for this activity reflects the critical role that the stress response plays in pain, and how our thoughts powerfully underlie its initiation. This is built on in Session 4, where patterns of thinking arising during stressful experiences are brought further into awareness with introducing the "Unhelpful Habits of Mind" handout, which, as in traditional CBT, is used to name styles of automatic thoughts (e.g., fortune telling)—akin to the use of the Automatic Thoughts Questionnaire in the original protocol for depression. In Session 5, this training in awareness is taken further in this text for pain to enhance awareness of unhelpful pain-related intermediate and core beliefs with an exercise (which was adapted from the CBT protocol we used in Beverly Thorn's RCT; Thorn et al., 2011) called "Getting Down to the Root of Our Thoughts and Beliefs about Pain."

The role of emotions feeding into thoughts is presented in Session 6. Also in this session is an exercise to build clients' awareness of their own unique warning signals (changes in mind, body, emotion, and behavior) that stress and pain might be beginning to take over. And finally, in Session 7, using activity as a way to self-manage pain effectively is covered and clients are given specific exercises to help increase the amount of nourishing, energizing activities in their day as well as those that build a sense of mastery, and to concurrently decrease time spent in depleting activities—again, this exercise has roots in behavioral activation (Jacobson, Martell, & Dimidjian, 2001). This, along with the identification of their own unique red flags is used to build a Mindfulness Maintenance Plan for relapse prevention, which is settled upon in Session 8. Essentially each session has at least one CBT-oriented exercise and sometimes more.

The Mindfulness Component

Although the CBT and mindfulness aspects of the adapted MBCT for chronic pain protocol are described relatively separately here, as in the original protocol, the practical exploration of the mind and body through a series of formal and informal mindfulness meditation practices is seamlessly integrated with the CBT-oriented exercises in each of the MBCT for chronic pain sessions. The mindfulness meditation practices that are taught function to augment the CBT-oriented exercises (or vice versa!) in further training the mind to cultivate insightful awareness into the transient, changing nature of experience/thinking, as well as the capacity to switch mental modes at will, to be in "being mode" more often. Specifically, the mindfulness meditation practices train the mind to (1) first be aware of unhelpful automatic patterns of thinking, feeling, and reacting to pain, and then to (2) step back and disengage from automatically getting hooked into these patterns, and instead (3) to simply observe and notice such experiences, and to then (4) purposefully, with kindness and a nonjudgmental attitude, place attention on anchoring bodily sensations (e.g., the breath) and other perceptive experiences (e.g., sounds).

The included mindfulness meditation practices in the MBCT for pain protocol are highly consistent with the practices taught in the original protocol and MBSR approaches. However, one main exception to this is the mindful movement practice in the MBCT for pain approach, which (given the potential risk for injury in the context of this being delivered for chronic pain) comprises very basic movements for both the in-session practice and the assigned at-home practice. This is in contrast to the hatha yoga sequences included in the original protocol and in MBSR. Of note, the second edition of Segal, Williams, and Teasdale's text described much simpler movements for the in-session practice, similar to those presented here, although yoga was still assigned for the take-home practice. The Mindful Movement practice along with Mindful Walking is delivered in Session 4 of this program as opposed to the third session in the original protocol. The reason for this is that we found in our experience that Session 3 needed more time to devote to a guided inquiry of client's experiences with the first Seated Meditation taught (prior to this session, clients had only practiced the Body Scan). Moreover, the third session was also when client's most typically described increasing difficulty in establishing and maintaining an at-home daily practice and working through this in-session took time, and was a priority as the at-home practice is the heart and soul of the program. We also found that the movement-based meditations fit well with the Session 4 theme of staying present, as when our mind is most stirred up a movement-focused meditation is a very effective practice to stay with experience. The other key difference in this program specifically delivered for pain (in comparison to Segal and colleagues' original version) for the formal meditation practices is that an extended sitting in silence practice is included in Session 5; given this is later assigned for an at-home practice, clients experiencing it first in the supportive environment of the class has worked well.

You will notice that the 3-Minute Breathing Space is delivered in the very first session of this protocol, in contrast to in the third session of the original protocol for depressive relapse prevention. This is a change that was unanimously advocated for by the patients themselves who have participated in the MBCT for chronic pain program, and we have found that presenting this brief practice early in treatment enhances confidence and a sense of self-efficacy: the belief that meditation is "do-able." Moreover, for those who struggle early on to practice formally each day for 45 min, having this practice available means they will at least practice *something*, and gives them a sense of success (as opposed to "complete failure," as some clients reported feeling when they did not engage in the longer practice). As in the original protocol, the application of the regular 3-Minute Breathing Space is extended in Session 4 as a "responsive" step when uncomfortable, stressful, or otherwise unpleasant experiences occur in daily life and this is taken further in Session 5 where instruction is added to bring mindfulness to the body as a way to stay present and open to the difficulty. In Session 6, the 3-Minute Breathing Space is taught as a first step prior to implementing other strategies to cope with unhelpful, negative thoughts. Finally, in Session 7, participants are encouraged to practice a breathing space, followed by a nourishing, self-care activity.

Overall, the meditation practices included in the MBCT for pain approach provide experiential training in learning to respond to pain, stress, negative thinking, and aversive emotions in a nonjudgmental, nonreactive, accepting manner. As in the original protocol, the meditation practices foster learning to let go of attachment and aversion, and self-imposed standards and expectations of how one's body, thoughts, emotions, and pain *should* be, and instead bringing a sense of curiosity and "allowing" to whatever is present. For the most part, the meditation structure itself as taught in MBCT for chronic pain really is not much different from many of the techniques that have been practiced for thousands of years in the East.

Beyond the structure and the various "technique" or form of meditation taught however, at the heart of meditation practice is what we ourselves bring into it. So in the context we are describing here, it is not just our bodies that we bring to the meditation cushion; what we also bring into the practice is a lifetime of experiences, memories, ideas, emotions, ego structures, and of course within all of this and infinitely more, in this context, there is also pain. Pain is an overriding stimulus that demands attention, and will inevitably be one of the most popular destinations that the mind wanders to during meditation for most individuals with chronic pain. Thus, the meditation practices in MBCT become adapted for pain not necessarily through any change in their structure, but in how the therapist responds to these pain-related challenges that will come up during the guided inquiry following the in-session practice, and how the mindfulness practice itself is related back to living with chronic pain.

The Therapist as an Instrument of Mindfulness

The approach of MBCT is collaborative in nature, and this is personified within the guided inquiry where the therapist invites clients to engage in a joint and interactive discussion of their moment-to-moment experience with the practice, placing the client firmly in the role of the expert of their own experience. In the guided inquiry, the therapist brings a sense of dynamic curiosity and openness to client's direct experience with the practice, without needing to jump in and fix, change, or problem solve in any way. The intention of the guided inquiry is to provide a space for clients to explore and experientially learn from their direct experience, guiding them to link the practices to a fresh understanding of their relationship to pain and suffering, and how we can shift this relationship to be more adaptive. There are a number of excellent, detailed descriptions available in the literature of the guided inquiry (Felder et al., 2012; Sears, 2015; Segal et al., 2013), however the basic instruction for guidance on this process across all of these descriptions is the metaphor of three concentric circles or layers of inquiry.

Starting at the center "personal" circle or layer, the therapist begins by first asking about direct experience, perhaps by a question such as: "What did you notice during that practice?" And in reflecting back and responding to what clients describe noticing, the therapist guides the focus of this discussion to emphasize exploration of direct experience, decoupled from judgment (inquiring into accompanying feelings, sensations, thoughts, fluctuations, reactions etc.). Thus, as a natural extension of this exploration, in the second "contextual" circle, the discussion is expanded outwards as the therapist asks a question along the theme of: "How was this practice different from the way you might normally eat?" (i.e., "normally eat" is what the therapist would inquire about following the raisin exercise; if it was the Body Scan meditation practiced, instead of "eat," it would be "relate to your body" etc.). This guides clients to personally contextualize their experience with the practice, and to deepen their exploration of the contrast between automatic ways of reacting and how the practice of mindfulness might be integrated into daily living. In the third, "pain-specific" circle, the mindfulness practice is placed within the larger purpose of why clients are participating in the program, most typically, to learn ways to manage pain. So the therapist might start this discussion by asking a question around: "In what ways do you think this practice relates to living with chronic pain?" The purpose of this third circle is not to delve into mindfulness as a "solution" to "the problem" of chronic pain, as if there is a right or a wrong way to go about it; rather, the idea is for the learning to be expanded to the application of living with pain. So the intention of this third circle or layer is to facilitate clients making the connection between their experiences with the practice, with the key themes of the session, and to explore how to use the practice as a pain management tool.

During the guided inquiry, one of the most critical elements is not necessarily following this question pattern of widening concentric circles. Rather, the most important aspect is actually the *quality* of the approach that the therapist takes in engaging clients in this discussion of their experience. This is where it is essential that the therapist embody and genuinely model for clients the qualities of mindfulness they are inviting clients to adopt and cultivate in the practice: presence in the moment, empathic attention (i.e., *being* with patients and attuned to their inner experiences as they describe their experience, as opposed to a sharp clinical attention devoid of warmth), a nonjudgmental attitude, a sense of non-striving, trust, beginner's mind, patience, acceptance, and kindness (Kabat-Zinn, 2013; Shapiro & Carlson, 2009). This may seem like a long list, but it is not exhaustive! Moreover, it is not just during the guided inquiry that these qualities are needed, but during the whole session, even while guiding the meditation practices.

Given the importance of embodying these therapist qualities during MBCT, it makes sense that a view held almost unanimously across all the experts in the field—Kabat-Zinn, Segal, Williams, Teasdale, Shapiro, Carlson—is that therapists are strongly encouraged to have their own established, regular daily personal mindfulness practice. After all, how else to better cultivate these qualities as an MBCT therapist than with meditation? In teaching workshops on MBCT for pain to therapists and other professionals, this is one aspect I have found myself sometimes discussing almost tentatively (goodness knows that time spent sitting, essentially *doing nothing* seems a big ask in today's fast-paced world, and indeed I am "guilty" myself of not keeping up a regular practice at times in my life). However, for me personally, beyond the benefits of a personal practice naturally leading to you as the therapist embodying the qualities of mindfulness, having my own personal practice means I am entirely *genuine* in delivering MBCT. The term "genuine" may seem rather boring in comparison to the above long list of typical qualities of embodied mindfulness, but our clients and we ourselves know (or at least later we might realize) when we are *not* genuinely in the moment, and instead speak from an "intellectualized" understanding as opposed to an internalized felt experience. Although currently there is not a lot of hard and fast data available to empirically inform recommendations on how long therapists need to practice for and how much of a difference it truly makes, preliminary research does suggest that it influences client outcomes. In a series of studies, Grepmair and colleagues found that client self-reported outcomes are consistently better across multiple domains when the MBI was delivered by a practicing therapist, compared to a nonpracticing therapist (Grepmair, Mitterlehner, Loew, Bachler, et al., 2007; Grepmair, Mitterlehner, Loew, & Nickel, 2007).

Besides the likely beneficial effects that having your own personal practice has on the quality of your delivery of MBCT (and possibly on client outcomes), as an added benefit, meditation is particularly helpful for one's own self-care as a therapist, and to prevent burnout. Research shows that burnout—typically defined as consisting of emotional exhaustion, depersonalization, and a reduced sense of personal accomplishment—is common among therapists and health professionals, with some estimates as high as 60–75% (Wallace, Lemaire, & Ghali, 2009). Adding insult to injury, burnout has been shown to lead to symptoms of depression and anxiety, lower mental quality of life, higher career turnover, decreased quality of psychological care, and in some cases, inadequate care (Dunn, Iglewicz, & Moutier, 2008; Shanafelt et al., 2012). As therapists, empathy is a cornerstone of what we do. Functionally, this means that we absorb a lot of emotion in therapy sessions as we focus on understanding our clients' distress and suffering and as we work with them to find ways to shift them towards more adaptive, valued patterns of functioning. Multiply this empathic absorption factor by multiple sessions a day, by multiple days in a year, and by multiple years in a career and it is easy to see why burnout is so common in our profession. Critical to preventing burnout and functioning optimally is *self-awareness* of stress and distress. At the core of meditation is training in self-awareness, and research with a group of healthcare providers found that training in mindfulness led to improved burnout symptoms, mood stability, mindfulness, and conscientiousness (Krasner et al., 2009). Thus, in this context, a personal mindfulness meditation practice will likely not only make one a more effective MBCT therapist, but it also represents an ideal, evidence-based tool that we can use to enhance our well-being and to promote career longevity.

MBCT for Pain: Emerging Empirical Evidence

Evaluating the Efficacy of MBCT for Chronic Pain

The empirical investigation of the potential benefit of applying MBCT to chronic pain is only in the early stages, and indeed, one of my hopes in writing this book is that it will make this approach more accessible to clinicians and researchers so that we can build an evidence base for this treatment. Looking back, the very first test of this approach was based on humble beginnings. At that time, I was a project manager on one of Beverly Thorn's NIH grants examining a literacy adapted CBT protocol compared to pain education within a rural, low-SES, mostly African American community (Thorn et al., 2011). This trial was mostly conducted at a healthcare center run by nuns in Pine Apple (that's two words!), Alabama, in the heart of the Black Belt region, and Beverly and I were travelling there weekly to deliver treatment. As it so happened, following our intensive MBCT training at Joshua Tree, there was a group of five African American women who had just completed the trial, and were eager to learn more pain management strategies. Since both Beverly and I were in Pine Apple anyway, we figured it represented a great opportunity to conduct a pilot run of the MBCT for chronic pain manual.

So it was with this group of five wonderful women with heterogeneous chronic pain conditions that we conducted our first feasibility pilot trial of the MBCT for chronic pain approach. Hesitant and wary to hope (after all, we were teaching a technique many associate with Buddhism in the "bible belt" of the deep South!), by the end of the 8 weeks with this brave group of women, we were amazed that the initial protocol was so well received and the qualitative feedback so overwhelmingly positive (Day & Thorn, 2011). It was not long after we finished this pilot feasibility trial that we received word from the Anthony Marchionne

Foundation informing us our MBCT for chronic pain grant was successful, and that they wanted to fund our research trial comparing MBCT to a treatment as usual, delayed treatment control within a headache pain population. Soon after, the National Headache Foundation notified us that they too were interested in the approach and funded our grant to additionally collect qualitative data to obtain first-person patient accounts of the treatment, as part of the larger trial. At this point, we had the initial version of the manual, and the resources, and it was time to hit the ground running.

So in our first RCT of the approach, we were interested in not only the efficacy of MBCT, but also the feasibility of recruitment and patient tolerability and acceptability of the approach (Day, Thorn, et al., 2014). Results of the intent to treat efficacy analyses ($n = 36$) showed that compared to the control, MBCT resulted in significantly greater improvement in pain interference, headache pain management self-efficacy, and pain acceptance, and a tendency toward greater reductions in pain catastrophizing ($ps < .05$). In those who completed the MBCT program or the wait-list period ($n = 24$), the findings were similar with significant effects across all of the aforementioned outcomes, as well as the MBCT group resulting in significantly greater improvements in pain catastrophizing and a trend toward a steeper decline in daily peak headache pain intensity ratings. These effect sizes within the completers indicated MBCT resulted in large, clinically meaningful effect size improvements in pain intensity ($ds = .80$ for both average and peak intensity), pain interference ($d = 1.29$), pain acceptance ($d = 1.22$), pain catastrophizing ($d = .94$), and headache pain management self-efficacy ($d = 1.65$), which is comparable to the range of effect sizes seen with other psychosocial interventions, such as CBT (Williams et al., 2012). Moreover, results showed that MBCT was feasible, tolerable, and acceptable to participants. The recruitment to enrolment rate was high, drop-out rates were similar to those published with other approaches, and participants reported (using standardized, validated measures) positive MBCT treatment expectations and motivation, high satisfaction with treatment, and a strong working alliance with the therapist. Although preliminary, these results certainly showed that the MBCT approach may be particularly promising in the context of chronic pain.

Unbeknown to us at the time, as we were conducting our initial RCT, researchers in Spain were also conducting a RCT to examine the efficacy of MBCT in reducing the impact of fibromyalgia in females, and included in their secondary analyses was examination of this approach in concurrently improving depressive symptoms and pain (Parra-Delgado & Latorre-Postigo, 2013). Parra-Delgado and Latorre-Postigo also employed a delayed treatment control condition, and results of their intent to treat analyses ($n = 33$) produced a pattern of findings similar to what we found with MBCT resulting in significantly greater improvements in the impact of fibromyalgia and depressive symptoms. These effects were maintained at the 3-month follow-up. They also found a slight decrease in pain intensity at post-treatment in the MBCT group, but this effect was not significant, and they did not include any other pain-specific outcomes. Possibly the nonsignificant pain outcome in this trial was due to pain management not being the primary focus in their MBCT protocol, rather the emphasis was on reducing the impact of fibromyalgia more broadly.

To date, I am aware of only one other trial that has been published examining the MBCT approach for pain, conducted by Dowd and colleagues (Dowd et al., 2015). In this study, a computerized, internet-delivered MBCT program was compared to a psychoeducation control condition within a heterogeneous, non-cancer pain population. Results of their intent to treat analyses ($n = 124$) showed that compared with the psychoeducation control, MBCT resulted in greater pre- to post-treatment improvements in subjective well-being, present pain intensity, and emotion regulation indicators. Both groups showed similarly significant improvements across pain interference, pain acceptance, pain catastrophizing, and average pain intensity outcomes, and most of these observed effects were maintained at 6-month follow-up. These findings are particularly exciting as innovations in internet-delivered therapies have the potential to overcome treatment access barriers for many individuals (e.g., lack of services, cost, rurality, lack of transportation, or physical disability that hinders mobility, just to name a few) (Day & Thorn, 2010; Tait & Chibnall, 2005). Although internet-delivered therapy in clinical practice brings with it a host of unique considerations (i.e., cost and reimbursement issues, management of suicidality, capacity to build alliance etc.), research suggests there is an increasing demand for access to such services (Griffiths et al., 2006). Hence, future translational research building upon Dowd and colleagues' findings is needed to determine how this approach might best be integrated and sustained in community-based clinics and for whom such approaches might be best suitable for and under what circumstances.

Preliminary Findings of the Mechanisms of MBCT for Chronic Pain

Although determining whether MBCT for chronic pain works is important, it is not enough. Research is also needed to further refine the theory of this approach for pain by identifying the mediators or processes of MBCT (i.e., *how* does the approach engender beneficial outcomes for pain?) as well as potential treatment moderators (i.e., for *whom* is this approach most suitable for under what circumstances?). My collaborators and I have commenced preliminary analyses investigating these questions using our proposed theoretical model of MBIs that I described earlier as a guide for a priori hypothesis generation. However, so far we are the only research group to have published data on the mechanisms of MBCT for chronic pain.

In one of our most recent studies, we examined the degree to which MCBT improves pain outcomes via the mechanisms specified by theory, that is, primarily through change in cognitive content *and* change in cognitive process (Day & Thorn, 2016). Results indicated that change in pain acceptance (conceptualized as a combined cognitive content and process construct) during MBCT was a driving force in reducing pain interference; however surprisingly, neither pain catastrophizing nor headache management self-efficacy predicted change in outcome, hence their mediational role could not be examined. Consistent with these findings, results of our mixed methods analysis that compared treatment responders (≥50% improvement in pain intensity and/or pain interference) to nonresponders (<50% improvement) identified that pain acceptance was a key differentiating factor, with responders reporting greater improvement than nonresponders in pain acceptance ($d = .64$) (Day, Thorn, & Rubin, 2014). Qualitatively, first-person accounts from the treatment responders reported that what helped their pain the most from the program was changes around themes of improved acceptance, mindfulness, and self-efficacy, and also a broader shift in relationship to thoughts and pain (Day, Thorn, & Rubin, 2014). These findings are consistent with theory and indicate that treatment-related improvement in pain acceptance during MBCT for chronic pain may be an especially critical pathway for treatment success. However, the sample size for these analyses was small and all of these results were with a headache pain sample. Larger, more definitive trials investigating the efficacy and mechanisms of MBCT with a diverse range of chronic pain conditions is needed.

Finally, one of the most robust effects reported in the pain and broad psychotherapy literature is that common factors of therapy are shared mechanisms across all efficacious treatments (Day et al., 2012). My collaborators and I have commenced a program of research aimed toward quantifying the role of such common factors in MBCT for chronic pain specifically. As described earlier, a strong therapeutic alliance is one common factor that may function as a foundation for all other treatment effects, and in our mixed methods analysis study (described above) we examined if differences in alliance might also be a differentiating factor between treatment responders and nonresponders. Results indicated that treatment responders did in fact report higher working alliance with the therapist than nonresponders, with the size of this effect being medium in nature (Day, Thorn, & Rubin, 2014). In another study we also found that higher working alliance, therapist adherence to protocol, and therapist quality (as assessed via the fidelity measure provided in Appendix E on the website) were all significantly correlated with higher client satisfaction at post-treatment; and those with more positive pre-treatment expectations and motivation showed greater improvement in pain interference (Day et al., 2016). Clearly an important line of future research will be to identify the ways in which specific and common factors work together in MBCT, and how to optimally target a synergistic combination of these factors to produce the greatest and most efficient benefit for clients living with chronic pain.

Summary

The MBCT for chronic approach was developed with the guiding premise of remaining true to the original protocol, and of integrating within this the rich history of theoretical, empirical, and clinical understandings of chronic pain and its optimal management. As more evidence and clinical experience accumulates on the MBCT for chronic pain approach, it will be essential that the theory evolve and be flexibly refined to integrate the evidence generated. Science, technology, innovation, and advancement of any kind are typically the accumulation of any number of prior individual's efforts, failures, contributions, and incremental steps toward eventual success. I say this as the development of the MBCT approach for chronic pain has been just like that; from the outset of our developing this protocol, it has been a team effort. And of course, current and future planned trials my collaborators and I are currently running to gain further evidence and insights on this approach is also very much a team effort. I am most humbled to be the one to describe this approach in detail in Part II. The overarching intention of the MBCT approach for chronic pain is to provide a way for our clients to be liberated from the cage of pain and suffering, and to live a meaningful life even in the face of pain.

Note

1 Note, pain catastrophizing and pain acceptance are considered to represent both cognitive content and cognitive processes due to the nature of the current most widely used assessment instruments measuring these variables containing item content that taps both.

References

Cahn, B. R., & Polich, J. (2006). Meditation states and traits: EEG, ERP, and neuroimaging studies. *Psychological Bulletin, 132*, 180–211.

Carmody, J., Baer, R. A., Lykins, E. L. B., & Olendzki, N. (2009). An empirical study of the mechanisms of mindfulness in a mindfulness-based stress reduction program. *Journal of Clinical Psychology, 65*(6), 613–626.

Chiesa, A., & Serretti, A. (2010). A systematic review of neurobiological and clinical features of mindfulness meditations. *Psychological Medicine, 40*(8), 1239–1252.

Day, M. A., Halpin, J., & Thorn, B. E. (2016). An empirical examination of the role of common factors of therapy during a mindfulness-based cognitive therapy intervention for headache pain. *Clinical Journal of Pain, 32*(5), 420–427.

Day, M. A., Jensen, M. P., Ehde, D. M., & Thorn, B. E. (2014). Towards a theoretical model for mindfulness-based pain management. *Journal of Pain, 15*(7), 691–703.

Day, M. A., & Thorn, B. E. (2010). The relationship of demographic and psychosocial variables to pain-related outcomes in a rural chronic pain population. *Pain, 151*(2), 467–474.

Day, M. A., & Thorn, B. E. (2011). *Mindfulness-based cognitive therapy for chronic pain in rural Alabama: A pilot study*. Paper presented at the 12th Annual Rural Health Conference, the University of Alabama, Tuscaloosa, Alabama, USA.

Day, M. A., & Thorn, B. E. (2016). The mediating role of pain acceptance during mindfulness-based cognitive therapy for headache. *Complementary Therapies in Medicine, 25*, 51–54.

Day, M. A., Thorn, B. E., & Burns, J. (2012). The continuing evolution of biopsychosocial interventions for chronic pain. *Journal of Cognitive Psychotherapy: An International Quarterly, 26*(2), 114–129.

Day, M. A., Thorn, B. E., & Kapoor, S. (2011). A qualitative analysis of a randomized controlled trial comparing a cognitive-behavioral treatment with education. *Journal of Pain, 12*(9), 941–952.

Day, M. A., Thorn, B. E., & Rubin, N. (2014). Mindfulness-based cognitive therapy for the treatment of headache pain: A mixed-methods analysis comparing

treatment responders and treatment non-responders. *Complementary Therapies in Medicine, 15*(3), 278–285.
Day, M. A., Thorn, B. E., Ward, L. C., Rubin, N., Hickman, S. D., Scogin, F., & Kilgo, G. R. (2014). Mindfulness-based cognitive therapy for the treatment of headache pain: A pilot study. *Clinical Journal of Pain, 22*(2), 278–285.
Deikman, A. (1982). *The observing self.* Boston, MA: Beacon Press.
Dowd, H., Hogan, M. J., McGuire, B. E., Davis, M. C., Sarma, K. M., Fish, R. A., & Zautra, A. J. (2015). Comparison of an online mindfulness-based cognitive therapy intervention with online pain management psychoeducation: A randomized controlled study. *Clinical Journal of Pain, 31*(6), 517–527.
Dunn, L. B., Iglewicz, A., & Moutier, C. (2008). A conceptual model of medical student well-being: Promoting resilience and preventing burnout. *Academic Psychiatry, 32,* 44–53.
Felder, J. N., Dimidjian, S., & Segal, Z. (2012). Collaboration in mindfulness-based cognitive therapy. *Journal of Clinical Psychology: In Session, 68*(2), 179–186.
Garland, E. L., Gaylord, S. A., Palsson, O., Faurot, K., Mann, J. D., & Whitehead, W. E. (2012). Therapeutic mechanisms of a mindfulness-based treatment for IBS: Effects on visceral sensitivity, catastrophizing, and affective processing of pain sensations. *Journal of Behavioral Medicine, 35*(6), 591–602.
Goossens, M. E., Vlaeyen, J. W., Hidding, A., Kole-Snijders, A., & Evers, S. M. (2005). Treatment expectancy affects the outcome of cognitive-behavioral interventions in chronic pain. *Clinical Journal of Pain, 21,* 18–26.
Grepmair, L., Mitterlehner, F., Loew, T., Bachler, E., Rother, W., & Nickel, M. (2007). Promoting mindfulness in psychotherapists in training influences the treatment results of their patients: A randomized, double-blind, controlled study. *Psychotherapy and Psychosomatics, 76,* 332–338.
Grepmair, L., Mitterlehner, F., Loew, T., & Nickel, M. (2007). Promotion of mindfulness in psychotherapists in training: Preliminary study. *European Psychiatry, 22,* 485–489.
Griffiths, F., Lindenmeyer, A., Powell, J., Lowe, P., & Thorogood, M. (2006). Why are health care interventions delivered over the internet? A systematic review of the published literature. *Journal of Medical Internet Research, 8,* e10.
Hayes, S. C., Strosahl, K. D., & Wilson, K. G. (1999). *Acceptance and commitment therapy: An experiential approach to behavior change.* New York, NY: Guilford Press.
Hofmann, S. G., & Asmundson, G. J. G. (2008). Acceptance and mindfulness-based therapy: New wave or old hat? *Clinical Psychology Review, 28,* 1–16.
Jacobson, N. S., Martell, C. R., & Dimidjian, S. (2001). Behavioral activation treatment for depression: Returning to contextual roots. *Clinical Psychology: Science and Practice, 8,* 255–270.
Jensen, M. P. (2011). Psychosocial approaches to pain management: An organizational framework. *Pain, 152*(4), 717–725.
Jensen, M. P., Day, M.A., & Miró, J. (2014). Neuromodulatory treatments for chronic pain: Efficacy and mechanisms. *Nature Reviews Neurology, 10,* 167–168.
Kabat-Zinn, J. (1990). *Full catastrophe living: Using the wisdom of your body and mind to face stress, pain and illness.* New York, NY: Delacourt.
Kabat-Zinn, J. (2013). *Full catastrophe living (revised edition): Using the wisdom of your body and mind to face stress, pain, and illness.* New York, NY: Bantam Books.

Krasner, M. S., Epstein, R. M., Beckman, H., Suchman, A. L., Chapman, B., Mooney, C. J., & Quill, T. E. (2009). Association of an educational program in mindful communication with burnout, empathy, and attitudes among primary care physicians. *Journal of the American Medical Association, 302*(12), 1284–1293.

Kuhajda, M. C., Thorn, B. E., Gaskins, S. W., Day, M. A., & Cabbil, C. M. (2011). Literacy and cultural adaptations for cognitive behavioral therapy in a rural pain population. *Translational Behavioral Medicine, 1*(2), 216–223.

Parra-Delgado, P. M., & Latorre-Postigo, J. M. (2013). Effectiveness of mindfulness-based cognitive therapy in the treatment of fibromyalgia: A randomised trial. *Cognitive Therapy Research, 37*, 1015–1026.

Peerdeman, K. J., van Laarhoven, A. I. M., Keij, S. M., Vase, L., Rovers, M. M., Peters, M. L., & Evers, A. W. M. (2016). Relieving patients' pain with expectation interventions: A meta-analysis. *Pain, 157*(6), 1179–1191.

Russel, J. A., & Barrett, L. F. (1999). Core affect, prototypical emotional episodes, and other things called emotion: Dissecting the elephant. *Journal of Personality and Social Psychology, 76*, 805–819.

Sears, R. W. (2015). *Building competence in mindfulness-based cognitive therapy*. New York, NY: Routledge.

Segal, Z., Williams, J. M., & Teasdale, J. (2002). *Mindfulness-based cognitive therapy for depression: A new approach to preventing relapse*. New York, NY: Guilford Press.

Segal, Z. V., Williams, J. M. G., & Teasdale, J. D. (2013). *Mindfulness-based cognitive therapy for depression*. New York, NY: Guilford.

Shanafelt, T. D., Oreskovich, M. R., Dyrbye, L. N., Satele, D. V., Hanks, J. B., Sloan, J. A., & Balch, C. M. (2012). Avoiding burnout: The personal health habits and wellness practices of US surgeons. *Annals of Surgery, 225*(4), 625–633.

Shapiro, S. L., Brown, K. W., Thoresen, K., & Plante, T. J. (2011). The moderation of mindfulness-based stress reduction effects by trait mindfulness: Results from a randomized controlled trial. *Journal of Clinical Psychology, 67*, 267–277.

Shapiro, S. L., & Carlson, L. E. (2009). *The art and science of mindfulness: Integrating mindfulness into psychology and the helping professions*. Washington, DC: American Psychological Association.

Smeets, R. J., Beelen, S., Goossens, M. E., Schouten, E. G., Knottnerus, J. A., & Vlaeyen, J. W. (2008). Treatment expectancy and credibility are associated with the outcome of both physical and cognitive-behavioral treatment in chronic low back pain. *Clinical Journal of Pain, 24*, 305–315.

Tait, R. C., & Chibnall, J. T. (2005). Racial and ethnic disparities in the evaluation and treatment of pain: psychological perspectives. *Professional Psychology: Research and Practice, 36*(6), 595–601.

Teasdale, J. D. (1999). Metacognition, mindfulness, and the modification of mood disorders. *Clinical Psychology and Psychotherapy, 6*, 146–155.

Thorn, B. E. (2004). *Cognitive therapy for chronic pain: A step-by-step guide*. New York, NY: Guilford Press.

Thorn, B. E., Day, M. A., Burns, J., Kuhajda, M. C., Gaskins, S. W., Sweeney, K., … Cabbil, C. (2011). Randomized trial of group cognitive behavioral therapy compared with a pain education control for low-literacy rural people with chronic pain. *Pain, 152*(12), 2710–2720.

Williams, A. C., Eccleston, C., & Morley, S. (2012). Psychological therapies for the management of chronic pain (excluding headache) in adults. *Cochrane Database of Systematic Reviews, 11*, CD007407.
Wallace, J. E., Lemaire, J. B., & Ghali, W. A. (2009). Physician wellness: A missing quality indicator. *Lancet, 374*, 1714–1721.
Yalom, I. D., & Leszcz, M. (2005). *The theory and practice of group psychotherapy* (5th ed.). New York, NY: Basic Books.

Part II

MBCT for Chronic Pain

4

Overview of the Eight-Session Treatment

The overall aim of the MBCT for chronic pain approach is for individuals with pain to achieve freedom—not freedom from the pain per se, but freedom from all the "extra baggage" and suffering that often gets piled on top of the bare bones pain in the form of negative thoughts/judgments, emotion, and unhelpful behavior. In learning to let go of this extra baggage, the load of the pain becomes lighter and a whole spectrum of choices on how to respond to the pain opens up in each moment, and along with that comes a radical shift towards a new, fresh way of living and relating to what each moment presents. Perhaps most importantly, this shift in how one relates to experience parallels a neurological shift in the way the brain processes pain itself, which improves pain coping and management.

In this chapter, I will first discuss some considerations to help prepare you for your first MBCT for chronic pain group. I will discuss potential caveats to consider in deciding whether this approach is suitable to a given client, so that treatment outcome is optimized and premature drop-out prevented. I will also provide some suggestions on validated, psychometrically sound measures and tracking tools that you might consider using to monitor your client's progress that are appropriate for use in the context of mindfulness-based approaches. Further, I will describe considerations regarding treatment integrity, and will provide a treatment fidelity measure that I developed with Beverly Thorn that might be useful for research, program evaluation, and clinician training purposes. Starting in the next chapter, I will then guide you through the content of each MBCT session in detail, with supervisory support and troubleshooting tips along the way.

Preparing to Deliver MBCT for Chronic Pain

Therapist Qualifications and Training

The MBCT protocol, both in its original form and as adapted for chronic pain here, integrates psychological principles and techniques; therefore, it is important that in delivering this intervention you are qualified and licensed in your jurisdiction to provide mental health services (i.e., have recognized training as a

Mindfulness-Based Cognitive Therapy for Chronic Pain: A Clinical Manual and Guide,
First Edition. Melissa A. Day.

Companion website: www.wiley.com/go/day/mindfulness_based_cognitive_therapy

mental health professional in counseling, psychology etc.) and follow the code of ethics relevant to your profession. Further, in considering implementing MBCT, as in implementing any other intervention, evidence-based practice and standards, relevant codes of ethics, and professional regulations direct clinicians to first receive training to gain the clinical skills, knowledge, and expertise needed to competently deliver the approach in order to maximize benefit and minimize potential harm. While there are general clinical skills needed, just as in delivering any other approach (i.e., cultural competency in working with diverse populations, skills in managing group dynamics, building rapport), there are also other specific areas of skill and expertise to develop in order to competently deliver MBCT for chronic pain. Just reading this book, with a little (or even a lot of) experience in mindfulness is insufficient for ensuring you have the necessary competence to deliver this approach.

As described in Chapter 1, it is strongly recommended that practitioners delivering MBCT in the context of chronic pain have a strong working knowledge of pain, the underlying neurophysiology, as well as an understanding of the full territory of the condition, including the social, emotional, behavioral, and cognitive aspects of chronic pain. There are high rates of comorbid conditions that go along with chronic pain (e.g., depression and anxiety disorders are common), and therefore being competent and comfortable working with any number of such comorbid conditions is needed. Within the practice of meditation, when we ask clients to simply sit with themselves and observe what arises, often what can arise is any number of suppressed emotions, memories, thoughts ... and especially early on, this might feel overwhelming to clients. Thus, it is essential that the MBCT therapist understand not just how to relate to the pain, but how to relate to this full range of experiences. However, recent reports by the Institute of Medicine (IOM, 2011), the National Pain Strategy (NIH, 2011), and a needs assessment specific to psychology (Darnall et al., 2016), show most psychologists receive inadequate training in how to work with individuals with chronic pain; therefore, there is a critical need for professionals working (or wanting to work) with chronic pain populations to seek out continued education, and enhanced matriculate and nonmatriculate training opportunities for learning how to effectively respond to the complex presentation of chronic pain and related comorbidities.

Given that MBCT is structured around cognitive and behavioral therapy theory, principles, and techniques, it is important for therapists to understand the principles described in Chapter 2, and to have training in these approaches. Further, although rarely implemented as the sole psychological treatment approach for pain (and therefore not discussed in prior sections), competence in motivational interviewing (MI; Miller & Rollnick, 2013) is additionally recommended as a core skill set of the MBCT therapist to increase and maintain client's motivation for mindfulness meditation practice outside of the session. Training in MI enhances the capacity for clinicians to be attuned to any comments made by clients about the ease or difficulty of practicing meditation, fitting meditation practice into their schedules, or other issues related to their likelihood of using the MBCT skills after treatment ends. For example, active listening to reflect back to clients any positive statements made about their ability to use the MBCT skills to *manage* (i.e., not necessarily remove) pain helps to increase their sense of self-efficacy. This can occur both during the homework review and during the guided inquiry following the formal in-session meditation practice.

In terms of gaining competence in the nuts and bolts of the MBCT approach itself, the best way is to personally experience the program and gain experiential knowledge and nuanced expertise on the theory and techniques (Segal et al., 2013). Segal, Williams, and Teasdale (2013) recommend completion of a rigorous mindfulness-based teacher training or a 12-month supervised pathway that includes attending three 8-week courses (as a participant, then as a trainee, and then as a co-facilitator).While attending an 8-week MBCT program may not be realistic for many of us (due to access, time, and any number of other factors), there are 5-day intensive training retreats available at a number of centers that cover the entire curriculum. Although there is no formal certification process that is *required* for delivering MBCT for pain, again, ethical standards of health professions mandate that we practice within the bounds of competence (APA, 2010) and attending professional training, workshops, and familiarizing oneself with the MBCT literature is highly recommended. The University of California San Diego (UCSD) Center for Mindfulness, *Mindfulness-Based Professional Training Institute* website is a useful resource that is regularly updated that provides recommended reading materials relevant to a wide range of conditions and populations, professional training experiences, as well as the option of undertaking a certification process for advancing expertise in MBCT (UCSD, 2016).

Continuing supervision or consultation as you get ready to start your first MBCT program is also ideal, and it is a good idea to consider recording the session (with the patient's consent/approval) to get specific feedback and to perhaps utilize the fidelity form described later in this chapter to obtain an objective sense of your delivery of MBCT. Recent research by Chow and colleagues has shown that the time spent in such deliberate practice in improving therapeutic skills significantly predicts outcome (Chow et al., 2015). Moreover, Chow et al. (2015) also found that highly effective therapists indicated that they required more effort reviewing therapy recordings alone than did less effective therapists. Given therapist factors consistently account for a significant portion of variance in client outcome (some argue even more so than treatment modality; Wampold, 2005; Wampold & Brown, 2005), ensuring you are well trained and competent in the MBCT approach is of critical importance.

As discussed in Chapter 3, in addition to meeting ethical standards and competencies, an established, on-going personal meditation practice is recommended to place you (as an MBCT therapist) in a better position to genuinely embody the qualities and attitudes that we invite our clients to adopt. Further, Segal, Williams, and Teasdale (2013) describe how it helps to build into your schedule time before each session to have a brief period of pause, to shift yourself (as the therapist) from doing mode to being mode, thereby preparing you to start the session from this reference point. My personal experience in delivering MBCT is certainly consistent with the experiences that have been described by Segal and colleagues, where oftentimes right before leading a group we can be arriving from meetings, conversations, deadlines ... any number of activities.

However, in making time to have at least just 10 min to myself to settle, review the session materials, and to rest with my breath, I am much more in tune and "prepared" to lead the session.

One word of caution that I should mention however, is that although I also regularly practice yoga personally, I am not a certified yoga instructor (as most likely neither will be most of you, nor the majority of practicing therapists). Therefore, I do not feel I have the necessary expertise to safely lead individuals with various chronic pain conditions through the hatha yoga sequence included in the original MBCT protocol and in MBSR. Further, even if you *are* a certified yoga instructor, unless you have specific expertise and experience in teaching yoga among physically vulnerable/highly disabled populations, a modified sequence such as the one I suggest in the manual described later represents a safe approach that still conveys the intended core messages and learning experiences associated with the Mindful Movement component of the program. The series of basic movements I suggest here do not entail more than an individual with chronic pain might typically engage in during day-to-day living (e.g., noticing the tension in raising and lowering an arm, and the contrast once the arm is relaxed by one's side). However, the suggested movements still provide training in stepping out of one's head and into awareness of one's body (which provides an alternative viewpoint from which to observe experience), the opportunity to notice variations in sensations in various parts of the body, as well as a means to notice the contrasts between contraction and relaxation, movement and stillness.

Dispelling the Myths

MBCT, MBSR, and other MBIs have roots in Buddhism and Eastern practices, however, as delivered clinically, these treatments are taught from a secular perspective. This is a fundamental point as clients are not likely to be coming to an MBCT program to gain "enlightenment" (and if they are, this misconception needs to be corrected!). Most, if not all, will be coming because they are suffering and want relief and skills to help manage their pain. In this clinical context, MBCT is first and foremost delivered as a treatment for pain management. The secular nature of MBCT is important to clarify for clients as early as possible, as given mindfulness meditation did originally stem from Eastern traditions some clients may be wary of the meditation practices taught in MBCT for this reason, and therefore may be reluctant to do the practices asked for homework. It is essential that this potential misconception be addressed and that patients are explicitly informed that in this context, the techniques are taught for pain management and not as a spiritual practice; a good place to have this conversation is within the initial intake (i.e., pre-treatment) assessment, which I will discuss in more detail shortly.

So you might wonder, what does it mean that MBCT for pain is secular in approach? What does teaching the core meditation practices from this perspective actually "look like"? Well, first to say what delivering MBCT from a secular perspective does *not* look like: currently in the popular media mindfulness and meditation is a hot topic, and the image for meditation portrayed in the media (and that often comes to mind for most people) is someone looking serene, sitting cross-legged in lotus pose on a meditation cushion, perhaps with chimes and incense and statues of the Buddha and other spiritual elements present. This is not to say that this is a problem. Indeed many of us with our own personal practice might practice in this way (although I am not sure that I look so serene...!). However, in delivering MBCT clinically as an intervention for pain, it is essential that such spiritual elements (and any others) be kept separate from your role as clinician not only for reasons of cultural sensitivity, but also to keep the focus directed on what the program in this context is being delivered for: pain management.

Now for what MBCT as delivered from a secular perspective *does* look like. As delivered from this perspective, meditation is taught in MBCT using practical, jargon-free language. In doing this, we reach the patient and speak their language. I also have never used chimes of any form to signal the start and end of practice, as chimes are a spiritual tradition; instead, I simply invite patients to settle into the practice and then at the end, I use a reorienting procedure to guide their awareness back to the room. I do not use meditation cushions, rather, in session we simply practice in a chair or if preferred by clients, on a mat on the floor. I encourage patients to assume an alert, dignified sitting posture for the seated meditations, and to make themselves as comfortable as best they can, I do not guide them to sit cross-legged. Inevitably, some patients may describe having personal "insights" during their meditation practice, and I approach this in the guided inquiry with the same mindful curiosity as I would when a patient describes being distracted by an itch. One of my favorite meditation teachers, Pema Chödrön, describes the benefit of responding to the distractions, insights, and "breakthroughs" all in the same way, with an attitude of "no big deal." In responding this way, there arises no attachment to the insights, we are not disappointed when they don't happen, and an attitude of no expectations or sense of striving is cultivated. Another way to describe this may be responding with equanimity, approaching all experiences in an even-minded manner. Given the popularity of mindfulness in the general public and popular media, it can be easy to "get caught up in the hype." I have only described a few basic premises here to guide delivery of MBCT from a secular perspective. However, it may be helpful if you are considering "adding something extra" (such as chimes, for example) to what I describe in the MBCT approach, to ask yourself: *what does this add in terms of pain management?* And let the answer to this question be your guiding principle. As again, first and foremost, what we are delivering in this clinical context is a treatment approach for chronic pain.

Basic Treatment Structure and Practical Considerations

MBCT for chronic pain is typically delivered in-person, in a group setting. Although the size of the group will be somewhat constrained by the available facilities and any number of other factors, I have found that approximately 6–12 individuals is an ideal group size that allows for interactive discussion while still allowing each person sufficient "air time." I find that the group delivery format fosters learning and serves a support function, and also often allows people to realize that they are not alone in their experiences with pain—all of which positively influences their experience of the program. However, you can also deliver the program in individual therapy if this is more suitable to your client's needs and/or practice context, and considerations surrounding this delivery format will be discussed in more detail in Chapter 13.

As in the original MBCT approach, clients entering the program first start with an initial assessment interview to obtain a comprehensive pain history, and to assess baseline functioning and patterns of cognitions, emotions, and behavioral/social responses to pain. This assessment is also where you determine the suitability of the client to a group delivered MBCT approach. Later in this chapter I will provide some recommendations for specific assessment tools you might include in this battery, and will describe important considerations to keep in mind during this assessment to determine an individual's suitability and to prevent premature drop-out and treatment failure. A critical part of this initial assessment interview is the informed consent process and a discussion of the background of MBCT (including its secular nature), and how the treatment approach might be beneficial for the client. It is essential for the client to gain a strong sense of what the treatment entails and the time commitment in terms of both the sessions and at-home exercises so that realistic pre-treatment expectations of the MBCT approach can be formed. Although clients are encouraged to lay all expectations aside from the outset of the program and to bring an open sense of curiosity to the unfolding of their experience during treatment, at this stage it is still essential that clients are informed and have a realistic sense of the program. This cultivation of realistic expectations and on-going informed consent is further supported with the provision of a packet of reading materials that is provided following the initial assessment to patients who are suitable to enroll in the program. This pre-treatment client handbook is provided in Appendix A on the website and provides information on chronic pain (which should be adapted for the specific form of chronic pain the clinician is working with, e.g., headache, back pain, etc.), treatment of chronic pain (again, adapted to the specific pain population), the MBCT for pain rationale, the importance of homework/practicing meditation, and on potential difficulties that may be encountered with the practice.

In terms of the basic treatment structure, the MBCT for chronic pain approach closely resembles that of Segal, Williams, and Teasdale's (2013) original protocol. The manual described in the coming chapters consists of eight sessions, each of which lasts for 2 h. The sessions are generally planned as one session per week, but session times, frequency, and delivery format can vary, as appropriate to the needs of the clients and the clinic infrastructure. Within MBSR, an all-day retreat is held between Sessions 6 and 7 and past graduates are invited to return to these retreats; some practitioners and researchers have included this as a component of MBCT. However, personally I have not included this component in my work as it has not fit within the various research or clinical contexts in which I have facilitated MBCT. Thus, I do not describe it in detail here—you should consider if inclusion of this element might be suitable for your needs. Segal, Williams, and Teasdale (2013) provide an excellent description of the possible content to include during an all-day mindfulness retreat. Continuing contact following the program and possible booster sessions are also important aspects to consider, and on-going opportunities for clients to return to formal practice within a class setting will most likely always be valuable. I describe some of the options for on-going follow-up and longer-term therapy in Chapter 13.

In some practice and research settings, eight sessions may not be feasible for reimbursement procedures, patient population characteristics, access issues, or for other reasons. If this is the case, you might like to consider using the brief, four-session version of the manual, which may represent a more viable alternative, and this manual is presented in basic form in Appendix F on the website.[1] In Chapter 13, I will discuss the four-session version further, and will also describe how there are further areas of flexibility in the MBCT for chronic pain format and structure, and how some of the techniques may also be selectively integrated within other approaches. However, in considering if the brief treatment alternative is more appropriate for your needs or whether you want to make other adjustments, first it is useful to have a strong understanding of each treatment component in detail, which is what I will touch on now and in detail in the coming chapters.

The actual individual session structure is the same across all eight of the MBCT for pain sessions, following the format of: (1) pre-session process check (except for Session 1) and pain measure; (2) orientation and theme for session; (3) in-session practice of both cognitive-behavioral and meditation-based exercises, including a period of extended formal mindfulness meditation practice and a guided inquiry; (4) assign at-home daily practice and summary; and (5) post-session process check. Immediately following each of the in-session practices is a guided inquiry of clients' direct experience (the key elements of which are described in Chapter 3). A guided inquiry of the clients' expectations of treatment (Session 1) or experiences with the at-home daily practices since the last treatment session (Sessions 2–8) is also incorporated. The pre- and post-session process checks I will describe in more detail within the "Tracking Patient Progress" section below; the orientation, assigning of homework and concluding summary components entail agenda setting and basic therapeutic skills, which will not be elaborated upon further here, although suggested verbiage to include for each of these elements is provided within the therapist manual and guide, and accompanying client handouts.

Regarding the basic instruction on guiding clients in meditation throughout the program, as you read through each of the MBCT sessions, you will notice that the focus of the meditation will become increasingly less tangible as the program progresses, starting with a body-focused meditation, moving to sounds and thoughts, and then progressing to thoughts and some experienced/perceived difficulty. The key aspects to consider in delivering each of these meditations is described within the "Therapist Tips, Troubleshooting and Supervision" section in the coming chapters following the presentation of each session. Scripts for each of the meditations included in the program are provided in Appendix B on the website, however, these scripts are intended to provide a general guide only, and should not be "read" to the participants word for word. You should feel comfortable modifying the suggested wording and metaphors included in the scripts as needed to enhance the flow for your own clinical use and to make them culturally sensitive and relevant to the client population you are working with.

Further, in guiding the meditations, you are encouraged to also personally concurrently engage in the practice as you are guiding it, so that the meditation is guided from within. Thus, although on one level you are guiding the meditation and remembering where you are up to in the practice and monitoring the group members, you are also strongly encouraged to remain in tune with your own experience on another level, in a way that parallels what is being asked of the client. One final point on the meditations scripts: unlike in a guided relaxation where you as the clinician might adopt a special tone, or soften or deepen your voice to enhance a sense of relaxation, here, the intention is not for people to relax (although this does often happen), rather the intention is for people to bring a sense of alert attentiveness to the practice. Hence, the meditations should be guided with an engaging, yet somewhat more matter-of-fact tone of voice, using the present participle.

Each in-session guided mediation practice (apart from the Mindful Walking practice in Session 4) begins by inviting clients to take on a comfortable, yet alert and dignified sitting posture. Again, this is in contrast to a relaxation session, as meditation is not geared toward attempting to engender relaxation but to train the mind to more closely attend to what is taking place, moment by moment. Hence, to avoid sleepiness, keeping the spine erect (but not stiff) with the chin and shoulders slightly lowered sends a subtle message to the mind that it is time to switch gears out of "doing" mode and into "being" mode. The exception to this is the Body Scan meditation, which, although often done in a seated position in session, is typically practiced laying on one's back (i.e., flat on the back, with arms by the sides, palms facing upwards and feet falling slightly away from each other). While most clients typically elect to close their eyes during the practice, they may also elect to keep their eyes open, fixing their gaze on a spot a few feet down in front of them. If clients report a problem with sleepiness, indeed, encouraging him/her to practice with eyes open is a good remedy to this common problem. Once settled, you will then guide clients through the extended meditation practice, making sure that you allow spaces and stretches of silence for clients to actually experience what you are inviting them to experience (i.e., pause long enough for clients to have time to take stock and notice what emotions are present, for example). At the end of each guided meditation practice you will then encourage clients to begin to bring their awareness back to the room and to perhaps (if not working with a spinal cord injury population) gently wriggle their feet and hands. And, without hurrying anyone, as they are ready, inviting clients to open their eyes and come back to full alertness. Once everyone seems relatively re-alerted, the guided inquiry can then occur, making sure not to leap into this as soon as clients open their eyes though. Included in the manual is a basic three-layer structure for the inquiry, however, this is only a "skeleton," and the guided inquiry is most beneficial when delivered in the manner described earlier in Chapter 3. The extended in-session practices should typically last around 30 min, depending on the practice (as some meditations, such as the Mindful Movement and Walking meditations are briefer). You will need to adjust the length of the in-session practice according to the flow of the session, implementing good time management skills to keep the session on track, without a sense of "rushing."

In terms of the approach in delivering the psychoeducational and cognitive-behavioral therapy components of each session, it is often easy to drift into problem solving mode, or perhaps into more traditional cognitive therapy mode, especially when clients resist the notion of staying open to difficult experiences, thoughts, feelings. While an overview of the rationale for each of the included CBT-oriented exercises in the program was provided in Chapter 3, here I will just take a moment to reiterate that it is not only in the delivery and discussion of the mindfulness meditation that you as the therapist need to embody the qualities of mindfulness; these qualities are equally needed in the delivery of all components of the session. The idea is to harness the CBT-based exercises to collaboratively enhance *awareness* of the automatic tendencies of the mind and habitual patterns of thinking, judging, and responding to pain and stress with an approach of open, non-judgmental acceptance in response to this emerging awareness. And, perhaps somewhat paradoxically, while not using these activities to explicitly aim to *change* one's moment-to-moment experience, still the intention is to use these activities to develop the capacity to choose wisely how to best respond to ultimately make a shift towards better self-care. With awareness comes choice, and why not choose to respond in such a way that lets go of some of the extra baggage that often gets carried along for the ride with chronic pain and that only adds to pain and suffering? Included in the manual is suggested verbiage for how you can approach presenting and discussing the CBT-oriented exercises from within this MBCT delivery framework.

Beyond any of the in-session mindfulness and cognitive-behavioral exercises however, critical to our clients learning and assimilating the MBCT for pain management skills is the between-session at-home practice component. In order to learn, we need to do. Thus, each week clients will be asked to engage in brief cognitive and behavioral exercises, to listen to and practice with an audio-recording of the formal mindfulness meditation technique taught in session,[2] as well as practice brief and informal exercises to integrate mindfulness into everyday life, and to read the weekly reading materials within the client handbook. The client handbook is included in the coming chapters following the therapist outline, and is designed to reinforce the skills taught during the sessions, to facilitate homework, and to prepare clients for the next session.[3] Usually I provide the recording for each of the meditations to clients only after I have delivered it in session; otherwise, if clients have access to all the meditations up front, the temptation is to jump ahead. Similarly, I also provide the client handouts at each session, as opposed to all at once. Client handouts are included as online appendices as well, see Appendix G on the website.

Consistent with the original MBCT protocol, clients are encouraged to practice daily meditation in-between group sessions for 45 min, 6 days per week, ideally at the time of the day they feel more alert, avoiding using them before going to sleep. An exception to this though is that many of my clients report that listening to the recordings before going to bed actually helps them fall asleep sooner; and so this use is encouraged in the context of also recommending an additional practice during the day when alert (as one is not learning the technique and training the mind if asleep while "practicing"). Clients may choose to listen to the recordings more often, as they find helpful. However, a more commonly reported experience than wanting to practice *more* than the recommended 45 min a day is that this amount of time seems "too much" (due to pain, fatigue, etc.), "impossible to fit into my day" and it often becomes a barrier to engaging in the practice. Thus, it is recommended that clients also be given a 20-min version of each of the guided audio-recordings. This shorter version may be especially helpful early on in treatment, when clients are introducing a "new habit" of meditation into their daily routine, and over time they can then experiment with gradually building to the recommended 45-min daily dose. Mindfulness is a skill. And like any skill it requires regular practice to master.

Tracking Patient Progress during MBCT for Chronic Pain

Who is Most Suitable for the MBCT for Chronic Pain Approach?

One of the most important underlying reasons as to why it is critical to track patient progress during MBCT (and all other therapy) is that by doing this we hope to catch, early on, those clients who are not meaningfully responding to treatment and who may be on a trajectory of treatment failure or even worse, on the verge of prematurely dropping out so we never see them in our office again. Ideally then, once we catch this failure to meaningfully respond, we then intervene and have a transparent discussion with our clients about the lack of improvement, and collaboratively decide whether to continue pursuing the current treatment option for a set number of sessions and to monitor and then reevaluate, or whether there may be an alternative treatment option that is more preferred. This is current best practice. However, clinical efficiency and effectiveness would be further optimized if even before the flat (or perhaps even downward) outcome trajectory emerged, we could first have informed algorithms to match patients to the one treatment approach most likely to be of benefit. In 1969, Dr Gordon Paul put forth this statement, which succinctly summarizes what we (still!) need to know in order to reach this utopia of clinical practice: "What treatment, by whom, is most effective for this individual with that specific problem under which set of circumstances, and how does it come about" (p. 44) (Paul, 1969). Although we are yet to discover the golden ticket and develop algorithms that answer these questions, 40 years on, we have been making closer and closer successive approximations toward success. What we do now know is that there are a number of patient characteristics that potentially influence whether a given individual is more or less suitable to MBCT, underscoring the need for collaborative, careful decision-making that importantly takes into account patient preferences, characteristics, and readiness for change.

As discussed earlier, an abundance of research shows that clients who have more positive and realistic expectations of treatment are more likely to finish treatment and obtain meaningful benefit (e.g., Goossens et al., 2005; Peerdeman et al., 2016; Smeets et al., 2008). It has been theorized that individuals who do not expect to obtain benefit or who may be classified as "pre-contemplators" according to the transtheoretical model of behavioral change (i.e., who are not even thinking about making changes to pain management coping behaviors) may not be well suited to a pain self-management approach, including but not limited to MBCT (Jensen, Nielson, Romano, Hill, & Turner, 2000, Jensen, Nielson, Turner, Romano, & Hill, 2004; Prochaska & DiClemente, 1992). Data from our lab and others are consistent with this theory and research, and have shown that it is critical that clients hold a realistic understanding of the time commitment involved prior to enrolling in an MBCT program. In our headache pain trial, a number of participants prematurely terminated treatment (Day, Jensen, et al., 2014) and the time commitment of participating in treatment was reported as a common barrier (Day, Thorn, et al., 2014). Similarly, unpublished research by Carmody (as cited in Carmody & Baer, 2009) found that the primary reported barrier to enrolling in a mindfulness-based treatment was the time commitment, with 45% of eligible clients declining to participate for this reason. In such circumstances, a preparatory pre-MBCT intervention to enhance readiness to change and motivation to engage in treatment may be advisable.

Related to ensuring realistic expectations and motivation prior to treatment is ensuring that any of the "myths" surrounding mindfulness as a therapeutic intervention that I described earlier are appropriately addressed. Specifically, any concerns about meditation in this context being a spiritual practice, or other cultural or personal misconceptions should be allayed, and the secular nature of MBCT clearly explained prior to treatment starting to prevent therapeutic alliance from being deleteriously impacted (Day, 2016). This level of care and attention in the preparatory phase is critically important when considered in relation to recent findings from the broad psychotherapy literature which found that those clients (from heterogeneous populations reporting various disorders) who were unsure of what type of therapy they received, and/or who were not given enough information about the type of therapy before it started were significantly more likely to experience lasting negative effects from psychological interventions (Crawford et al., 2016).

Finally, despite the relatively low risk of MBCT, there is some suggestion in the literature that certain individuals might *not* be ideally suited to this treatment approach and, if they do commence MBCT for pain, should be monitored closely. Patient characteristics such as severe psychological dysfunction or dysregulation, significantly impaired cognition or attention, acute agitation, or active substance abuse may not benefit from some or all of the MBCT treatment components due to difficulties engaging cognitively, receiving group delivered treatment, or managing distraction (Day, Eyer, & Thorn, 2013). Further, there is some indication that meditation may trigger psychotic or manic symptoms in vulnerable individuals (Kuijpers et al., 2007; Yorsten, 2001). Thus, patients with a history of trauma may especially benefit from efforts at building safety and trust before attempting mindfulness meditation, and should be instructed on grounding techniques prior to commencing MBCT.

Recommended Pain Assessment Tools and Tracking Measures

When working with chronic pain, a multidimensional assessment approach is needed to identify distinctive maintenance factors of pain, stress, suffering, disability, and dysfunction. Typically clients will see an array of healthcare professionals prior to considering entering an MBCT program for their chronic pain;

thus, any available information regarding the physical pathology (i.e., pain type) and any alterations to the peripheral and central nervous system (i.e., sensitization) attributable to the onset of the pain should be gathered prior to treatment commencing. Further, the IASP recommends that the major pain site(s) should be assessed using 10 demarcated regions of the body: (1) head, face, and mouth; (2) cervical (i.e., neck) region; (3) upper shoulder and upper limbs; (4) thoracic (i.e., chest) region; (5) abdominal (i.e., stomach) region; (6) lower back/lumbar spine, sacrum (i.e., bone at the base of the spine) and coccyx (i.e., tail bone); (7) lower limbs; (8) pelvic region (i.e., hip region); (9) anal, perineal (i.e., area between genitals and anus), and genital region; and (10) more than three major sites.

It is also recommended that a comprehensive clinical interview, which is typically semi-structured, be included in all pain assessment batteries. Turk and Robinson (2010) recommend that the clinical interview should address: (1) experience of pain and related symptoms, including not only the aforementioned medical history variables, but also exacerbating and relieving factors and the client's pain beliefs and understanding of how thoughts, behaviors, and emotions might influence their pain; (2) treatments received and currently receiving (including current medications as well as complementary/alternative treatments) and how useful these have been/are, as well as reported adherence/compliance to these treatments and attitudes toward providers; (3) current or planned compensation and litigation status; (4) responses to symptoms as well as responses from significant others; (5) coping efforts, including the client's perceived role in managing pain, life stressors, and pleasant activities; (6) educational and vocational history and current employment status, and (if appropriate) any return to work plans; (7) social history, including a history of, or current, trauma, physical, emotional, or sexual abuse; (8) alcohol and substance use (where indicated as a source for concern, consider supplementing this assessment alongside the WHO-ASSIST, available at: http://www.who.int/substance_abuse/activities/assist/en/); (9) psychological dysfunction, including history of, or current, psychological symptoms/diagnosis (depending on responses, a more formal interview could be indicated, such as the recently developed Structured Clinical Interview for the DSM-5), past or current experiences with psychological treatment and if relevant, perceptions on how helpful this treatment was/is; (10) concerns and expectations, including explanatory models of pain the client holds; and (11) treatment goals. During this interview, close observation of any pain behaviors and how these convey information is also needed, along with attending to temporal associations between the pain and ways the client responds to the pain. Basic patient demographic information is also typically collected.

While the clinical interview is a crucial element of the initial assessment, supplementing this should be a carefully selected battery of standardized, psychometrically sound self-report measures that tap each of the multidimensional aspects of chronic pain. Such measures typically require less time, are easy to administer, and can be reliably used to track client progress through the MBCT for chronic pain treatment. Given the current climate of evidence-based practice and that many insurance and reimbursement bodies want to see evidence of efficacy, such measures are increasingly needed not only for research trials but also clinical practice. Although the topic of evidence-based practice and delivery of empirically supported treatments is one of much debate, quality assurance for clients receiving psychotherapy (of which patient-focused monitoring of outcomes is a central component) is a worldwide topic of importance and extends beyond the debate over providing particular treatments with "X" amount of evidence (Andrews, 2000; Lambert et al., 2003). However, there are a massive number of instruments available to assess various pain domains; therefore, it is often confusing which assessment tools are ideal for clinical practice and research purposes. Ultimately the selection of measures to include in your assessment battery is driven by a number of considerations such as patient population (including such factors as age, setting, cognitive, or communication deficits), pain type (i.e., low back pain, headache, fibromyalgia etc.) and the purpose of the evaluation (i.e., research trial, clinical practice etc.) (Dixon & Thorn, 2015). Thankfully, a great advancement of the past decade is the growing momentum behind the identification of key domains of assessment by renowned international experts in the field of pain, with the intention of standardizing the domains of assessment and the associated measures used in clinical and research settings.

The Initiative on Methods, Measurement, and Pain Assessment in Clinical Trials (IMMPACT) workgroup identified six core pain outcome domains (Turk et al., 2003), and made recommendations for the best practice assessment approach in measuring these domains (Dworkin et al., 2005):

1) *Pain*: an 11-point Numerical Rating Scale (NRS) for current, worst, least, and/or average pain intensity in the past 24 hr or week, depending on context (with anchors at 0 = "No pain" and 10 = "Pain as bad as you can imagine"); an 11-point NRS for pain quality (with anchors at 0 = "not unpleasant" and 10 = "most unpleasant feeling possible"[4]; the Short-Form McGill Pain Questionnaire is also recommended to assess sensory and affective pain (Melzack, 1987).
2) *Physical functioning*: disease-specific measures, where one is available that is suitable (i.e., the Roland–Morris Back Pain Disability Scale; Roland & Morris, 1983; Henry Ford Headache Disability Inventory; Jacobson, Ramadan, Aggarwal, & Newman, 1994), or otherwise the West Haven Yale Multidimensional Pain Inventory, Interference Scale (Kerns, Turk, & Rudy, 1985), or the Brief Pain Inventory, Interference Scale (Cleeland & Ryan, 1994); inclusion of a generic health-related quality of life (HRQoL) measure is also recommended, such as the SF-36 Health Survey (Ware & Sherbourne, 1992).
3) *Emotional functioning*: either the Beck Depression Inventory (Beck, Ward, Mendelson, Mock, & Erbaugh, 1961), which assesses depressive symptoms only, or the Profile of Mood States (McNair, Lorr, & Droppleman, 1971), which assesses six mood states (tension–anxiety, depression–dejection, anger–hostility, vigor–activity, fatigue–inertia, confusion–bewilderment) and provides a sum score of total mood disturbance.
4) *Participant ratings of global improvement* and *satisfaction with treatment*: the Patient Global Impressions of Change scale (PGIC; Farrar, 2003), which consists of a single-item rating assessing perceived improvement with treatment on a 7-point scale ranging from "Very much improved" to "Very much worse" and "No change" as the mid-point (we have assessed various other domains with this PGIC scale in our research, including pain intensity, pain interference, negative pain-related cognitions, fatigue, mindfulness, and pain acceptance).

5) *Symptoms* and *adverse events*: assessed passively via spontaneous capture of reported events using open-ended prompts, or more ideally via active capture methods which use structured interviews specifically assessing worsening of symptoms and adverse events that are relevant to the disorder/treatment (e.g., pain flare-ups, emergency department visits etc.). You will notice the template at-home practice record (provided in Appendix C on the website) includes an item assessing adverse effects.
6) *Participant disposition*: the recommendation is to follow the Consolidated Standards of Reporting Trials guidelines (Moher et al., 2010), gathering data such as recruitment to enrollment rates (and associated reasons for potential exclusion or declined participation), progression through the trial/program, adherence, reasons for premature withdrawal and/or loss to follow-up, and return to work rates following treatment.

The IMMPACT recommendations represent a substantial advancement in standardizing the pain assessment process. However, some of the measures recommended by IMMPACT are not available in the public domain, and the scope of the recommended assessment battery is relatively narrow and may not be sufficient in all clinical and research contexts. Thus, complementing the IMMPACT workgroup's efforts, the NIH funded an initiative in 2004 titled the "Patient Reported Outcomes Measurement Information System" (PROMIS), which saw the implementation of item response theory (IRT) to develop standardized, psychometrically sound assessment tools that tap broader domains of functioning. The PROMIS assessment instruments comprise calibrated item banks that can be used to derive short forms (typically 4–10 items per construct) or computerized adaptive tests (typically consisting of 4–7 items per concept, which provides a more precise measurement as this system adjusts the number of items within domains based on an individual's response to previous questions). There are pain-specific domains tapped in this battery, including pain intensity, pain interference, and pain behaviors (which was not included in IMMPACT and is a limitation of those recommendations), as well as a wide range of physical, emotional, HRQoL, and social domains. All of the PROMIS measures are available in the public domain, free of charge within the online Assessment Centre, and can be accessed at: http://www.assessmentcenter.net/. Further, this Assessment Centre also provides tools to assess neuropsychological function, which may be useful to assess in the context of chronic pain, depending on your clinical/research needs.

In our current and on-going MBCT trials, we are implementing the PROMIS assessment battery for measurement of our core outcome domains, supplemented by additional measures that map onto IMMPACT recommendations. In research settings, a priori selection of the *primary* outcome is required before commencement of a trial, and given that MBCT aims to target clients' *relationship* to the pain and not reduction in pain intensity per se (Day, Jensen, et al., 2014; Kabat-Zinn, 1990), pain interference is emerging in the literature as the recommended primary outcome to track during MBIs (Veehof et al., 2011) and is what we have used in our MBCT research. While IMMPACT recommendations do clearly state that their suggested outcome domains and recommended assessment tools can be augmented, a notable gap is a lack of attention toward measures of positive psychological outcomes (e.g., happiness) and cognitive content and cognitive process variables. Although the PROMIS battery includes measures of various forms of self-efficacy (i.e., self-efficacy in managing emotions, medications, social interactions etc.), currently the battery does not include a measure of pain management self-efficacy, pain catastrophizing, pain beliefs, and measures of other key cognitive processes (e.g., pain acceptance, mindfulness). Research led by Dr. Dagmar Amtmann is currently underway to extend the PROMIS battery to include items that tap pain self-efficacy and pain catastrophizing (Amtmann, 2016). However, even with this likely near-future expansion of the PROMIS item banks, other measures that specifically map onto the theoretical framework of the intervention under investigation are needed to be included in order to assess not only outcomes but also treatment processes/mechanisms.

Given the central role that cognitive factors are theorized to play in pain coping and management (in MBCT and across CBT, ACT, and many other frameworks), it is imperative that the assessment battery include measures of relevant cognitive variables. There are a number of valid measures of pain-related attitudes and self-efficacy commonly used in pain research (Anderson, Noel Dowds, Pelletz, Edwards, & Peeters-Asdourian, 1995; French et al., 2000; Jensen, Karoly, & Huger, 1987; Nicholas, 2007), and given how robust pain catastrophizing is in predicting outcomes, it is strongly recommended that this also be assessed by one of several validated, widely used measures (the Coping Strategies Questionnaire-Revised; Robinson et al., 1997; or the Pain Catastrophizing Scale; Sullivan, Bishop, & Pivik, 1995). Further, mindfulness and pain acceptance are theorized to be key mechanisms of MBCT, thus inclusion of measures designed to tap these processes is recommended. Although no current measure of mindfulness specific to pain exists (Day, Lang, Newton-John, Ehde, & Jensen, in press), the Five Facet Mindfulness Questionnaire (Baer et al., 2008; Bohlmeijer, ten Klooster, Fledderus, Veehof, & Baer, 2011), is one validated, psychometrically sound option, and is one of the currently most widely used measures of mindfulness in pain research. In terms of pain acceptance, although the Chronic Pain Acceptance Questionnaire (Fish, Hogan, Morrison, & Stewart, 2010; McCracken et al., 2004) is typically implemented, evaluations of the measure have identified that this questionnaire does not tap cognitive conceptualizations of acceptance (Lauwerier et al., 2015).[5] In a recent review of the most widely used pain-related cognitive process measures (Day et al., in press), the Brief Pain Coping Inventory, "Accepted Pain" scale (McCracken, Eccleston, & Bell, 2005) was found to provide a pure measure of cognitive process, although it consists of only one item, hence the clinical utility and treatment sensitivity of this still needs to be confirmed. Inclusion of assessment tools measuring other mechanism variables (e.g., measurement of changes in fear of pain/movement during MBCT; Asmundson, Bovell, Carleton, & McWilliams, 2008; Woby, Roach, Urmston, & Watson, 2005) might also be relevant, depending on your clinical setting and/or research objectives.

To address the current limitations of available measures of cognitive process, my colleagues and I recently developed and validated the Pain-Related Cognitive Processes Questionnaire (PCPQ), which provides a pure assessment of nine cognitive processes specific to pain: suppression, distraction, enhancement, dissociation, reappraisal, absorption, rumination, non-judgment, and acceptance (Day et al., in press). More research is needed to establish the capacity of this measure to assess the potential mechanism role of change in cognitive processes during MBCT (and other treatments) for chronic pain. For a more comprehensive discussion of cognitive content and cognitive process measures used in pain research, see DeGood and Cook's review, which provides an excellent coverage of cognitive content measures (DeGood & Cook, 2010), as well as our recent review of cognitive process measures (Day et al., in press).

Finally, two more critically important aspects to consider in tracking outcomes and client progress both clinically and in a research setting are: (1) the platform you use to collect the data, and (2) ensuring an adequate balance between obtaining useful information vs. patient burden (i.e., overloading patients with an excessively long assessment process). In MBCT, each of the sessions contains a lot of content, thus you will need the full 2 hr and will only have time for an exceptionally brief in-session assessment. To optimize the time in sessions such that it is spent actually delivering treatment, I typically opt for an exceptionally brief in-session weekly assessment focused primarily on common factors and engagement indicators (which I will discuss in the next section, below) complemented by an online weekly repeated assessment procedure that patients can do in the location of their choosing (i.e., outside of session using either a smartphone, desktop, laptop, or essentially any medium that is connected to the internet). On the market there are numerous technology forms and brands for such ecological momentary assessment or daily/weekly diary methods that you might choose to use, depending on your needs. In the past, we have used platforms such as Qualtrics and SurveyMonkey, which provide advanced encryption technology; however, it is still best to assign to clients nonidentifiable IDs for them to enter these data under, and not to collect any identifiable patient information via these platforms. One benefit of these platforms is that they contain built in technology to build graphs and other forms of visual and written feedback that you can (depending on your clinical context, research design etc.) provide to your patients, and, of course, providing feedback in and of itself has been shown to be associated with improved outcomes (Lambert et al., 2003). Further, in terms of the balance of obtaining useful information while not overly burdening clients with the assessment process, again, this is a consideration that must be made in the context of the level of functioning of the population you are working with. For example, if working with a highly disabled multiple sclerosis population, fatigue may be a major problem along with potential cognitive deficits, thus, a shorter battery is likely more appropriate (i.e., the PROMIS short forms may be particularly useful here, which consist of just four items to tap a given domain). However, in other higher functioning populations, a weekly assessment of around 15 min might be feasible. As you can see, choosing the right assessment battery for your purposes requires a great deal of thought and planning, especially if you are working in a research setting where the ability to change measures flexibly is highly limited once data collection commences.

Therapist Fidelity and Client Engagement

Fidelity (also termed treatment integrity) is a term that dates back over three decades as a central concept in program evaluation (Sechrest, West, Phillips, Redner, & Yeaton, 1979). A thorough history of the evolution of this concept is available elsewhere (Bond, Evans, Salyers, Williams, & Kim, 2000), however at base, as applied to the delivery of psychological treatments, fidelity entails two major elements: (1) therapist adherence to the treatment protocol, which refers to the degree to which the treatment was delivered as intended; and (2) therapist competence, which encompasses the overall quality of the delivery of treatment provided and includes nonspecific therapeutic factors such as empathy, congruence etc. Effective treatment delivery requires both of these elements as, although adherence is a necessary condition, it is not sufficient; on the other hand, a "competent" delivery of a treatment is not possible without adherence to that treatment model. A further component that is useful to consider is therapist "appropriateness" as in some circumstances, a therapist *not* adhering to a certain treatment component may actually be appropriate, culturally sensitive, and an indicator of strong therapeutic expertise and competence.

In a research setting, treatment fidelity is closely aligned with highly specified and detailed treatment manuals, therapist training, and other research practices designed to increase the internal validity of studies. Essentially, in the absence of ensuring that treatment was delivered as specified, any conclusions as to the efficacy of that treatment are tentative at best (Sechrest et al., 1979). However, a common misperception is the idea that fidelity is *only* relevant in such research contexts where a core constituent of RCTs is evaluation of whether therapists adhered to the manual. On the contrary, fidelity is equally important in clinical settings, especially in the current healthcare climate of clients and family members using the internet to research available treatment options and then actively seeking treatment practices supported by research, and indeed holding the expectation that this is what will be delivered in any healthcare system (Mowbray, Holter, Teague, & Bybee, 2003). Further, reimbursement procedures and policymakers often require assurances that treatments are implemented as intended and are reaching the target patient population (Orwin, 2000).

Research from the broad psychotherapy literature has found support for the importance of monitoring fidelity in both research and clinical settings, as when established treatment models are replicated in clinical practice, measures of fidelity have been found to predict outcome (Paulson, Post, Herinckx, & Risser, 2002), although findings are mixed (Perepletchikova & Kazdin, 2005; Perepletchikova, Treat, & Kazdin, 2007). In our own research, we have found a positive association between therapist adherence and quality with post-treatment client satisfaction during MBCT (Day et al., 2016). Other research has shown that high levels of treatment fidelity are associated with changes in mediating variables (i.e., mechanisms of change) theorized within the treatment model to underlie change in outcome (Ellis, Naar-King, Templin, Frey, & Cunningham, 2007; Hansen, Graham, Wolkenstein, & Rohrbach, 1991), and interventions that more closely adhere to the theoretical model have been shown to have stronger effects (Resnick et al., 2005). Thus, although not often discussed within the realm of fidelity, assessment of therapist adherence and competence also facilitates testing of theoretical models and establishment of treatment mechanisms.

The sine qua non of establishing treatment fidelity is precise specification of the treatment components, and then evaluation of whether the therapist adhered to these components and, if so, the quality or competence with which the therapist delivered the components. Typically this is achieved via independent (i.e., not the therapist) review of patient consented audio/video recordings of a random selection of sessions; however, some therapist self-rated fidelity protocols have also been implemented, although this approach does include inherent bias and has been shown to be less reliable and to have low correlations with objective measures (Carroll et al., 2000; Wickstrom, Jones, LaFleur, & Witt, 1998). While specific guidelines pertaining to the "optimum" level of adherence are lacking, current convention suggests that 80–100% integrity constitutes high fidelity, whereas 50% constitutes low fidelity (Borrelli, 2011). Further, depending on the context, assessment of therapist drift in delivering treatment components from other treatment approaches (i.e., termed "proscribed" treatment components) should be considered. Therapist competence ratings are more subjective, and therefore typically need to be undertaken by a coder who is an expert in the treatment being delivered.

Appendix E includes the "Mindfulness-Based Cognitive Therapy Adherence Appropriateness and Quality Scale (MBCT-AAQS)," which is adapted from the Cognitive Therapy Adherence and Competence Scale (Barber, Liese, & Abrams, 2003) and the MBCT-Adherence Scale (Segal, Teasdale, Williams, & Gemar, 2002). The MBCT-AAQS specifies the various treatment components of MBCT for chronic pain, and also includes a contextual consideration section, which is a critical element of fidelity (often *not* assessed) given that client-related variables might substantially impact a therapist's capacity to deliver all the treatment components of a given session (Waltz, Addis, Koerner, & Jacobson, 1993). If used for research purposes, you may find that adapting the MBCT-AAQS to include relevant proscribed elements central to a comparison treatment may also be useful.

Along with the aforementioned therapist adherence and competence factors, Lichstein and colleagues (Lichstein, Riedel, & Grieve, 1994) have highlighted that equally as critical for asserting an unbiased test of the treatment delivered is: (1) the client's mastery of the treatment skills (termed "client receipt"); and (2) the client's application of the treatment outside the bounds of the therapeutic setting (termed "client enactment"). Thus, in Lichstein and colleagues' (1994) model, the concept of fidelity is broadened beyond simply therapist delivery (i.e., adherence and competence) to also include client-related factors, which they termed "treatment implementation." In our research we have assessed treatment receipt and retention via weekly pre- and post-session process checks adapted from Thorn (2004). The pre-session check is completed before each session (except Session 1) and asks clients "What was the main point you got from last week's group?" The post-session process check is completed at the conclusion of each session and asks "What was the main point you got from today's group?" We have then quantified the response with 0 = Inaccurate and 1 = Attempted with at least moderate accuracy (Thorn et al., 2011). In terms of engagement, I include in my assessment battery a Daily Home Practice Record, which is provided in Appendix C, and asks clients daily whether they practiced, and if so, what form of meditation they practiced and for how long, and also what comments or questions they might have, which we can then follow up on in group. Finally, I include a therapist-rated "Checklist of Patient Engagement in Group" measure, which we developed in our original MBCT trial and is completed by the therapist(s) immediately following the conclusion of each session (Mignogna, Thorn, & Day, 2007). This checklist uses a 9-point scale (with anchors at 0 = None, 2 = A little, 4 = Some, 6 = Much, and 8 = A lot) and the items are: (1) "Overall, how much effort did the patient exert during group activities?" (2) "How much was the patient engaged in the review of last week's concepts?" (3) "How much was the patient engaged in the discussion of homework?" (4) "How much was the patient engaged in the discussion of this week's new material?" and (5) "How much was the patient engaged in the in-session learning activity?" In our original MBCT trial, this measure significantly predicted both session attendance and how much clients practiced meditation *outside* of session (Day et al., 2016), and therefore may prove to be a useful tracking measure of client engagement. Most recently, the client-related factors highlighted by Lichstein and colleagues (1994) have been integrated within the NIH Behavior Change Consortium's Best Practice and Recommendations for enhancing treatment fidelity, and these recommendations (all of which have been covered in this section) also represent a potentially useful resource (Borrelli, 2011).

Summary

There are a number of preparatory steps that are worth considering prior to jumping into delivering your first MBCT for chronic pain program. In this chapter I have outlined the essential and primary considerations that you should reflect upon if you are wanting to implement the MBCT program described in the coming chapters. You might find it useful to return to this chapter after orienting yourself to the MBCT for chronic pain session-by-session manual and guide. Taking the time to contemplate, and to initially orient yourself to the model and processes in this way will likely be helpful in ensuring that your experience in implementing the approach is a smooth and rewarding process that is of benefit to your clients. Further, you may likely benefit from reading the original and updated MBCT texts by Segal, Williams, and Teasdale, and to acquaintance yourself with the other useful resources I suggest in the Conclusion section to further your training, expertise, and skill, and to build competence in this approach. As your familiarity with the "nuts and bolts" of the treatment components develops and you have a sense of your own "felt experience" of delivering the techniques, my hope is that many of the MBCT theoretical and practical concepts will feel natural and will give not only your clients, but also you as the clinician a fresh way of relating to experience, and enhancing well-being.

Notes

1 Appendix F contains a basic outline and instructional material; however, it is recommended that if you are considering using this brief approach to first be highly familiar with the detailed information provided herein with the eight-session manual, as this will comprehensively inform your delivery of the four-session version.

2 Guided audio recordings are available for download as MP3 files from the companion webpage.
3 The client handouts from within the handbook are also available in electronic form for ease of distribution to clients, downloadable at the companion webpage.
4 Some population groups have been shown to have difficulty accurately completing NRS ratings of pain intensity, including individuals with cognitive impairment (Jensen & Karoly, 2011), communication, and understanding deficits (Herr & Garand, 2001), and the elderly (Chibnall & Tait, 2001). IMMPACT suggests that in such circumstances a Verbal Rating Scale may be appropriate. Dixon and Thorn (2015) suggest also considering using the Non-Communicative Patient's Pain Assessment Instrument (Snow et al., 2004) as an additional alternative.
5 The "Activity Engagement" scale of the CPAQ measures behavioral notions of acceptance, and all of the items of the "Pain Willingness" scale are reverse scored items that actually assess a perceived need or desire for pain control, and as such it has been recommended that this scale be relabeled "Pain Control" (Lauwerier et al., 2015).

References

American Psychology Association (APA) (2010). Ethical principles of psychologists and code of conduct: 2010 amendments. Retrieved from http://www.apa.org/ethics/code/

Amtmann, D. (2016). Extending PROMIS pain item banks: Pain self-efficacy and pain catastrophizing. Retrieved from http://www.pcori.org/research-results/2014/extending-promis-pain-item-banks-pain-self-efficacy-and-pain-catastrophizing

Anderson, K. O., Noel Dowds, B., Pelletz, R. E., Edwards, W. T., & Peeters-Asdourian, C. (1995). Development and initial validation of a scale to measure self-efficacy beliefs in patients with chronic pain. *Pain, 63,* 77–84.

Andrews, G. (2000). A focus on empirically supported outcomes: A commentary on the search for empirically supported treatments. *Clinical Psychology: Science and Practice, 7,* 264–268.

Asmundson, G. J. G., Bovell, C. V., Carleton, R. N., & McWilliams, L. A. (2008). The fear of pain questionnaire—short form (FPQ-SF): Factorial validity and psychometric properties. *Pain, 134,* 51–58.

Baer, R. A., Smith, G. T., Lykins, E., Button, D., Krietemeyer, J., Sauer, S., ... Williams, J. M. G. (2008). Construct validity of the five facet mindfulness questionnaire in meditating and nonmeditating samples. *Assessment, 15*(3), 329–342.

Barber, J. P., Liese, B. S., & Abrams, M. J. (2003). Development of the cognitive therapy adherence and competence scale. *Psychotherapy Research, 13*(2), 205–221.

Beck, A. T., Ward, C. H., Mendelson, M., Mock, J., & Erbaugh, J. (1961). An inventory for measuring depression. *Archives of General Psychiatry, 4,* 561–571.

Bohlmeijer, E., ten Klooster, P. M., Fledderus, M., Veehof, M., & Baer, R. A. (2011). Psychometric properties of the five facet mindfulness questionnaire in depressed adults and development of a Short Form. *Assessment, 18*(3), 308–320.

Bond, G. R., Evans, L., Salyers, M. P., Williams, J., & Kim, H. W. (2000). Measurement of fidelity in psychiatric rehabilitation. *Mental Health Services Research, 2*(2), 75–87.

Borrelli, B. (2011). The assessment, monitoring, and enhancement of treatment fidelity in public health clinical trials. *Journal of Public Health Dentistry, 71*(S1), S52–S63.

Carmody, J., & Baer, R. A. (2009). How long does a mindfulness-based stress reduction program need to be? A review of class contact hours and effect sizes for psychological distress. *Journal of Clinical Psychology, 65*(6), 627–638.

Carroll, K. M., Nich, C., Sifry, R. L., Nuro, K. F., Frankforter, T. L., Ball, S. A., ... Rounsaville, B. J. (2000). A general system for evaluating therapist adherence and competence in psychotherapy research in the addictions. *Drug and Alcohol Dependence, 57*(3), 225–238.

Chibnall, J. T., & Tait, R. C. (2001). Pain assessment in cognitively impaired and unimpaired older adults: A comparison of four scales. *Pain, 92*, 173–186.

Chow, D. L., Miller, S. D., Seidel, J. A., Kane, R. T., Thornton, J. A., & Andrews, W. P. (2015). The role of deliberate practice in the development of highly effective psychotherapists. *Psychotherapy, 52*(3), 337–345.

Cleeland, C. S., & Ryan, K. M. (1994). Pain assessment: Global use of the Brief Pain Inventory. *Annals of the Academy of Medicine, Singapore, 23*(2), 129–138.

Crawford, M. J., Thana, L., Farquharson, L., Palmer, L., Hancock, E., Bassett, P., ... Parry, G. D. (2016). Patient experience of negative effects of psychological treatment: Results of a national survey. *British Journal of Psychiatry, 208*(3), 260–265.

Darnall, B. D., Scheman, J., Davin, S., Burns, J. W., Murphy, J. L., Wilson, A. C., ... Mackey, S. C. (2016). Pain psychology: A global needs assessment and national call to action. *Pain Medicine, 17*, 250–263.

Day, M. A. (2016). The application of mindfulness-based cognitive therapy for chronic pain. In S. Eisendrath (Ed.), *Mindfulness-based cognitive therapy: Innovative applications*. Springer, 65–74.

Day, M. A., Eyer, J., & Thorn, B.E. (2013). Therapeutic relaxation. In S. G. Hofmann (Ed.), *The Wiley Handbook of Cognitive Behavioral Therapy: A Complete Reference Guide. Volume 1: CBT General Strategies* (Vol. *1*, pp. 157–180). Oxford: Wiley-Blackwell.

Day, M. A., Halpin, J., & Thorn, B. E. (2016). An empirical examination of the role of common factors of therapy during a mindfulness-based cognitive therapy intervention for headache pain. *Clinical Journal of Pain, 32*(5), 420–427.

Day, M. A., Jensen, M. P., Ehde, D. M., & Thorn, B. E. (2014). Towards a theoretical model for mindfulness-based pain management. *Journal of Pain, 15*(7), 691–703.

Day, M. A., Lang, C., Newton-John, T. R. O., Ehde, D. M., & Jensen, M. P. (in press). A content review of cognitive process measures used in pain research with adult populations. *European Journal of Pain.*

Day, M. A., Thorn, B. E., Ward, L. C., Rubin, N., Hickman, S. D., Scogin, F., & Kilgo, G. R. (2014). Mindfulness-based cognitive therapy for the treatment of headache pain: A pilot study. *Clinical Journal of Pain, 22*(2), 278–285.

Day, M. A., Ward, L. C., Thorn, B. E., Lang, C. P., Newton-John, T. R. O., Ehde, D. M., & Jensen, M. P. (in press). The Pain-Related Cognitive Processes Questionnaire (PCPQ): Development and validation. *Pain Medicine.*

DeGood, D. E., & Cook, A. J. (2010). Psychosocial Assessment: Comprehensive measures and measures specific to pain beliefs and coping. In D. C. Turk & R. Melzack (Eds.), *Handbook of Pain Assessment* (3rd ed., pp. 67–97). New York, NY: Guilford.

Dixon, K. E., & Thorn, B. E. (2015). Pain assessment: A practical guide for researchers and clinicians. *Journal of Rational-Emotive Cognitive-Behavioral Therapy, 33*, 202–217.

Dworkin, R. H., Turk, D. C., Farrar, J. T., Haythornthwaite, J. A., Jensen, M. P., Katz, N. P., ... Witter, J. (2005). Core outcome measures for chronic pain clinical trials: IMMPACT recommendations. *Pain, 113*, 9–19.

Ellis, D. A., Naar-King, S., Templin, T., Frey, M. A., & Cunningham, P. B. (2007). Improving health outcomes among youth with poorly controlled type I diabetes: The role of treatment fidelity in a randomized clinical trial of multisystemic therapy. *Journal of Family Psychology, 21*(3), 363–371.

Farrar, J. T. (2003). *The global assessment of pain and related symptoms.* Paper presented at the second meeting of the Initiative on Methods, Measurement, and Pain Assessment in Clinical Trials (IMMPACT-II). Retrieved from www.immpact.org/meetings.html

Fish, R. M. B., Hogan, M., Morrison, T., & Stewart, I. (2010). Validation of the Chronic Pain Acceptance Questionnaire (CPAQ) in an internet sample and development and preliminary validation of the CPAQ-8. *Pain, 149*, 435–443.

French, D. J., Holroyd, K. A., Pinell, C., Malinoski, P. T., O'Donnell, F., & Hill, K. R. (2000). Perceived self-efficacy and headache related disability. *Headache, 40*, 647–656.

Goossens, M. E., Vlaeyen, J. W., Hidding, A., Kole-Snijders, A., & Evers, S. M. (2005). Treatment expectancy affects the outcome of cognitive-behavioral interventions in chronic pain. *Clinical Journal of Pain, 21*, 18–26.

Herr, K. A., & Garand, L. (2001). Assessment and measurement of pain in older adults. *Clinics in Geriatric Medicine, 17*, 457–478.

Hansen, W. B., Graham, J. W., Wolkenstein, B. H., & Rohrbach, L. A. (1991). Program integrity as a moderator of prevention program effectiveness: Results for fifth-grade students in the adolescent alcohol prevention trial. *Journal of Studies on Alcohol, 52*(6), 568–579.

IOM. (2011). *Relieving pain in America: A blueprint for transforming prevention, care, education, and research.* Washington, DC: The National Academics Press.

Jacobson, G. P., Ramadan, N. M., Aggarwal, S. K., & Newman, C. W. (1994). The Henry Ford Hospital Headache Disability Inventory (HDI). *Neurology, 44*(5), 837–842.

Jensen, M. P., & Karoly, P. (2011). Self-report scales and procedures for assessing pain in adults. In D. C. Turk & R. Melzack (Eds.), *Handbook of pain assessment* (Vol. 3, pp. 19–44). New York, NY: Guilford Press.

Jensen, M. P., Karoly, P., & Huger, R. (1987). The development and reliminary validation of an instrument to assess patients' attitudes toward pain. *Journal of Psychosomatic Research, 31*, 393–400.

Jensen, M., Nielson, W. R., Romano, J. M., Hill, M. L., & Turner, J. A. (2000). Further evaluation of the Pain Stages of Change Questionnaire: Is the transtheoretical model useful for patients with chronic pain? *Pain, 86*, 255–264.

Jensen, M., Nielson, W. R., Turner, J. A., Romano, J. M., & Hill, M. L. (2004). Changes in readiness to self-manage pain are associated with improvement in multidisciplinary pain treatment and pain coping. *Pain, 111*, 84–95.

Kabat-Zinn, J. (1990). *Full catastrophe living: Using the wisdom of your body and mind to face stress, pain and illness.* New York, NY: Delacourt.

Kerns, R. D., Turk, D. C., & Rudy, T. E. (1985). The West Haven-Yale multidimensional pain inventory (WHYMPI). *Pain, 23*, 345–356.

Kuijpers, H. J. H., van der Heijden, F. M. M. A., Tuinier, S., & Verhoeven, W. M. A. (2007). Meditation-induced psychosis. *Psychopathology, 40*(6), 461–464.

Lambert, M. J., Whipple, J. L., Hawkins, E. J., Vermeersch, D. A., Nielsen, S. L., & Smart, D. W. (2003). Is it time for clinicians to routinely track patient outcome? A meta-analysis. *Clinical Psychology: Science and Practice, 10*, 288–301.

Lauwerier, E., Caes, L., Van Damme, S., Goubert, L., Rosseel, Y., & Crombez, G. (2015). Acceptance: What's in a name? A content analysis of acceptance instruments in individuals with chronic pain. *Journal of Pain, 16*(4), 306–317.

Lichstein, K. L., Riedel, B. W., & Grieve, R. (1994). Fair tests of clinical trials: A treatment implementation model. *Advances in Behavior Research and Therapy, 16*, 1–29.

McCracken, L. M., Eccleston, C., & Bell, L. (2005). Clinical assessment of behavioral coping responses: Preliminary results from a brief inventory. *European Journal of Pain, 9*, 69–78.

McCracken, L. M., Vowles, K. E., & Eccleston, C. (2004). The Chronic Pain Acceptance Questionnaire. *Pain, 107*(1), 271–277.

McNair, D. M., Lorr, M., & Droppleman, L. F. (1971). *Profile of mood states.* San Diego, CA: Educational and Industrial Testing Service.

Melzack, R. (1987). The short-form McGill Pain Questionnaire. *Pain, 30*(2), 191–197.

Mignogna, J., Thorn, B. E., & Day, M. A. (2007). *The checklist of patient engagement in group form.* The University of Alabama, Tuscaloosa.

Miller, W. R., & Rollnick, S. (2013). *Motivational interviewing : Helping people change* (3rd ed.). New York, NY: Guilford Press.

Moher, D., Hopewell, S., Schulz, K. F., Montori, V., Gotzsche, P. C., Devereaux, P. J., ... Altman, D. G. (2010). CONSORT 2010 explanation and elaboration: Updated guidelines for reporting parallel group randomised trials. *British Medical Journal, 340*, c869.

Mowbray, C. T., Holter, M. C., Teague, G. B., & Bybee, D. (2003). Fidelity criteria: Development, measurement and validation. *American Journal of Evaluation, 24*(3), 315–340.

Nicholas, M. K. (2007). The pain self-efficacy questionnaire: Taking pain into account. *European Journal of Pain, 11*, 153–163.

NIH. (2011). *Interagency pain research coordinating committee: National Pain Strategy.* Retrieved from https://iprcc.nih.gov/docs/DraftHHSNationalPain Strategy.pdf#

Orwin, R. G. (2000). Assessing program fidelity in substance abuse health services research. *Addiction, 95*(S3), S309–S327.

Paul, G. L. (1969). Behavior modification research: Design and tactics. In C. M. Franks (Ed.), *Behavior therapy: Appraisal and status* (pp. 29–62). New York, NY: McGraw-Hill.
Paulson, R. I., Post, R. L., Herinckx, H. A., & Risser, P. (2002). Beyond components: Using fidelity scales to measure and assure choice in program implementation and quality assurance. *Community Mental Health Journal, 38*, 119–128.
Peerdeman, K. J., van Laarhoven, A. I. M., Keij, S. M., Vase, L., Rovers, M. M., Peters, M. L., & Evers, A. W. M. (2016). Relieving patients' pain with expectation interventions: A meta-analysis. *Pain, 157*(6), 1179–1191.
Perepletchikova, F., & Kazdin, A. E. (2005). Treatment integrity and therapeutic change: Issues and recommendations. *Clinical Psychology Science and Practice, 12*, 365–383.
Perepletchikova, F., Treat, T. A., & Kazdin, A. E. (2007). Treatment integrity in psychotherapy research: Analysis of the studies and examination of the associated factors. *Journal of Consulting and Clinical Psychology, 75*(6), 829–841.
Prochaska, J. O., & DiClemente, C. C. (1992). Stages of change in the modification of problem behaviors. *Progress in Behavior Modification, 28*, 183–218.
Resnick, B., Bellg, A. J., Borrelli, B., Defrancesco, C., Breger, R., Hecht, J., ... Czajkowski, S. (2005). Examples of implementation and evaluation of treatment fidelity in the BCC studies: Where we are and where we need to go. *Annals of Behavioral Medicine, 29*, 46–54.
Robinson, M. E., Riley, J., Myers, C., Sadler, I., Kvaal, S., Geisser, M. E., & Keefe, F. J. (1997). The coping strategies questionnaire: A large sample, item level factor analysis. *The Clinical Journal of Pain, 13*(1), 43–49.
Roland, M., & Morris, R. (1983). A study of the natural history of back pain, part I: Development of a reliable and sensitive measure of disability in low back pain. *Spine, 8*, 141–144.
Sechrest, L., West, S. G., Phillips, M. A., Redner, R., & Yeaton, W. (1979). Some neglected problems in evaluation research: Strength and integrity of treatments. In L. Sechrest, S. G. West, M. A. Phillips, R. Redner, & W. Yeaton (Eds.), *Evaluation studies review annual, Volume 4*. Thousand Oaks, CA: Sage.
Segal, Z., Teasdale, J. D., Williams, J. M., & Gemar, M. C. (2002). The mindfulness-based cognitive therapy adherence scale: Inter-rater reliability, adherence to protocol and treatment distinctiveness. *Clinical Psychology and Psychotherapy, 9*(2), 131–138.
Segal, Z. V., Williams, J. M. G., & Teasdale, J. D. (2013). *Mindfulness-based cognitive therapy for depression*. New York, NY: Guilford.
Smeets, R. J., Beelen, S., Goossens, M. E., Schouten, E. G., Knottnerus, J. A., & Vlaeyen, J. W. (2008). Treatment expectancy and credibility are associated with the outcome of both physical and cognitive-behavioral treatment in chronic low back pain. *Clinical Journal of Pain, 24*, 305–315.
Snow, A. L., Weber, J. B., O'Malley, K. J., Cody, M., Beck, C., Bruera, E., ... Kunik, M. E. (2004). NOPPAIN: A nursing assistant-administered pain assessment instrument for use in dementia. *Dementia and Geriatric Cognitive Disorders, 17*(3), 240–246.
Sullivan, M. J. L., Bishop, S., & Pivik, J. (1995). The Pain Catastrophizing Scale: Development and validation. *Psychological Assessment, 7*, 524–532.

Thorn, B. E. (2004). *Cognitive therapy for chronic pain: A step-by-step guide.* New York, NY: Guilford Press.

Thorn, B. E., Day, M. A., Burns, J., Kuhajda, M. C., Gaskins, S. W., Sweeney, K., ... Cabbil, C. (2011). Randomized trial of group cognitive behavioral therapy compared with a pain education control for low-literacy rural people with chronic pain. *Pain, 152*(12), 2710–2720.

Turk, D. C., Dworkin, R. H., Allen, R. R., Bellamy, N., Brandenburg, N., Carr, D. B., ... Witter, J. (2003). Core outcome domains for chronic pain clinical trials: IMMPACT recommendations. *Pain, 106*, 337–345.

Turk, D. C., & Robinson, J. P. (2010). Multidisciplinary assessment of patients with chronic pain. In S. Fishman, J. C. Ballantyne, & J. P. Rathmell (Eds.), *Bonica's management of pain* (4th ed.). Philadelphia, PA: Lippincott Williams & Wilkins, 288–301.

UCSD. (2016). Mindfulness-Based Professional Training Institute. Retrieved from http://mbpti.org/

Veehof, M. M., Oskam, M. J., Schreurs, K. M., & Bohlmeijer, E. T. (2011). Acceptance-based interventions for the treatment of chronic pain: A systematic review and meta-analysis. *Pain, 152*(3), 533–542.

Waltz, J., Addis, M. E., Koerner, K., & Jacobson, N. S. (1993). Testing the integrity of a psychotherapy protocol: Assessment of adherence and competence. *Journal of Consulting and Clinical Psychology, 61*(4), 620–630.

Wampold, B. E. (2005). Establishing specificity in psychotherapy scientifically: Design and evidence issues. *Clinical Psychology: Science and Practice, 12*, 194–197.

Wampold, B. E., & Brown, G. S. (2005). Estimating variability in outcomes attributable to therapists: A naturalistic study of outcomes in managed care. *Journal of Consulting and Clinical Psychology, 73*, 914–923.

Ware, J. E., & Sherbourne, C. D. (1992). The MOS 36-item short form health survey (SF-36). *Medical Care, 30*, 473–483.

Wickstrom, K., Jones, K., LaFleur, L., & Witt, J. (1998). An analysis of treatment integrity in school-based behavioral consultation. *School Psychology Quarterly, 13*, 141–154.

Woby, S. R., Roach, N. K., Urmston, M., & Watson, P. J. (2005). Psychometric properties of the TSK-11: A shortened version of the Tampa Scale for Kinesiophobia. *Pain, 117*(1–2), 137–144.

Yorsten, G. A. (2001). Mania precipitated by meditation: A case report and literature review. *Mental Health, Religion, and Culture, 4*(2), 209–213.

5

Session 1: Stepping Out of Automatic Pain Habits

Therapist Introduction

In the beginning of this first session, you should encourage clients to treat the next 8 weeks "like an experiment." The approach is one of nonstriving, so participants are invited to set aside any goals or expectations they may have coming into this program (as in a sense these set limits and parameters around what might happen), and instead approach the program with an open curiosity. The idea that there is "more right than wrong with you" should be conveyed.

It is important to discuss confidentiality, the nature of group therapy, roles, and responsibilities. The idea is to emphasize that with practice, this program provides skills clients can use to feel empowered and to have a sense of control. During the opening introductions and discussion is an important time to foster a sense of group cohesion and alliance, and to balance the group dynamics to ensure everyone has the opportunity to share their experiences.

To enhance buy-in, it is essential that the message be clearly conveyed that the client's pain is real, and to provide a rationale as to why this approach will be beneficial for their pain (i.e., the Gate Control Theory). Mindfulness is introduced in a practical, concrete, jargon-free way with a discussion of Automatic Pilot, and this is connected back to the experience of pain. The raisin exercise illustrates how an activity as simple as eating can become a means to engage all of the senses when we simply bring attention to the process. The first formal meditation, the Body Scan, is used to begin to train the mind to have the capacity to move attention at will. Finally, the 3-Minute Breathing Space is taught as a means to further generalize the practice.

Mindfulness-Based Cognitive Therapy for Chronic Pain: A Clinical Manual and Guide,
First Edition. Melissa A. Day.

Companion website: www.wiley.com/go/day/mindfulness_based_cognitive_therapy

Therapist Outline

Welcome

We're delighted that you are taking the time for yourself to be a part of this group. Our intention is to make this room a safe and supportive place where you can learn that there is more right with you than wrong with you. If at any time in the sessions you need to move around or re-position yourself to be comfortable, please feel free to do so. We invite you to think of the next eight group classes as an experiment. We're inviting you to learn how to quiet your body and mind by exploring different ways of thinking, feeling, behaving, and responding to pain. At first, you might not see the connection between what we're inviting you to do and your chronic pain. But we're asking you to place your trust in us, stick it out, and see what you find at the end. After all, what do you have to lose?

Assessment

Have clients fill out weekly assessment measures. Provide assistance as needed.

Confidentiality and Privacy

As the group leaders, we will not disclose names/identifying information or tell anything discussed within our group to other people outside the group. However, to ensure safety, the law is that we must break this rule if we think you are in imminent danger of hurting yourself or someone else, or if a child or elderly person is being abused. Out of respect for your other group members, and so that we each feel comfortable sharing our experience, please do not talk about members of your group outside of this group. You may feel free to discuss the skills you are learning and your experiences with meditation, but we ask that you please not disclose the names or other identifying information of your group members. Does that sound okay to everyone?

Working Together: Empowering Ourselves and Empowering Each Other

This program will give you skills you can use to manage your pain. As your group leaders, we will teach you active pain management skills and will work together with you, as a team. This teamwork approach is likely radically different to other approaches you have used for your pain, such as medication, where you were a passive recipient. In this treatment, you are an active, engaging force for your own well-being and in changing the way you respond to your pain and direct experience. What this means is that it is important that you show up for each group session. Further, you are not just a team with us as your group leaders: this whole group is a team, a community, and what you say in group is important. Taking an active role in group and speaking up about your direct experiences not only empowers you, but also may spark learning and motivation for your other group members. Further, the key to this treatment is learning by doing, in order to learn you need to do; just like any other skill, you need to practice to become masterful. So after each session we will be inviting you to practice at home what you learn in group. Each week we will discuss your experiences with this at-home practice, sharing experiences with what you have begun to practice, including any successes you may have as well as any challenges. Treatment works best when you take part in each group. *But remember that you only need to share as much information as you are comfortable sharing.*

Introductions: Tell the Group about You

- What is your name?
- What do you like to do? What is your hobby?
- Tell the group briefly about what made you decide to participate in this program.

Overview of Group Treatment Approach

Over the course of the eight group classes, you will learn about a new way to live with chronic pain, and you will learn new ways to relate to the new ways to relate to how pain may influence your thoughts, feelings and relationships. You will learn how to pay attention, on purpose, in each moment, and without judgment. This program will provide you with a highly portable pain management skill set that will always be available to you to cope with pain and whatever comes along with it.

You will learn:

- How your thoughts affect your feelings, your behavior, and your pain.
- How to focus your attention, and be in the moment.
- How to become aware of, and simply let go of thoughts and feelings.
- How to work with stress and pain so that it causes less suffering.
- You will learn other skills to cope with your chronic pain:
  - for example, you will learn how to practice meditation and how to recognize difficult situations early and see more clearly how best to respond.

No matter how much pain you feel or for how long, and no matter how hopeless you are feeling right now, you will learn to focus and quiet your mind and body. No matter what your situation is right now, we will start with you where you are. You will learn that each moment is a new opportunity for a fresh start and a new beginning. The aim of the program is freedom; not freedom from chronic pain, but freedom from the extra baggage we pile on top of the pain, which increases suffering. We're going to encourage you not to strive for anything in particular throughout the course of this program and to use this class as an experiment, and to be curious about what might happen during this course. So as best you can, lay aside any goals or expectations you may have for now, practice with us, and see what happens.

Our Starting Point

This room is filled with XX people, and we suspect that everyone feels at least a little like chronic pain has robbed them of part of their life. Everyone has felt concerned and scared about the pain, and everyone has tried lots of ways to get rid of the pain. If we spent our time together focusing on *these* feelings, it would only increase pain and suffering by increasing our attention toward what we can't do because of the pain or what has been lost. Since you've already spent so much time discussing your pain and symptoms with health-care practitioners, friends, family, loved ones … here, we will be taking a radically different approach and will not be focusing on "what's wrong with you," instead we want to help you focus on "what's right with you."

With this in mind, during our time together, we won't focus directly on discussing your pain and how to alleviate it. Instead, when we do pay attention to pain, it will be to help you develop a different relationship to the pain, to learn to respond to it in a very different way, and to learn an approach that allows your mind and body to not be totally taken over by the pain. This approach does not ask you to deny what is wrong with you, or to pretend the pain does not exist—the pain is real, and it is here. Learning to focus on what is right with you rather than what is wrong with you though helps free you from the cage of an identity of a "chronic pain patient." In other words, this approach helps you to realize that in this moment, you are a whole person, pain and all.

Our Theme

Mindfulness means simply learning how to pay attention to the present moment without judging it and without being swept away by it. You will see in your reading materials a popular definition of mindfulness from Dr. Jon Kabat-Zinn, a pioneer in the development of mindfulness interventions for various health conditions. This approach of mindfulness begins when we realize that we are often not fully aware of what we are doing, what we are feeling, or what we are thinking from one moment to the next. There is nothing mystical about mindfulness, and in this program we will not be approaching meditation from the context of any particular religious tradition, as it may sometimes be practiced. In this program, we are teaching mindfulness as a way to manage chronic pain and live a fulfilled life even in the presence of pain. We typically go through our day on "automatic pilot," which means we just go through the motions without contacting our direct experience of what we are doing, feeling, or thinking from one moment to the next. Once we recognize our tendency to be on "autopilot," we can make a commitment to learn how to step out of automatic habits and ways of reacting to pain, and to step into being fully present and in direct contact with each moment.

The Brain is in Charge: Learning about the Gate Control Theory

You might be wondering, what has all this being in the moment business got to do with my pain? Early models and understandings of pain considered the pain we feel is in direct proportion to the amount of tissue damage or the stage of the disease; the brain was thought to play a passive, receiving role of pain signals coming from the injured area, telling us we have pain. However, actual experience and evidence fails to support this model.

We have probably all heard stories of this, such as the severely wounded soldier carrying out heroic feats on the battlefield, who at the time was not aware of any pain. Perhaps you have experienced something similar yourself, when you are completely absorbed in a cherished moment with your child or loved one, for example, where pain somewhat fades and becomes more like background static. With the advent of modern brain imaging techniques such as MRI, a wealth of evidence has now shown that the brain plays an active role in processing pain. Indeed, the brain is "in charge" and the amount of pain we feel has a lot more to do with what happens above the level of the spine (i.e., in the brain) than below it.

Current models and evidence show that the brain acts like a pain filter, and the experience of pain (i.e., the way pain signals are processed in the brain) is influenced by the way we think, feel, behave. Think of it like the volume on the stereo: some thoughts, feelings, and actions can turn the volume up on pain and lead to more pain signals being processed, and make the pain feel worse; other thoughts, feelings, and actions can turn down the volume on pain, and reduce the amount of pain signals processed in the brain—modulating and reducing the amount of pain you feel. This model was originally called the Gate Control Theory of pain, and more recently has been updated to the Neuromatrix Model, reflective of the highly interconnected nature of thoughts, feelings/emotions, actions, and other sensory pain processing areas of the brain.

Draw a schematic of the spinal cord and brain to illustrate the gate control theory, direct clients to their handout on this in their handbook. Point out that:

Research has shown that when people in pain have their brains scanned, these thought and feeling areas light up and show activity. These areas are closely intertwined with the experience of pain, and affect how the brain processes pain, and how much pain we feel. The types of thoughts we have, and how we relate to them, play a critical role in determining how much pain we experience, how we feel emotionally, and what we do. According to current scientific understanding, thoughts can either "open up the gate" and let more pain signals through to the brain (increasing the amount of pain we feel) or they can "close the gate," lessening the amount of pain signals processed in the brain. So our thoughts are very important, but often our mind functions automatically, and we often are not even aware of what it is we are telling ourselves.

What have you noticed in your experience that seems to "open the gate" and let more pain signals be processed in the brain, and increase your pain? *Discuss, ask for examples, and write these on the flip chart next to the schematic:*

- no exercise, sitting around a lot *or* overdoing;
- feeling depressed, anxious, angry, fearful, or other negative moods;
- unhelpful, catastrophic, negative thoughts;
- too much pain medicine over a long period of time.

And what have you noticed seems to "close the gate" and reduce the number of pain signals processed in the brain, or in other words, make your pain decrease? *Discuss, ask for examples, and write these on the flip chart next to the schematic*:

- meditation, yoga, and physical activity;
- mindfulness;
- present-moment awareness;
- pacing activities, without underdoing or overdoing.

Typically we react to pain automatically, out of what have become pre-programmed, habitual reactions. When we're on this automatic pilot mode, our thoughts are affecting our emotions, body, actions, and pain, although we are not even aware of it.

Learning about Automatic Pilot

From time to time, we all experience the effects of absentmindedness, or of being on autopilot. What comes to mind for you when you hear the term "automatic pilot"? *Generate discussion based on the clients' responses.*

For example, we may be driving home along our route that we take each day, and we manage to stay on the right side of the road and follow all the driving rules, but only occasionally do we arrive at our destination with any actual memory of the drive along the way. We drive along and our mind wanders and skips along from memories, to planning what to cook for dinner, to conversations had during the day and what we should have said … perhaps a certain emotion was triggered along the way: anxiety, anger, excitement, or happiness. Or, we might have been distracted by feelings of discomfort in our bodies, and been carried away by the negative emotions and thoughts that can go along with increased pain.

When our mind wanders in this way, we may or may not be aware of where our attention goes exactly: we are "on automatic pilot," and the process of traveling from one place to another gets lost in a sea of thoughts, body sensations, and emotions. And we are not just on autopilot when we are driving! For much of our lives we often "go through the motions" without really being present, without really being in the moment.

When we are in automatic pilot mode…

- Our body is performing an action of some kind, while the mind is miles away doing something else.
- Our attention is carried away by physical sensations, emotions, thoughts, memories, or plans.
- The present moment fades into the background and so we are only dimly aware of our thoughts, feelings, and sensations associated with what is happening around us. Because of this, we are much more likely to react reflexively.

- We tend to react reflexively and have a "short fuse," which can look quite different for each of us, and each of us has our own particular triggers—some of us may lash out, others may withdraw. When we near the end of our fuse though or even "blow it," before we know it we are overtaken with a cascade of thoughts and emotions that can trigger our own particular flavor of old habits or behaviors that are unhelpful and may cause those neurological "gates" we just discussed to open wide, leading to worsening pain and suffering.

The good news is though, that each time we bring our mind back to the present moment, and become aware of our thoughts, feelings, and body sensations, we give ourselves the possibility of responding with greater freedom and choice. We don't reflexively react with habitual ways of thinking and acting, and what emerges or opens up from this is that we realize we have the choice to respond in a new way.

The Raisin Exercise (*or, if in Australia or Other Parts: "The Sultana Exercise"*)

To experience a first "taste" of mindfulness, and how you can begin to train your mind to be more present, more often, we are going to experiment with doing something very routine, something that you do every day, in a new and different way—slowing it down, and bringing careful attention to each part of the process. *Lead the group through the raisin meditation; see Appendix B on the website for a script for this meditation.*

Guided Inquiry

- What did you notice during this exercise?
- How was this experience different from the way you would normally eat?
- How do you think this exercise might be related to living with chronic pain?

When we slow down and bring careful attention to everyday things that we do—knowing what you are doing as you are doing it—we begin to see how often we are *not* paying attention, and are simply automatically going through the motions. Most often when we eat we are on autopilot and may not actually taste, let alone savor the taste, of what it is we are eating. In bringing awareness to the process of eating, not only are we more in tune with the messages of hunger and satiation from our body, but the meal or snack or whatever it is we are eating is typically much more satisfying. This exercise shows how anything we do, even eating, can become an opportunity to practice mindfulness—again highlighting how there is nothing mystical about mindfulness, it is simply bringing a quality of open observation and attentiveness to whatever it is we do, think and feel from moment to moment.

People with chronic pain often say that it is difficult to pay attention to anything other than the pain, and that once pain captures their attention, it is hard to direct their attention away from it. This exercise is a way of showing how attention can be deliberately directed to something very specific. As you learn to pay careful attention in this way, and as you become more skillful at directing your attention at will, your relationship to pain may change. In reality, all we have is the present moment—the past is a memory, the future simply a concept of mind—the present is all we have to work with. When we are fully *in* and present *with* each moment, then we open up for ourselves a different way of relating to life and all that it brings us.

Body Scan

This next exercise is called a Body Scan meditation, and the essence of this practice is to train your mind to purposefully bring detailed awareness to each part of the body in turn. Tuning into the sensations that are present, not stopping at any labels, and going further into the sensations, exploring what you find with gentleness, kindness, and an open sense of curiosity. There is no right or wrong way to do this practice, whatever your experience is, that is okay.

You may find that your mind wanders, and that's no problem. Whenever you notice that your mind has drifted, that awareness *is* mindfulness! You have become aware that you are thinking and the technique is to simply label this mind activity: "thinking," and then to gently return your attention back to the body part currently being explored with meditation. A key point is to apply kindness when you discover your mind has wandered. So, rather than saying to yourself, "Argh, I blew it! I am a bad meditator!", instead use a gentle inner tone of voice to yourself when you say "thinking" and then simply bring your mind back, over and over again, gently, patiently, and kindly training your mind to stay present.

During this practice, the words you hear may or may not match your experience. It is perfectly fine if your experience is different from the words you hear. For example, I may say some words that may characterize your experience, such as sensations or feelings. However, if you are noticing different sensations or feelings, or noticing different parts of your body from what I am talking about, this is perfectly fine. This in no way changes the effectiveness of the practice. If you find yourself falling asleep, you might find it helpful to open your eyes during part or all of the practice. And if at any point you need to readjust your posture to make yourself more comfortable, that is also perfectly fine—if you do wish to make a readjustment, perhaps experiment with making that a mindful process as well: first being aware of the urge to shift or readjust, then aware of the intention to make some adjustment, and then mindfully making whatever adjustment you need to do to be kind to yourself, and then returning to the instruction.

Body Scan practice: *Lead the group through the Body Scan meditation; see Appendix B on the website for a script for this meditation.*

Guided Inquiry

- What did you notice with that experience?
- How was this exercise different from how you normally experience your body?
- In what ways do you think the Body Scan relates to living with chronic pain?

Greater awareness of your body as a whole, not just the area that you might typically label as "painful," will be helpful not only in learning to notice those places where we might be holding tension, but will also help in learning how to relate to, and manage, both physical and emotional pain. If a strong emotion arises, or perhaps your mind keeps getting drawn to a particular pattern of thought, experiment with asking yourself, "How am I feeling this in my body?" This will give you another place to stand to observe your experience that does not continue to feed into the emotion or thought. At first, you might be so focused on the part of your body that is in pain that you have trouble concentrating on any other region of your body. If this happens, it's okay. Rather than fight against it, you may choose to intentionally bring your awareness to the discomfort, to breathe with the sensations: breathing in space on the inbreath, letting go on the outbreath. Another way to think about this idea of "breathing with the sensation"—which can sometimes seem abstract—is to think of it as though you are holding the movements of the breath in the foreground of your awareness while still aware in the background of the sensation, and in this way, you are gently staying with the sensation, breathing with it. And then, as it feels right to you, gently returning your awareness back to the focus of the meditation, to whatever part of the body we are up to.

Meditation for the Real World: The 3-Minute Breathing Space

This last practice we are going to do together today is highly portable; everywhere you go, this practice will be available to you and so it will allow you to bring the mindfulness skills you are learning into any situation you find yourself. It is exhausting to carry around regret about the past, and/or anticipation about what needs to be done today, this week, this month, this year ... which turns into a lifetime of anticipated to-do lists. It is a burden that doesn't need to be carried. The present moment is all we ever have; and tuning into it during your daily life allows energy to flow through into the task, conversation—whatever experience you may be facing—and allows you to complete just this moment's task. In engaging in learning about and practicing meditation, it is not that we ultimately want to become "good meditators." This practice is training the mind to be openly attentive, nonjudgmental, accepting, and mindful during the moments of our lives "out in the real world"—not just when we are on the mat or sitting in meditation. It is not unusual though for people to forget about infusing this practice into their day-to-day lives. Today though, we have been practicing bringing mindfulness into everyday tasks, starting with eating the raisin mindfully, and this will be an on-going theme in the program. We are now going to build on this, to take it a little further...

There are three basic steps to this exercise, as shown in one of your handouts in your reading materials:

1) Awareness. As this is a brief practice, you bring yourself into a dignified sitting posture to signal to your mind you are switching into "being" mode. Closing your eyes, bringing awareness to what is happening in this moment,

asking yourself what thoughts are around? Emotions? Sensations? Just acknowledging your experience in this moment, whether it be seen as pleasant, unpleasant, or neutral, with a sense of equanimity.

2) Anchoring. Having acknowledged your experience, focusing your attention, narrowing it like a spotlight just as you did in the Body Scan, and focusing it fully on the breath, aware as you breathe in, and as you breathe out. Not controlling the breath, simply tuning into the felt sensations of the breath. Using the breath as an anchor to the present moment, to reconnect with awareness and a sense of stillness and spaciousness.
3) Opening. Having returned to, and anchored yourself to your breathing and the present moment, then let your attention expand outwards to openly include not only the breath, but also the body as a whole—holding it all in this open, more spacious awareness.

This exercise, the Breathing Space, ventilates situations, allows you to step out of automatic pilot, and brings you back to present-moment awareness. If you notice your mind wanders, that's no problem, it is what minds do! As many times as you notice it, simply observe it, perhaps label it "thinking," and then each time, nonjudgmentally return your awareness back to your breath.

Breathing Space practice: *Lead the group through the 3-Minute Breathing Space meditation; see Appendix B on the website for a script for this meditation.*

Guided Inquiry

- What did you notice with that brief practice? (*Depending on time, you may wish to further this discussion, inquiring into how this was different from how we might typically spend a spare 3 min, and/or how this practice relates to living with chronic pain.*)

At-Home Daily Practice

Just as no one else can exercise for you in order for you to benefit, no one else can practice meditation for you either! The key in these 8 weeks together is to learn by doing; like learning any new skill, learning and mastering the pain management techniques taught in this program takes regular daily practice. During the coming week, your daily practice, as shown in your handout will be… *Go over client handout describing at-home practice following Session 1. Note: the daily at-home practice record is provided in Appendix C on the website.*

What obstacles or challenges do you possibly foresee in looking at this at-home practice schedule? (*Generate discussion.*) How might you best navigate overcoming these possible obstacles?

At first you may think it "impossible" to fit this practice into your schedule. What we have found is that it helps to practice consistently in the same place at the same time each day, and in this way, it becomes habit. So exploring what times are best for you, and then sticking with it. There may be difficulties, and we will work with those together and will talk about what you learned in the next group meeting. You will also see in one of your handouts a description of the experience of a woman who went through this program, who described feeling many of the same challenges when she first started the Body Scan as what you have noted from today's practice. But over time, her experience—as is nearly always the case—shifted. So just hang in there. It may not seem relevant to your pain right now, but just stick with it and see what you find.

Distribute Session 1 guided meditation audio files and Session 1 client handouts.

Summary

What we have been learning today is that... *Go over client summary handout: "Stepping out of Automatic Pain Habits."*

Client Handbook

Session 1 Summary: Stepping out of Automatic Pain Habits

The Gate Control Theory—more recently updated to the Neuromatrix Model—of pain indicates that our thoughts and feelings have a direct connection to our experience of chronic pain. Therefore, we need to become aware of our thoughts and feelings, so that we can have them work for us rather than against us in managing pain.

We often go through much of our day on "automatic pilot," without really being aware of what we are doing. So moment by moment, day by day, we wind up not really being "present" for much of our lives. When we are on automatic pilot, we tend to react reflexively and have a "short fuse." Accompanying this is usually a stream of negative thoughts and feelings that may "open the gates" and lead to worsening pain.

During this program we will be learning skills to become more aware of the moment-by-moment experiences of our lives so that we can then *choose* how we wish to respond, rather than react in our typical, kneejerk fashion. The practices you are learning train the mind to become more aware (more often!) of where attention has drifted to, and then, nonjudgmentally acknowledging that our mind has wandered, we practice in deliberately, and kindly, bringing that focus of attention back to the present moment. And we do this over and over again.

We start by bringing attention to different parts of the body as a focus to anchor our awareness in the moment. We train in deliberately moving our attention, practicing in tuning into each part of the body, and then letting go as we move our attention to the next part of the body in turn. This is the intention of engaging in the Body Scan exercise, which is the main practice you will be engaging in at home from today's session.

What is Mindfulness?

> Mindfulness means paying attention in a particular way:
> on purpose, in the present moment, and nonjudgmentally.
>
> *Jon Kabat-Zinn*

The Brain is in Charge

Current models of pain show that the brain acts like a pain filter, and the experience of pain is influenced by the way we think, feel, behave. This model was originally called the Gate Control Theory, and is now known as the Neuromatrix Model of Pain. Some thoughts, feelings, and actions *open the gate*, which increases the amount of pain signals processed in the brain, worsening our pain. Other thoughts, feelings, and actions *close the gate* and reduce the amount of pain signals processed in the brain, leading to improved pain and coping.

Gate Openers

- no exercise, sitting around a lot, overdoing;
- feeling depressed, anxious, angry, fearful, or other negative moods;
- unhelpful, catastrophic, negative thoughts;
- too much pain medicine over a long period of time.

Gate Closers

- meditation, yoga, physical activity;
- mindfulness;
- present-moment awareness;
- pacing your activities without underdoing or overdoing.

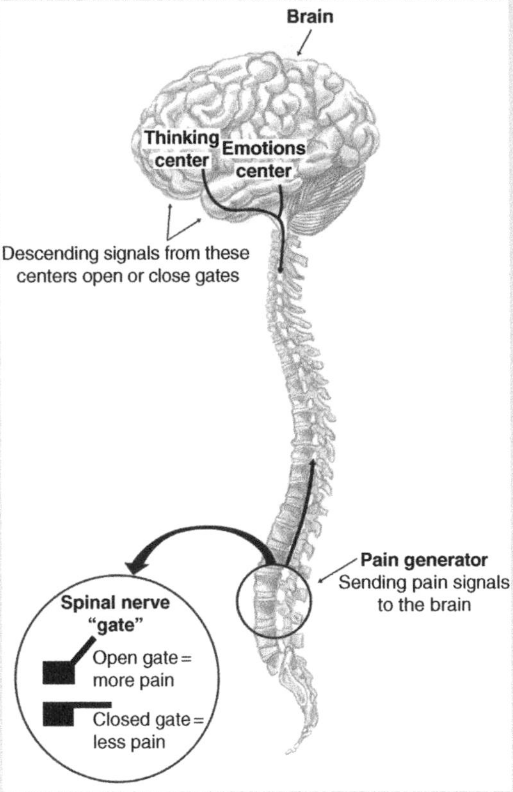

Helpful Hints for the Body Scan

1) There is no right or wrong way to do this practice. As best you can, let go of any ideas of what a "good" meditation period "should be" (e.g., that you should be able to "empty your mind," maintain near-constant focus and attention with no mind wandering), and just do the practice with an open sense of curiosity and see what happens. There is nothing to strive for, except to do the practice regularly and frequently.
2) No matter what happens (e.g., if you keep falling asleep, lose track of what body part you are up to, are distracted and your mind feels like it is trailing off in a hundred different directions all at once, feel bored…), as best you can, just keep practicing each day. That you even notice that you are distracted or thinking *is* mindfulness itself, and with practice, you will become more aware more often of your experiences as they are happening in the moment.
3) If you do find that your mind is extremely active and is wandering a lot, practice labelling any and all thoughts (no matter how "important" your mind might be telling you that the thought is) simply as "thinking," with a kind and gentle inner tone of voice, and then patiently but firmly, ushering your mind back to the Body Scan.
4) Similarly, let go of any ideas about what you will get out of the practice (i.e., a sense of relaxation, noticeable reduction in pain etc.). Each time you practice will inevitably be different; the idea is to let go of expectations, and be patient and constant with your practice. You are developing a new skill, and like any new skill, it takes practice over time in order to become masterful and reap the benefit.
5) Approach whatever you encounter in each moment with a sense of open acceptance, perhaps saying to yourself: "Okay, this is how things are right now." Letting go of any attempts to fix, change, fight, control, or make your experience go away, as each of these forms of resistance consumes your energy and your focus. Again and again, returning to training your mind to be aware, precise, nonstriving, accepting, and increasingly to rest in the present moment.

Meditation for the Real World: The 3-Minute Breathing Space Practice[1]

The Breathing Space ventilates situations, allows you to step out of automatic pilot, and brings you back to present-moment awareness. There are three steps to this exercise:

Step 1: Awareness

As this is a brief practice, you bring yourself into a dignified sitting posture to signal to your mind you are switching into "being" mode. Closing your eyes, bringing awareness to what is happening in this moment, asking yourself: what thoughts are around? Emotions? Sensations?

Just acknowledging your experience in this moment, whether it be seen as pleasant, unpleasant, or neutral, with a sense of equanimity.

Step 2: Anchoring

Having acknowledged your experience, focusing your attention, narrowing it like a spotlight just as you did in the Body Scan, and focusing it fully on the breath, aware as you breathe in, and as you breathe out. Not controlling the breath, simply tuning into the felt sensations of the breath.

Using the breath as an anchor to the present moment, to reconnect with awareness and a sense of stillness and spaciousness.

Step 3: Opening

Having returned to, and anchored yourself to your breathing and the present moment, now letting your attention expand outwards to openly include not only the breath, but also the body as a whole—holding it all in this open, more spacious awareness, as you go about your day.

Reflections from a Past Group Member

This person had suffered with chronic pain for over 10 years. She was forced to retire early on disability due to missing too many days at work due to her pain, causing more financial strain for the family. She was also unable to do some of the housework and family activities that she had done earlier in her life; if she ever did go to social activities, she also carried with her the fear of experiencing a pain flare-up while there. She came into the group feeling that pain had robbed her of her life. She started to practice with the guided Body Scan audio without much of a sense that it would help her pain, but she figured if nothing else, it might help her to relax. These were her comments looking back after eight group meetings:

> At first it was just one more thing I had to do. I wanted so badly for this to help my pain, but the whole notion of not striving for anything in particular and just accepting my experience seemed totally unreasonable. Before I started the program I had always said I was a "bad meditator" and my experience for the first week matched that. My mind was wandering all over the place, and much of the time I felt like I was fighting against it, trying to force my mind to focus.
>
> After a while, I relaxed more and just listened to the guided audio and just expected that my mind would wander, and over time I realized that actually that was no big deal—I found that I noticed my mind drifting earlier and earlier in the process, and gradually the pause between one thought ending and the next beginning got longer and longer. And when my mind did wander, I stopped beating myself up for it, and just picked up on the guided audio again when I noticed it.
>
> After that first week, I stopped wrestling with my mind and I found I was happy to listen to the guided audio, it wasn't a burden anymore; I began to look forward to it. Soon I had developed it to where I could feel my breath going around my body, breathing with the sensations. I began to find my experience of the pain was changing. The pain was still there, but I no longer felt trapped by it.
>
> In structuring in the time to practice with the guided audio each day, I began to find it easier to structure other things in my life as well. The Body Scan really does have to be a daily thing; it is not something you can do just half a dozen times. The key is to just stick with it!

At-Home Daily Practice for Following Session 1

1) Practice with the Body Scan guided meditation audio each day. Letting go of any expectations about how you might feel during or after this practice, and any judgments about "how well" you might have done, just let your experience each day *be* your experience. Bringing an open curiosity to what it might be like each time. Included in your reading materials are some helpful hints for engaging in the Body Scan.
2) Engage in at least three short 3-Minute Breathing Spaces every day at set times that you have decided in advance. Some people find it helps to schedule these in by perhaps setting reminders on your phone for yourself, or linking the practice to activities of your day (e.g., morning tea, after meals, before going to bed etc.). We intentionally do not give you a guided audio for this practice as the key is to hone this skill to be highly portable, not needing an audio player, or anything else for that matter, in order to practice it. There is a handout in your reading materials with reminders about the steps to this brief, highly portable practice.
3) Practice bringing present-moment awareness to everyday activities such as washing your face, getting dressed, grocery shopping, washing dishes—any activity at all you can use as a means to practice, simply knowing what you are doing as you are doing it. Also practice eating at least one meal "mindfully," just as we did today with the raisin.
4) Read your handouts over the next few days. One of your handouts provides a description of the experience of one woman who went through this program, and her experiences in first practicing with the Body Scan, and what helped her as she kept up the daily practice over time.
5) Complete your daily at-home practice record; it helps to fill this in as close to finishing your practice as possible. Make a note in the comment box of anything that comes up during your meditation and we can talk about it next week.

Therapist Tips, Troubleshooting, and Supervision for Session 1

The Gate Control Theory

Following covering the content regarding confidentiality and the nature of the program, the Gate Control Theory is introduced. This model describes how the brain actively receives messages from the "pain generator" (e.g., the injury or source of pain) and the rest of the body, and also sends descending signals down the spinal cord, which can increase or decrease pain transmission—opening or closing metaphorical gates. As mentioned earlier, this content in the manual provides clients with a sound rationale for why a psychological treatment is effective for *real* pain and conveys your belief (as the therapist) in your client's pain as real, and that it is not "all in their head." During this discussion you may also provide clarifying statements and additional information to clarify any expectations or goals that are inconsistent with the nature of the MBCT program (e.g., "to cure my pain," or "to cure my multiple sclerosis"). Introducing the Gate Control Theory is best done by engaging clients in a highly interactive way, inviting clients to describe what they have noticed are "gate openers" and "gate closers" in their experience, making sure to touch on examples of thinking, feeling, and behaving. Typically clients have no problems at all identifying things that they have noticed make their pain worse, and things that make their pain better. This discussion places the client firmly in the expert role from the outset of the program, reinforcing that they themselves are the expert on their pain, and we are here to work together with them to provide a skill set they can hone and use to better manage the pain.

Learning about Automatic Pilot

The discussion of automatic pilot segues on from the Gate Control Theory and illustrates how often we are having thoughts and feelings and are acting in particular ways that can "open the gate" and increase pain, without even being aware of it. The concept of mindfulness is introduced in a very practical way as a means to train the mind to step out of automatic pilot simply by bringing a quality of nonjudgmental awareness and attention to what it is we are doing, feeling, and thinking moment by moment. Again, it is best to make this discussion interactive, asking clients to provide examples of times they find themselves on autopilot and connecting this back to pain.

Mindfulness Exercises

The specific skill of mindfulness meditation will be taught in depth throughout the program as a "mindfulness muscle building tool" to cultivate nonstriving, nonjudgmental present-moment awareness that includes awareness not only of painful sensations, but also of a rich life that is available, even in the presence of pain. The Raisin Exercise (or "The Sultana Exercise" if in Australia or other similar cultures) is the first "taste" of mindfulness for clients in the program, and illustrates that there is nothing mystical about mindfulness, it is simply engaging all of our senses and bringing attention to our experience as we are experiencing.

This exercise is best done without a great deal of introductory remarks, indeed, the less said the better! The idea is for this to be an experiential learning exercise, not a didactic learning exercise. A script is provided but you should feel free to let your own experience with the raisin guide how you deliver this exercise as you should also engage in doing this exercise with the raisin, just as you invite your clients to do so. Most clients will report a sense of how, through their own direct experience of eating the raisin in this way (i.e., not from what you as the therapist said or did not say), that the nature or quality of their experience changed, and most will readily relate this to their experience of pain. Generalizing the practice of mindfulness to daily tasks such as eating, having a shower, washing the dishes etc. is part of the assigned learning activities for the week.

The Body Scan is the first formal meditation taught, and is delivered in the first, second, and last session (i.e., Sessions 1, 2, and 8). As with the other meditations taught in the program, the aim of the Body Scan is not to necessarily feel relaxed, calm, or different in any way; rather, the aim is to bring a gentle, open curiosity to each part of the body in turn, training the mind to attend in a nonjudgmental manner to whatever is present, moment by moment. There are at least three primary advantages to teaching the Body Scan as the first meditation taught: (1) the body is tangible, and therefore relatively "easy" to bring direct attention to; (2) wherever we go, there we are—the body is always with us and it can be a useful check-in point to touch in with our emotions and to learn to notice what thoughts arise; and (3) it helps get clients "out of their head" and back in touch with their body. Clients should be encouraged to practice with the Body Scan guided meditation audio for 45 min each day following Session 1, although I find it helps to also provide a shorter, 20-min version. It is important to provide the rationale to clients for why the longer version is considered particularly helpful. Specifically (besides it being a larger dose), in the 45-min version, there are longer "gaps" or pauses in the verbal instruction, hence, the "leash" on the mind as represented by the verbal instruction is not so tight (i.e., the voice is not there to regularly bring the focus of attention back). The longer pauses, therefore, typically provide more opportunity to experientially notice—without necessarily the voice on the guided audio being the impetus *driving the noticing*—that the mind has wandered, and also to notice the ways in which the mind entertains itself in such gaps, often wandering off in various well-worn pathways... Along with this, then, is also more opportunity to practice gently, patiently, and firmly, bringing the mind back, over and over again, to the object of the meditation.

The final exercise taught is the 3-Minute Breathing Space, which was developed by Segal, Williams, and Teasdale (2013) as a cognitive-therapy infused meditation practice in the sense that it is highly structured, is practiced repeatedly (to foster therapeutic learning), and is explicit in its focus of generalizing mindfulness, and bringing the practice of mindfulness into day-to-day living. This practice is included in all subsequent sessions throughout the program, and Segal et al. (2013) refer to this practice as the "spine" of the MBCT program (p. 384). While initially this practice is assigned as a take-home activity with instruction that it should be programmed into client's days at set times (again, to provide explicit structure), later in the program this instruction will be expanded to include application of this practice when stress, pain, or difficulty in some form arises, and as an action step. One of my clients recently called this practice a "mindfulness pit stop" where he pauses and "tops up on mindfulness," shifting mental gears into being mode intermittently during the day. I find that introducing clients to this practice in the first session (as opposed to Session 3 as in Segal and colleagues' original protocol) builds a client's sense of self-efficacy that they can do this, and conveys the important message that the essence of this pain management approach is to bring mindfulness into your day-to-day life, not to become a "good meditator." Finally, it is useful to be explicit in telling clients that, although it is called a "3-Minute" exercise, they do not need to practice it with a stop watch! The idea is to practice each of the three steps, without worrying about the exact amount of time involved.

Although increased awareness is the foundation of decentering, concurrent consideration of the attitude one brings to what is observed in meditation is critical. While not often thought of in this way, it is actually very possible (and I would venture even common, at least for beginning meditators) to use this technique as another form of ammunition toward oneself: whether it be by berating a wandering mind, to view the thoughts and/or feelings one has with a sense of harshness or self-criticism, to engage in rumination (perhaps under the guise of "observing" experience), or even to use meditation as a form of suppression (i.e., in not wanting to feel something, conveniently using the technique of returning to the breath to "not go there," to stop the feeling from being present). As an example of suppression creeping into the technique, the thought might come up "I don't like this feeling of sadness" and then perhaps "let me return my awareness to my breathing," with the subtext being "so that I can make this feeling go away and distract myself with my breath." Alternatively, the thought might come up "I don't like this feeling of sadness," and underneath this, "let me breathe with this feeling, open to it, give it space," which entails a radically different approach of staying open to the difficulty (in the form of thoughts, emotions, sensations), and observing it with acceptance and kindness toward oneself. I hope I am making it clear here that awareness *without* the attitude of a nonjudgmental acceptance and kindness toward oneself is *not* mindfulness—the critical ingredient in mindfulness is self-compassion.

After guiding clients through each of the meditation practices, it is most helpful to keep the discussion during the ensuing guided inquiry as close as possible to the practice that has just ended (i.e., as opposed to clients' experiences with meditation in the past etc.). This models present-focused attention. Further, asking open-ended questions about the practice keeps the discussion grounded in moment-to-moment experience. It is important to always explicitly link the practice back to a connection with chronic pain and to discuss how it relates to pain coping. As discussed in detail in Chapter 3, the quality of the way in which you conduct the inquiry is central; as the therapist you need to embody and model a sense of curiosity, openness, and a nonjudgmental attentiveness to the feedback provided by clients. Your job is not to fix or problem solve, but to facilitate deeper exploration. Any difficulties, obstacles, or challenges that came up during the practice should also be discussed (e.g., "What, if any, difficulties or challenges did you experience?"). This is also an opportunity to increase motivation for participation and engagement, as well as to demonstrate the mindfulness model. For example, an inevitable perceived "difficulty" that will come up is mind wandering. Here, you might respond by reinforcing that just *noticing* that the mind has wandered is mindfulness itself, and is the practice. Even if we are only able to notice one time during the whole meditation period that our mind wandered (perhaps when we suddenly realize that the guided audio has stopped and we were thinking the whole time!), this one moment of awareness *is* mindfulness. I like to use the analogy that training our mind with meditation to be present in the moment is just like training a puppy to stay: it takes kindness, patience, and practice, and gradually the puppy learns to flexibly follow your instruction and to stay. The troubleshooting section following Session 2 covers in more detail many of the most common experiences that clients will report with meditation, and how you might approach exploring these experiences in the guided inquiry.

Note

1 Adapted from Segal, Williams, and Teasdale (2013).

Reference

Segal, Z. V., Williams, J. M. G., & Teasdale, J. D. (2013). *Mindfulness-based cognitive therapy for depression*. New York, NY: Guilford.

6

Session 2: Facing the Challenge

Therapist Introduction

We start this session by returning to the Body Scan, to shift clients from "doing" mode to "being" mode. A guided inquiry following this practice is then used to transition to a discussion of the at-home formal and informal practices (as usually there is a lot of overlap in the difficulties reported for the two), and although experience will be varied, it is important to explicitly discuss any challenges that clients faced during the week (e.g., pain as a distraction, finding time to practice). A key element to this discussion of their practice is for you to bring a nonjudgmental, open curiosity to client's experiences, and to guide them to explore the themes that came up during the week (as it is likely they will be recurring) with those same qualities.

Another focus of this session is to continue to enhance the client's awareness of the connection between their thoughts, pain, and functioning through CBT-oriented exercises. The second half of the session includes a brief thoughts and feelings exercise that illustrates how we typically see our thoughts as the truth, and how our judgments of situations colour how we perceive those situations. Discussion of this exercise segues to the connection between stress and pain, and how an essential first step in breaking the stress–pain cycle is increasing our awareness. To further build awareness of the connection between how we judge experience and how we feel, the Pleasant Experiences Diary is introduced as a take-home activity—this also tunes clients into noticing any "good things" that might be present in their day-to-day experience, even if only small. The session concludes with a 10-min breath-focused seated meditation.

Mindfulness-Based Cognitive Therapy for Chronic Pain: A Clinical Manual and Guide,
First Edition. Melissa A. Day.

Companion website: www.wiley.com/go/day/mindfulness_based_cognitive_therapy

Therapist Outline

Assessment Measures

Have clients fill out the assessment measures. Provide assistance as needed.

Orientation

Welcome back! We appreciate that you are willing to experiment with this process and to see what happens with the group sessions and the daily practice.

Theme

Today we are going to practice meditation together and further explore the connection between our thoughts, emotions, and pain. We will also have an extended discussion about your at-home practice during the week. Let's start the session today by doing a Body Scan meditation, which will help shift us from all the "doing" that we're used to, into a mode of just "being."

Body Scan practice: *Lead the group through the Body Scan meditation; see Appendix B on the website for a script for this meditation.*

Guided Inquiry

- What did you notice during that practice?
- How was taking this time for your body in this way different from the time you would normally take for your body?
- In what ways do you think this practice relates to living with chronic pain?

Guided inquiry of experience with at-home practice: *Body Scan, 3-Minute Breathing Space, Routine Activity, Mindful Eating, Client's Report Handouts. Review practice logs and make copies if part of a research project (i.e., to track treatment dose).*

- Now let's move on to a discussion of your at-home practice. What was that experience like for you?
- How was engaging in the 3-Minute Breathing Space different from the longer sitting practice?
- What challenges did you experience? How might you overcome them?

Breathing Space practice: As a means to anchor us back in the present, let's practice a 3-Minute Breathing Space. *Lead the group through the 3-Minute Breathing Space meditation; see Appendix B on the website for a script.*

Guided Inquiry

- What did you notice with that brief practice? (*Depending on time, you may wish to further this discussion, inquiring into how this was different from how we might typically spend a spare 3 min, and/or how this practice relates to living with chronic pain.*)

Exploring the Thoughts and Feelings Connection

We are going to experiment with a somewhat different exercise now from what we have done so far. Settle into a comfortable seated position, and once you feel reasonably settled, close your eyes and imagine the following scenario:

You receive an invitation to attend a party that will be held at a local restaurant this Thursday evening. As you are imagining this scenario, become aware of what is going through your mind, including any thoughts, and what feelings, or bodily sensations you may have.

Now open your eyes, and when you are ready, describe to the group any feelings or bodily sensations you experienced and any thoughts or images that went through your mind (*list on the flip chart, note if it is a thought, feeling, or sensation in the body*).

What we see here from all these responses on the flip chart is that we are all judging and interpreting this same event differently, through our own particular lens, and closely following on the heels of that are all these different feelings and changes in the body. Some of you saw this invitation as a welcome opportunity to socialize and have fun, and described feeling a sense of eager anticipation. And if the invitation was seen as another strain on your schedule and one more thing to add to your busy life, along with that we see this sense of anxiety or irritation arising.

What's interesting is that we believe our thoughts—we view them as the Truth—but, the truth usually only has one version. Given all these different interpretations of the same event, we see that neither one of them can be absolutely certain. By noticing all the different versions and interpretations we have listed here, it is easy to see that our appraisals of the situation and judgments of events (and the feelings they evoke) reflect what we bring to them as much as the "objective" situation does. What effect do you see each of these ways of thinking likely having on your experience of painful sensations? *Discuss.*

It is important to note that the body doesn't know the difference between a thought and external reality—the body doesn't have the innate intelligence of mind to just label thoughts as thinking—so the body reacts to all thoughts as if they are actually happening. When we perceive something as a threat, our body gears up as if it is about to fight off a lion! As this exercise shows, our emotions and even body sensations are often powerfully determined by our interpretations of events and our thoughts that spin off that interpretation. The event in this exercise was neither inherently good nor bad—it was neutral. But depending on how you interpreted the event, this powerfully influences what happens next. So what we are learning to do is to become more aware of these intervening automatic appraisals, judgments, and thoughts.

The Stress–Pain Thermometer: "Hot" Thoughts Raise the Temperature

The exercise we just completed demonstrates that our emotions, and even our sense of physical well-being, are consequences of a situation plus an interpretation, appraisal, or judgment. How we judge a situation (and then react) is more important than the actual situation. But often our thoughts are happening below the surface, and we are not aware of what we are telling ourselves or when our tension and stress levels may be on the rise. How does this impact your pain you may wonder? Well, a big part of how our thoughts influence our pain is through initiating and maintaining a prolonged stress response that opens the pain gates.

Introducing the Stress–Pain Connection

It should be said that not all stress is inherently bad; indeed, stress is a natural part of life and in "balanced" doses, leads to optimal performance. However, long-term stress, as is often the case in chronic pain, has a harmful effect on our well-being. When we have chronic pain, this often puts us "on edge" and produces a prolonged stress response that feeds back around and produces even more pain, creating a vicious cycle. Breaking this stress–pain cycle and learning skills to lower the stress–pain thermometer improves your pain.

What is the Stress Response?

The stress response is a four-part reaction to something (a situation/event, emotion, physical feeling) that people think they cannot cope with, and which taxes their resources. These are the four parts of the reaction *(ask clients for examples under each of these components and list on a flip chart)*:

1) *Physical/biological reactions*: examples include increased blood pressure, muscle tension, stress hormones, lowered immune response.
2) *Feelings/emotions*: examples include anxiety, sadness, anger, embarrassment, shame, depression.
3) *Behavior/what you do*: examples include withdrawing, underdoing or over-doing with activity, lashing out at other people.
4) *Cognitive/your thoughts*: examples include trouble thinking/concentrating, difficulty making decisions, thoughts and images about the event and about the self and other people.

Anything that triggers these reactions and the stress response is a "stressor." Chronic pain itself can be a major on-going stressor. Sometimes we are not even aware that we are having these reactions and that the stress–pain thermometer is rising; it might be that we finally notice how others are reacting to us, and this is what lets us know we are stressed. Physical changes, emotions, behaviors, and thoughts can all be (nonpain) stressors that can trigger pain flare-ups.

Research shows that, a lot of the time, we react to stressful events or feelings by labeling them as a threat, a loss, or a challenge. Once we label something as a threat, loss, or challenge, that judgment of "good" or "bad" triggers the mind to get swept away in thoughts and emotions. Becoming more fully aware of the way a situation is classified by the mind as "pleasant" or "stressful" takes practice.

Introduce the ABC Cognitive Model

Often we find ourselves in a situation (A), perhaps a traffic jam, for example, when we need to get across to the other side of town for an appointment, and at some point we become aware of feeling a certain way (C), perhaps anxiety at running late, or anger toward other drivers, or perhaps muscle tension as we grip the steering wheel, or perhaps increased pain. Usually, we are most aware of the feelings. Often, we are not aware of a thought that links the situation and the feeling (B), perhaps "My doctor is not going to see me if I am late, and I am going to have to wait a whole more two months for another appointment…" *It helps to use the flip chart with this example, writing A (and the example), then C (and the example), then inserting B.*

This is called the ABC model. Most often we find ourselves in a situation, the "activating event" or "antecedent" (A), and then end up with a feeling, the "consequence" (C), and we are not usually aware of the powerful role of thinking that connects the two, our "beliefs" (B). Often thoughts are just neutral, like "what's for dinner?" You can think of these sorts of thoughts as "cold cognitions" that don't raise the stress–pain thermometer. "Hot cognitions," however, are those thoughts and beliefs that really grab you and that raise the stress–pain thermometer. Hot thoughts actually drive the emotions we feel, and how strongly we feel them and also contribute to our experience of painful sensations in the body. When we are stressed and in pain, we tend to have more "hot cognitions" more often, which continues to feed into the stress–pain cycle. This connection between stress, pain, and automatic appraisals or judgments is also sometimes referred to as the stress–pain–appraisal connection.

Automatic "hot thoughts" have powerful effects on your chronic pain by drawing your attention to the pain to the point where it becomes hard to think of anything *but* the pain. When your mind is caught up in the pain it can lead you to feel helpless and overwhelmed, which feeds in to more "hot thoughts" such as the pain is "ruining my life," and "it is unbearable." One automatic thought that is a "frequent flier" for many people with chronic pain is the thought that because of their pain they are no longer "whole," or they are "disabled," "worthless," or "dysfunctional" in some way. However, if you think about your entire body and how many things have to work right just to breathe, and eat, remove waste etc., you might come to realize that there is more right with your body than wrong with it.

Noticing these hot thoughts and judgments is important, but it is not what we typically do—usually they happen quite automatically, without us even realizing that we are getting carried away by them. One minute we are thinking about the upcoming party and the next minute we are feeling anxious and overwhelmed with life's demands … and having greater pain. As we saw with the party scenario just before though, our judgments of the same situation vary amongst us and also over time (e.g., with changes in mood or pain); this provides further evidence that *thoughts are not facts.*

Catching and skillfully responding to hot thoughts and judgments are easier if we spot them early in the process of their unfolding. By learning to be aware of these automatic thoughts, we become more skilled at not being swept away by the flood of our emotions. Also, just as we learned in the raisin exercise, we may begin to notice new things about our thoughts and feelings that we had not seen before. In this way, the "C" in the ABC model can be shifted from "consequence" to "choice." With awareness, we can then *choose* how to respond, gaining freedom from reflexive automatic reactions. This is what we are going to continue to work with and develop throughout this program.

Mindfulness of Pleasant Experiences

Chronic pain can oftentimes consume all available mental resources; it's almost like the pain and stress puts the blinders on and many people with chronic pain can become so focused on the pain that they are no longer fully aware of what is happening outside of their pain. The pain and the stress in their lives trap their mind in a sense, locking it onto the pain, and the simple things in life, the little things that bring pleasure, may be overlooked or not even acknowledged in awareness. This next exercise is intended to guide your attention toward awareness of pleasant experiences (no matter how big or small)—those things that bring a smile to your face, warm your heart, bring you some sense of gladness. Bringing our awareness to pleasant experiences, however, is sometimes enough to break the stress–pain cycle.

As we have been learning today, usually the process of judging something as "pleasant" or "unpleasant" happens automatically, and without this awareness we are swept away in a sea of emotions and thoughts that go along with that first judgment; so intentionally bringing awareness to the mind classifying something as pleasant takes practice. As part of this practice, this week we are inviting you to intentionally bring awareness to at least one thing you experience as pleasant each day (and preferably by noticing that you are experiencing it as pleasant as it is happening in the moment). Included in your handouts this week is the Pleasant Experiences Diary, which has spaces in it each day to write down, as closely as possible in time to any pleasant experience, the thoughts, feelings, and body sensations that accompany the event. It can sometimes be difficult to distinguish between thoughts and emotions; one way to think of it is that emotions can usually be described in one word, whereas thoughts take more than one word to describe. It can be helpful to write down thoughts as though they were spoken out loud. Explore and describe the emotions and feelings in the body that arise with as much detail as possible; this helps you to really closely examine how you are relating to the pleasant experience.

Brief Breath-Focused Seated Meditation

In our last practice today we are going to engage in a brief breath-focused meditation. As we have been exploring in working with the 3-Minute Breathing Space, bringing our awareness to the movements of the breath can be a useful tool for tuning into our experience and for settling our mind by anchoring it on just one thing: the breath. We are going to continue to explore this throughout the program. *Guide participants in a brief, 10-min meditation of their breath, first with instruction on posture, and then guiding them to tune into the movement of the breath, noticing and labeling thoughts as "thinking" and guiding awareness back to the breath. See the breathing space transcript in Appendix B on the website for suggestions on guiding this practice.*

At-Home Daily Practice

During the coming week, your daily at-home practice, as shown in your handouts, will be… *Go over client handout describing at-home practice following Session 2.*

Distribute Session 2 client handouts.

Summary

What we have been learning today is that… *Go over the client summary handout: "Facing the Challenge."*

Client Handbook

Session 2 Summary: Facing the Challenge

The skills you are practicing train the mind to step out of automatic pilot and into awareness of the present moment. One of the most typical ways we get hooked and taken out of the "now" is our basic tendency to want things to be other than they are, to make an automatic judgment of "things not being okay" in some way, shape, or form, which raises our stress–pain thermometer. Stress arises when we resist our direct experience, judging whatever is happening as "too much," "not fine," "unacceptable."

When our mind trails off in such directions, we are more likely to behave in automatic, habitual ways and, in doing this, we have closed the door on *choosing* if that is indeed what we want to do and whether it is the most helpful thing to do given the circumstances.

With practice (meditation practice, that is), we learn to slow down this chain reaction, to observe what is happening, and to hold it all in nonjudgmental awareness. With this awareness, we find we have a choice and this frees us from old mental and emotional "hooks" that grab us and take us along on a ride—we learn to *respond* rather than *react*. We might also begin to notice little things in our life that bring a smile to our face, warm our heart, and bring some sense of gladness.

The Body Scan meditation you will be working with again this week cultivates the capacity of our mind to be with experience just as it is, letting go of the need to change or fix things. Our task is to bring a friendly curiosity to exploring what is present, whether that be happiness or sadness, calm or wandering mind, tension or no tension, pain or no pain.

Pleasant Experiences Diary

Practice noticing a pleasant experience *as it is happening* in the moment. Use this handout to guide your awareness to take stock of what the pleasant experience is, and how you are reacting to this event in your body, emotions, and mind as it is happening. Fill this diary out as close to the event as you can.

What was the pleasant experience?	Describe in detail what sensations were present in your body during this experience	What moods/ emotions did you notice arising?	What thoughts were present?	What are you thinking as you write about this experience now?
Example. *Being warm, sitting inside listening to the rain gently landing on the tin roof, while I read my book.*	*My brow is smooth, unfurrowed, the muscles in my neck feel loose and relaxed, and a soft smile rests on my face.*	*A sense of ease, calm, grateful for being inside in the warm.*	*"This feels good." "I could stay here like this all day."*	*It was such a simple thing, but in being aware as it was happening I was able to really savor it.*

Source: Adapted from Segal, Williams, and Teasdale, 2013.

At-Home Daily Practice for Following Session 2

1) Practice with the Body Scan guided meditation audio each day. Again, letting go of any expectations or judgments about how you might feel during or after this practice, and just let your experience each day *be* your experience.
2) Engage in at least three short 3-Minute Breathing Spaces every day at set times that you have decided in advance.
3) Practice mindfulness of your breath for 10 to 15 min each day. Remember, just as in the Breathing Space, it helps to take on a dignified sitting posture and to remind yourself that there is no need to control the breath in any way; no need to do, fix, or change anything—the idea is to simply rest your awareness on the movements of your breath.
4) Complete one entry each day in your Pleasant Experiences Diary. This activity hones your awareness of those little (or perhaps big!) things in life that, when noticed, might bring you a sense of ease, joy, calmness, happiness, or otherwise pleasant experience. It helps to make these entries as close to the event as you can and record in detail your reactions, noting the precise thoughts and images that came to mind, and the exact location and nature of changes in your body.
5) Practice bringing present-moment awareness to one new everyday, routine activity such as washing your face, getting dressed, grocery shopping, washing dishes … any activity at all you can use as a means to practice, simply knowing what you are doing as you are doing it.
6) Complete your daily at-home practice record; it helps to fill this in as close to finishing your practice as possible. Make note in the comment box of anything that comes up in the at-home practice so that we can talk about it at the next meeting.

Therapist Tips, Troubleshooting, and Supervision for Session 2

Discussion of the Experiences with Practicing Mindfulness

In the guided inquiry regarding clients' in-session and at-home practice there are some common recurring difficulties that at least some clients will report. Although primarily our response here is to nonjudgmentally guide clients to explore their experience (as opposed to jumping into problem solving mode), for troubleshooting purposes, here are some example ways that you as the therapist may choose to respond following/during this inquiry while embodying the core principles of mindfulness. The idea here is not for you to "memorize" these example responses, but simply to be familiar with them, letting the theme of these responses be in the back of your mind as you lead the guided inquiry. Of course, not every form of client response is possible to cover here, however Segal, Williams, and Teasdale (2002, 2013) offer further excellent examples, and Dr. Richard Sears has written an informative book that includes transcripts from his MBCT sessions and is a further valuable resource (Sears, 2015).

Also, remember, first and foremost, *we use open-ended questions to guide client's self-exploration of their experience,* and the three basic questions included in the manual within the guided inquiry sections are only a starting point, and should not be mechanically followed. Following up (i.e., inquiring into what thoughts, emotions, reactions arose in the context of experience) and reflecting what clients share as their experience is the essence of the inquiry; although it is often not possible to get to every experience, so sometimes a simple "thank you" is enough. As in motivational interviewing, there are a number of reflections possible (reflection of feelings, thoughts, content, underlying meaning etc.), and around particularly sensitive topics, asking permission to explore further is recommended. In exploring experience this way, and in using the guided inquiry to contextualize and relate clients' experience back to pain, it is then sometimes useful to provide teaching to further facilitate clients making these connections. So, the examples that follow are intended to be possible "teaching" responses that arise and follow on from such exploration—not to replace it.

Pain was Distracting

Some participants might report they had difficulty with the meditation as their mind kept getting pulled away from the technique to a painful sensation calling for their attention.

Possible Therapist Teaching Response

> When we engage in mindfulness practice, we may likely become more aware of bodily sensations, like an itch, twitch, tightness ... that we weren't necessarily as aware of before practicing. And many people who live with chronic pain find that painful sensations often have a particularly strong pull on our attention. It may be helpful to approach this with the same

> basic instruction as you approach your mind wandering to any other experience: to nonjudgmentally acknowledge that your mind has wandered, to perhaps gently label what is calling for your attention, "Ahh, there's tension and irritation," and then to patiently escort your attention back to scanning the body. If you choose, you might also like to mindfully make any adjustments to your posture that would make you feel more comfortable; so first being aware of the urge to shift your position, then aware of the intention to make an adjustment of whatever form, and then mindfully making whatever adjustment you need to be kind to yourself, and then simply returning back to the Body Scan. And when you do move through the problem area during the Body Scan practice, just experimenting with relating to that area just as you would any other part of the body, exploring what sensations are present, breathing into them on the inbreath, and breathing back out from them on the outbreath as you soften and relax your body. Nonjudgmentally aware of any thoughts or emotions that arise, acknowledging those too, without needing for your experience to be other than it is. And then gently letting go when it becomes time to move your awareness to the next region of the body.

In some instances clients may report that the pain was so intense that it was "impossible" to focus on anything but the pain.

Possible Therapist Teaching Response

> During times of intense pain when you find you mind is "captured" by the pain, the practice is to let go of resistance to the pain. So at times of a severe pain flare-up, let go of the Body Scan practice (turning off the guided audio if you are listening to it), and rather than thinking *about* the pain, bring an open awareness and curiosity *into* the painful sensations that arise: Is it hot? Cold? Burning? Tingling? Sharp? Dull? What is underneath and beyond this label of "pain?" Rather than forcing yourself to attempt to stick to the instructions on the guided audio, let your attention go deeply into the region of greatest intensity. Breathe into and out from the pain itself. Imagine or feel the breath going deeper and deeper into the pain, breathing into it on the inbreath, and breathing back out, ventilating that region on the outbreath. As you do this, pay close attention to any subtle changes in the quality of the sensation. As best you can, letting go of any expectations or hopes that this will alleviate the intensity of the pain in some way (this may or may not happen), and just bringing a sense of open, gentle attention to the sensations, and in this way, perhaps becoming aware of fluctuations in the sensation that you hadn't noticed before. Just breathing with the sensations. And if it becomes too intense, perhaps choosing to work just at the edges of the sensation, without going all the way into it; moving closer, or giving it space and moving back away from that edge, breathing, and then perhaps gently approaching once more… And if you find that after a time the grip of the pain on your attention has loosened somewhat, then perhaps choosing to gently return back to the Body Scan meditation.

Why Would I Want to be Mindful of Pain?

The natural response to pain is aversion; we want to get rid of it, so being mindful and open to the pain is a radically different approach and most likely at least one client will have the thought, "Why am I doing this? I don't want to observe the pain, I just want it gone."

Possible Therapist Teaching Response

> It is often the case that people doing this program wonder "Why on earth would anyone want to pay attention to pain?" The more typical response is loathing the pain and just wanting it to go away, with a strong preference to attempt to ignore the pain, distract yourself from it, or "just push through." This may work for a little while, but not always and not particularly well for very long; chronic pain has a habit of sticking around and sometimes the pain may be so intense that you can't just take your mind off it. At those times, it is helpful to have another approach that you can use, besides just enduring it or depending on pain medications. And even if you can successfully use distraction as a way to alleviate your pain, experimenting with this approach of mindfully *entering into* pain, might lead to new levels of understanding about your body, possible triggers, and places of "holding"—something distraction can never do. This will move you in the direction of learning how to live with pain, not just get through it. Sometimes though, it's a balancing act between going into the pain, and getting completely overwhelmed by it. This is where the kindness component of mindfulness is so important. Having a certain lightness of touch, touching in with pain, working at that edge, and then returning back to the object of meditation may provide another way to steady yourself and not be "blown away" by the pain.

I Don't Understand the Point of This

The idea of letting go of expectations and goals, and of striving to find a "solution" to the problem of pain seems like a foreign concept to many clients.

Possible Therapist Teaching Response

> The idea that there are no goals with the meditation practice may seem like a strange concept. You may well ask, "Why bother practicing this meditation every day if there is nothing I can expect to get out of it?" As you have likely experienced for yourself from time to time, attempting to fix, change, or escape pain takes a great deal of effort and energy; the notion of nonstriving is to let go of these efforts, efforts that, in the context of chronic pain, typically do not result in any long-term solutions and just add baggage to the pain in the form of thoughts, emotions, and unhelpful behaviors. Moreover, what gets lost in striving for whatever it might be that you set your mind to is what is already available to us in the present moment. Expectations and striving in a sense place boundaries around what is possible, whereas nonstriving attentiveness opens us up to explore what *is* possible and available to us in this moment. Striving for any one thing in particular drains our

inherent capacity to learn, grow, change, and tune into what is available to us. And what is available, when you tune in with mindfulness, may surprise you! The idea is to stick with the practice daily, and to see what form "progress" takes with this fresh type of "effortless effort" that comes with settling into the present, without aiming to achieve anything in particular.

Strong Emotions Arise During Meditation

When we finally slow down and just sit with ourselves in meditation and stay open to our experience, clients may find that this "opens the flood gates" and suppressed emotions and strong feelings may bubble up to the surface. For clients with comorbid post-traumatic stress symptoms, this often comes up when they bring attention to a particular part of the body in the Body Scan.

Possible Therapist Teaching Response

> When we feel strong emotions, particularly when the emotion is unpleasant in some way, our automatic tendency is to want to *do* something about it, to "fix it" or change it in some way. What we are inviting you to experience in meditation is a different way of *responding* to the feeling, vs. having a kneejerk *reaction,* which only adds to stress and pain. Instead of fighting *against* the strong emotion, pushing it away or wanting it to be different, what we are inviting you to experiment with here is working *with* it, by holding it mindfully in awareness without having to act on it. We can say to ourselves: "Oh, anger is here" rather than adding to the anger with "I am really fed up with this pain and what it's done to me," or "Here is fear" rather than adding baggage in the form of something along the lines of "I am terrified that if I fall I will be an invalid," or "Here is vulnerability" rather than closing in around that and covering it over with "I am so weak and useless." Our task remains the same, simply to notice what arises, gently and with kindness to label it, and as best you can, to guide your awareness back to the object of meditation.

There will be occasions when clients will report that the emotion was too overwhelming for them to effectively implement this technique. Although later in the program (once the mind is more stabilized in meditation) we will be teaching a practice specifically to work with such difficult emotions, another option here would be to suggest (just as with the example of when pain was too overwhelming) that the client gently bring their awareness into the emotion, breathing with it, ventilating it.

Possible Therapist Teaching Response

> If it seems you are overwhelmed by the emotion and are so caught up that it feels your mind is hostage to the emotion, and you just cannot seem to guide your mind back to the Body Scan, instead of resisting your experience, dip your toe in, so to speak, and breathe with it. Breathing into the emotion on the inbreath, and breathing back out from it on the outbreath ... and if at any point this feels too much, being kind to yourself

> and resting your attention fully on the breath as it enters and leaves your body ... anchoring your awareness firmly on the breath ... and as you feel reasonably settled, simply returning back to the Body Scan practice. When we can be with emotions in this way, we no longer identify with them—they are present, but they are not all defining.

No "Ideal" Place to Practice

Many of us have an image in our mind of what meditation "should" be—quiet, calm, uninterrupted by external noises, events, or circumstances. However, such ideals are usually not compatible with our actual experience and if we keep waiting for these ideal circumstances then this typically turns into a barrier to regular practice.

Possible Therapist Teaching Response

> It is natural that we have a sense of what an "ideal" environment for meditation might look like: quiet, comfortable temperature, no other place we need to be... And then the phone rings, our partner yells out our name looking for us, someone knocks at the door, the thought: "Did I remember to turn the oven off?" This may upset us or have an impact on us in some way or another. However, unexpected distractions and imperfect circumstances make for a great opportunity to see what we do when things don't go as planned. When conditions are not what we want them to be, an experiment you might like to try is to bring a sense of curiosity to what happens next? Do we spin off? Do we prematurely end our practice? Do we persist practicing but then hold onto a grudge after the practice ends? Isn't it funny how all this happens because we have an idea of what and how things should be. We can use this experience itself as a part of the exercise of mindfulness. Distractions are noted as a part of our experience, "Ah, dog barking across the street" and then any need for conditions to be other than they are is simply let go ... over and over again if need be.

"Lack of Time" as a Barrier

This challenge will always come up. It is human nature to have difficulty changing habits, and introducing mindfulness practice for most of us represents a significant shift in how we habitually go about our days, and inevitably some patients will report they did not do the meditation practice. It helps to provide "tough love" in responding to this, as learning by doing is at the heart of this program. Be firm but nonjudgmental, encourage clients who have difficulty doing the homework to see this also as an opportunity to bring a sense of curiosity to this experience.

Possible Therapist Teaching Response

> What we have found is that it really helps to find a regular time each day for your meditation practice; in doing it at the same time each day, meditation practice will itself become a habit, and a healthy one! (*Explore with clients when might be a good time of day for them.*) And if from time to time you still find yourself battling with your alarm clock, and the warmth of a

> comfortable bed is seductively winning out over getting up to meditate, why not just meditate in bed? You are lying there observing your mental dialogue anyway: "I need to get up and meditate, but I am so tired and ooooh it is so nice just lying here ... but I *should* get up..." So why not shift that experience ever so slightly and bring to that a quality of mindfulness and practice on the spot? There is nothing special about practicing on a mat, meditation cushion, or in a certain location. The key point with this program, though, is that you will really get out of it what you put into it; the approach we are exploring is to learn by doing, and in order to learn we need to do.

Fell Asleep or Found it Relaxing

For some people the Body Scan may make them fall asleep, and they might welcome that as for many people with chronic pain, getting to sleep can often be difficult. Similarly, another "positive" may be that clients report feeling more relaxed after the Body Scan. "Positive" responses are not necessarily problematic in their own right, however often what comes with such responses is a sense that "Yes, I got it right! It worked!" and then the next time, when relaxation doesn't happen: "Arghhh, why can't I do it right?!" So we train in nonjudgmentally noticing these "positive" experiences, and return to approach the practice with an attitude of nonstriving.

Possible Therapist Teaching Response

> Isn't that interesting? As you continue to practice, we hope that this skill will actually train you to "wake up" to what is present, in your body, emotions, and mind-state. So while it's no problem that you found it relaxing and fell asleep, perhaps it is useful to remind ourselves that the practice is to train the mind in alert attentiveness, to train in simply observing what happens with gentleness and acceptance. If you sit down to practice mindfulness and you think, "I am going to feel relaxed" or "This is going to take my pain away" or "make me sleep" or "make me a better person," then you have raised the idea to yourself that this is what you *should* achieve, which sets limits on what may actually be achievable. And along with that, is the idea that how you are right now is not okay in some way and needs to change. Holding the thought of "not being okay" is a trap that limits you from getting the most out of your life. The idea is to bring a nonjudgmental, open curiosity to each practice, as it is likely that each time you practice your experience will be unique. Whatever happens, the practice is to simply just be aware of it and accept it as your experience in this moment, without needing it to *be* anything in particular.

I can't do it Right, I am a Bad Meditator

Again, most of us have some idea of what meditation *should* look like—ideas such as emptying the mind, switching it off, or achieving some special state—and when we have a meditation period where we were just thinking, thinking, thinking ... lost in discursive thought the whole time, a common response is to feel like "I blew it!"

Possible Therapist Teaching Response

> Just noticing the tendencies of our mind, and even now, that you have noticed this thought "I am a bad meditator"—that is the practice itself! We train in becoming more aware more often. So as best you can, begin to let go of ideas of "success" or "failure" or "doing it right" and just stick with it. As long as you are practicing the mindfulness exercises regularly, with an attitude of curiosity and openness to your experiences, you are doing it right.

Mind Wandering

Many of the above challenges are actually various forms of mind wandering—an inevitable, and indeed essential, part of the mindfulness practice—that takes on many subtle and often disguised forms.

Possible Therapist Teaching Response

> Mind wandering is no problem: it is what minds do, whether during or outside of meditation practice, our minds tend to drift, skip, or race along, even in our sleep our minds are still actively dreaming! In practicing meditation, however, you are training in becoming more aware of this running internal stream of commentary, and this noticing *is* the practice; this is mindfulness itself. It is actually a sign that the observer quality of your mind is waking up, so the fact that you are aware that you were often thinking in meditation is very good news! Left unchecked, thoughts can quickly build momentum, increasing our stress and pain and controlling how we react to life's circumstances. Even long-term meditators report having thoughts passing through their minds much of the time; the difference is they get "hooked" by the content of the thoughts far less often, and are able to let the thoughts just pass through. So we practice in noticing when our mind wanders and with gentleness and kindness toward ourselves, we return, over and over again, back to the object of meditation. And if our experience is "struggling" to maintain this awareness, we can notice this sense of struggle as simply another feeling, and we note that, and return back to our object of meditation.

Thoughts and Feelings and the Stress–Pain Thermometer

For those of you who are therapists trained in CBT for pain, the cognitive exercises of this session likely feel highly familiar. The thoughts and feelings exercise provides an opportunity for experiential learning of the role our thoughts and judgments play in powerfully determining how we relate to the circumstances in which we find ourselves. This learning is then further bolstered by a (ideally) highly interactive discussion of the stress–pain–appraisal connection and the associated ABC model. A key difference in delivering these exercises from an MBCT theoretical framework, in comparison to in traditional CBT, is that stress, "negative" thoughts, and emotions are not inherently in need of *changing*; the focus of these exercises is simply on enhancing *awareness* of stress and automatic "hot" cognitions.

The Pleasant Experiences Diary

The Pleasant Experiences Diary is also included this week in clients' at-home activities. This activity reinforces the idea that how we think about and view our experiences influences our body, mood, and later subsequent thoughts. The idea of this exercise, unlike in CBT, is not to *schedule* pleasant events, rather at this stage in the program, the intention is simply to enhance our awareness. It is helpful to go over the example included on this handout in session, and to allow time for clients to ask any questions. We will return to this handout in Session 7 as a means to help clients identify activities, practices, and experiences that are nourishing, pleasant, and/or provide a sense of mastery, to foster self-care and work toward developing a relapse prevention plan.

Brief Breath-Focused Seated Meditation

The final practice in Session 2 is a 10-min breath-focused seated meditation, which is also assigned as a take-home activity. This practice is intended to ease the transition to engaging in an extended seated meditation in Session 3 by providing clients with the opportunity to practice with just one object of meditation, the movements of the breath. When awareness drifts away from the breath to thoughts, emotions, physical sensations, or anything else, the practice (as in the Body Scan) is simply to notice this, perhaps nonjudgmentally label it, and then as many times as the mind wanders, patiently and with kindness, bring the attention back to the breath.

References

Sears, R. W. (2015). *Building competence in mindfulness-based cognitive therapy*. New York, NY: Routledge.

Segal, Z., Williams, J. M., & Teasdale, J. (2002). *Mindfulness-based cognitive therapy for depression: A new approach to preventing relapse*. New York, NY: Guilford Press.

Segal, Z. V., Williams, J. M. G., & Teasdale, J. D. (2013). *Mindfulness-based cognitive therapy for depression*. New York, NY: Guilford.

7

Session 3: The Breath as an Anchor

Therapist Introduction

After a brief orientation to the key themes of Session 3, the first practice is introduced, which is a brief, 5-min "seeing" meditation (if there is a window in the therapy space available) or "hearing" meditation (if no window is available). This exercise generalizes the training in mindfulness to our everyday, automatic perceptive experience to enhance the observer capacity of our mind to learn to step out of automatic thinking and into awareness. The breath is then introduced as a powerful anchor to the present, and this is reinforced with the first Seated Meditation of the program, with a breath and body focus. Built into this Seated Meditation practice is instruction on how to stay with difficult physical sensations (such as pain, or an urge to readjust one's position), and the breath is used as a supportive anchor in working with uncomfortable sensations in this way; this activity is assigned for at-home practice.

Following the guided inquiry of the in-session Seated Meditation practice, the discussion is expanded outwards to include also a discussion of clients' experiences with their at-home practice, including with the Pleasant Experiences Diary. This exercise is then built on with the Stressful Experiences Diary, which will be assigned for at-home practice. Session 3 is typically a time when initial enthusiasm may be wearing off, and clients are coming to realize that mindfulness is not a quick fix solution; thus, during the discussion of homework it is important to inquire about challenges and to encourage steadfastness with daily practice.

Mindfulness-Based Cognitive Therapy for Chronic Pain: A Clinical Manual and Guide,
First Edition. Melissa A. Day.

Companion website: www.wiley.com/go/day/mindfulness_based_cognitive_therapy

Therapist Outline

Assessment Measures

Have clients fill out the Assessment Measures. Provide assistance as needed.

Orientation

Our minds automatically parse the world into "good" and "bad," "right" and "wrong," "pleasant" and "unpleasant," "dangerous" and "safe," etc. The ability to use our mind to think, make judgments, and solve problems is a valuable part of our minds, and it helps us make sense of the world around us. It is natural for us to extend this to believe that thinking can also solve our pain, perhaps thinking "If I could just find the right doctor..." or some other solution-focused train of thought—with the clear end point being a desire to get rid of pain, unhappiness, suffering in a variety of forms, and to obtain perhaps a "pain-free" body and a lasting, unwavering sense of happiness. This drive to be "pain-free" and to escape unhappiness turns out to be a big problem for us, as it puts our mind into overdrive where it is constantly thinking, thinking, thinking ... and paradoxically, all those thoughts create more feelings and behaviors that are unhelpful because they simply spiral (usually downward) without producing the desired outcome.

The skills you are learning in this class provide you with the option of going beyond the automatic, problem solving approach and to experience and nurture a different mode of mind, one of *staying with the pain*. Letting go of extra baggage in terms of judgment or a need to urgently want to control or fix the pain, letting go of immediately wanting the pain to be other than it is. Bringing a sense of space to the situation by breathing with the tendency to want solutions to the "problem" of pain, we begin to see how much of what we do, how we feel, and what we think is motivated by a deep-seated need to avoid unpleasantness, and a strong desire to hold on to that which is pleasant. So we are training in bringing these powerful, automatic tendencies into conscious awareness, and are learning to gently pause, choosing to breathe with the difficulty. Over time and with patient practice, what we find is that this opens up space and choice, giving you options for how to respond wisely.

Theme

To step out of our usual striving, goal-oriented, problem solving tendencies, we need to find a balance between calmness and wakefulness. With a greater awareness of the patterns of our mind and its tendencies, learning to focus on one thing—your breath—supports a sense of feeling grounded and more focused.

Mindful Seeing (or Hearing)

As a way to generalize our practice further, and to sample additional ways of stepping out of unhelpful, analytical, or judgmental mind patterns, we are going to start today's session by experimenting with bringing awareness to one of our most basic senses that we rarely bring attention to, unless it gives us some difficulty or another: seeing/hearing. So we are going to take this most automatic of our senses, and see what happens when we bring a quality of mindfulness to the matter that constitutes the raw material of our day-to-day experience. *Lead the group through a 5-min awareness of sights (if a window is available) or sounds mindfulness exercise.*

Guided Inquiry

- What did you notice with that practice?
- How was this brief exercise different from how you might normally experience seeing/hearing?
- In what ways do you think this exercise relates to living with chronic pain?

Bringing Mindfulness to Breathing

Noticing changes in your breathing is a helpful way to get another perspective on how you are feeling. Has anyone noticed what happens to the breath when we are tense and in pain (*short and shallow, perhaps almost disappearing*), or when we are relaxed and happy (*slower and full*)? We can actually harness this awareness of changes in our breath as a way to help us notice any changes in our mood and how we feel, and to then use the breath to bring the mind and body back, anchored to a stable place. Usually we are not aware of our breathing, it is much like our vision (*or hearing*) that we experienced in that seeing (*or hearing*) exercise just now, or our heart beating, or our digestive system—it is just happening of its own accord, without our thinking about it. But when we tune into our breath, and become aware of it (which we can do at any time as it is always with us), we can create this stability in our mind, emotions, and body. Paying attention to your breathing doesn't mean that you need to control, slow down, deepen, or force the breath in any way: it just means paying *bare* attention.

The practice is to bring a light touch to being aware of the movements of the breath, the *feeling* of the breath moving into the body on each inbreath, and moving back out on each outbreath. And in doing this practice, we become increasingly more in tune with how our breath mirrors our mind, body, and mood state. With practice, we learn to use the breath as an anchor to the present. To harness the breath in this way, we practice precisely attending with a singular focus on the movements of the breath, and letting any arising distractions—whether they be thoughts, feelings, sensations—just come and go as they do without grasping or holding on to them. Just letting them pass through you, without hooking you and demanding attention. Over the course of our time together we will be exploring the ways we can harness the breath as a means to cope with pain and to anchor ourselves to the present moment.

The Breath as an Anchor

Tuning into the breath provides a way to switch gears and to move out of "doing" mode and into "being" mode. Mindfulness of the breath provides a way to ground yourself in the moment; it provides an anchor that will keep bringing you back to your moment-to-moment experience, steadying you. There are five key benefits to using the breath as your anchor, described in your handouts. *Go over the "The Benefits of Using the Breath as Your Anchor" handout.*

Seated Meditation practice, Mindfulness of the Breath and Body: *lead the group through the Mindfulness of the Breath and Body Seated Meditation, which has an emphasis on how to respond to uncomfortable sensations; see Appendix B on the website for a script.*

Guided Inquiry

- What did you notice during that practice? *If no one raises any difficulties, explicitly inquire:*
  - What, if any difficulties or challenges did you notice?
- How was bringing your awareness to your breath different from bringing your awareness to each part of the body, as you have been doing with the Body Scan?
- How do you think this practice relates to living with chronic pain?

Guided inquiry of experience with at-home practice: *Body Scan, 3-Minute Breathing Space, Routine Activity, The Pleasant Experiences Diary. Review practice logs and make copies if it is part of a research project (i.e., to track treatment dose).*

- Now let's move on to a discussion of your at-home practice. What was that experience like for you?
- How was taking this time for your body in this way different from the time you would normally take for your body?
- How was engaging in a routine activity in a mindful way different from your usual experience?
- Having experienced the daily practice for 2 weeks now, what thoughts do you have regarding how the Body Scan relates to living with chronic pain?
- What was the experience of filling out the Pleasant Experiences Diary like for you?

Give everyone the chance to reflect with each other on what happened when they tried to record such moments on the Pleasant Experiences Diary, and to record exactly the thoughts, emotions, and body sensations that occurred in the moments they describe. Record responses on the flip chart, differentiating between thoughts, bodily sensations, and emotions by listing them in separate columns.

Isn't it interesting how all these changes in emotion and body and thoughts spin off this initial judgment of something being pleasant? This is useful to notice as we can use these changes as "portals" into deeper awareness of how we are responding to experience—usually we are not aware of the subtle messages our body is sending us.

A common experience for people living with chronic pain who do this exercise is that they often say they are surprised to find there actually *is* something pleasant, no matter how big or small, that can be noticed and treasured each and every day, even if that something pleasant is only one dimension of something larger that might be a mix of experiences. Usually it is as though the pain and the stress and the depressed or irritable mood that often goes along with pain take over and we can't see past the pain, and pleasant moments go overlooked—unregistered in the pain landscape.

Something else to experiment with in doing this exercise is to pay particular attention when the pleasant event may be finishing: do you have a sense of "attachment" to the pleasant thoughts, feelings, and sensations? Wanting them to last? Stay the same? Perhaps you can also notice how this might be closely followed by aversion when it ends or changes (and along with this, a desire for things to be different from how they are), and then attachment again (when something else pleasant comes up) and then aversion all over again when that too does not last—over and over again—creating a vicious cycle.

The key to stepping out of this cycle is awareness. With awareness we won't get automatically swept away in a sea of thoughts and emotions that usually closely follow initial judgments of "pleasant," "unpleasant," and ensuing attachment and aversion. With awareness we are simply present with these judgments, holding them in awareness, and then mindfully *choosing* what, if any, action we may wish to respond with. With mindful awareness we learn to savor pleasant experiences as they are happening without feeling an overwhelming sadness when they shift; and when unpleasant experiences arise, we won't get swallowed up in them as we know those too, shall pass.

Breathing Space practice: The 3-Minute Breathing Space is an excellent way to check in throughout the day and see what thoughts might be present, and to observe whether the stress–pain thermometer might be rising. Let's practice that skill now. *Lead the group through the 3-Minute Breathing Space meditation; see Appendix B on the website for a script for this meditation.*

Guided Inquiry

- What did you notice with that brief practice? (*Depending on time, you may wish to further this discussion, inquiring into how this was different from how we might typically spend a spare 3 min, and/or how this practice relates to living with chronic pain.*)

Awareness of Stressful Experiences

Building on what we have been learning about the connection between our thoughts, judgments, emotions, body, and pain, part of your at-home practice following this session is to be aware of at least one stressful event that occurs each day (and preferably to become aware of it while it is occurring) and also of any triggers of "good" and "bad" labels.

You will see in your handouts a Stressful Experiences Diary, with spaces in it to write down, as closely as possible in time to any stressful event, the feelings, body sensations, and "hot" thoughts that accompany the event.

- It may be helpful to write any thoughts down as if they were spoken out loud, perhaps using quotation marks if that helps.
- Describe the feelings and body sensations in as much detail as you possibly can.

At-Home Daily Practice

During the coming week, your daily practice will be, as outlined in your handout… *Go over client handout describing at-home practice following Session 3. Distribute guided meditation audio files and Session 3 client handouts.*

Summary

What we have been learning today is that… *Go over client summary handout: "The Breath as an Anchor."*

Client Handbook

Session 3 Summary: The Breath as an Anchor

Returning your awareness back to the breath reconnects you with your immediate experience of this very moment—the *here and now*. Wherever you go, the breath will be there, so it is a portable tool that can be used as an anchor to stabilize your mind, no matter where you are. Simply bringing awareness to our anchor brings a sense of spaciousness to experience, allowing you to step back and to view things from a wider perspective.

Practicing meditation is like learning any new skill: it takes patient persistence, even during times of greatest pain and difficulty or when you might not be seeing quick "results," especially when you don't feel you are experiencing a reduction in pain. Unlike pain medication, when practicing meditation, you will not necessarily feel "immediate symptom relief." However, just as you need to *take* medication for it to benefit, so too do you need to *practice* meditation for it to do its work. Gradually, with patient persistence and kindness to yourself, you may be surprised to see what you do experience from meditation over the course of this program and beyond.

Mindfulness does not bulldoze through pain, or through resistance to practice. Slow and steady, working gently at the edges, not pushing too hard to break through. Letting go of the baggage you may have piled on top of the pain, in thoughts, emotions, baggage you no longer have to carry. Letting go, a little here, a little there, with gentleness, patience, kindness, and curiosity. Letting the breakthroughs happen on their own schedule, in good time.

The Benefits of Using the Breath as Your Anchor

There are five key benefits to using the breath as your anchor:

1) Breathing can't happen in the future. It can't happen in the past. It happens now. So focusing on the breath focuses you and grounds you in the now.
2) Wherever you go, your breath is always with you, so it is always available as a window into your emotions, physical sensations, and thoughts.
3) As we learned in the Gate Control Theory, the brain can only process so much at any given time—if mental resources are devoted to attending to the breath, this means fewer mental resources devoted to processing pain, which "closes the gates." This is not another clever problem solving approach though as we are not doing this to *tune out*, we are engaging in this practice to *tune in*.
4) Mindfulness of the breath embodies the nonstriving approach we are cultivating, with no goals to be achieved: you don't need to *do* anything for the breath to breathe itself. Attending to this breath, to this moment, has the potential to bring a quality of spaciousness to experience, to transform experience by letting go of the need to problem solve and "fix" or control it. Tuning in with this attitude of *allowing*—simply allowing the breath to do its thing—while you watch the process as an observer allows you to experience a wider approach on how you can respond to pain, strong emotions, and troublesome thoughts.
5) Finally, attending to the breath as an anchor to the present means that we won't get "hooked" by old unhelpful patterns of mind that lead to emotions such as anxiety, depression, and anger that make pain worse. Attending to the felt sensation of the breath allows us to catch ourselves when we are drifting into unhelpful mind patterns, and to flexibly shift our focus before we get hooked (or stuck). This may actually reduce the amount of pain signals that are processed by the brain, reducing the amount of pain we feel.

Stressful Experiences Diary

Practice noticing stressful experiences *as they are happening* in the moment. Use this handout to guide your awareness to take stock of what the stressful event is, and how you are reacting to this event in your body, emotions, and mind as it is happening. Fill this diary out as close to the event as you can.

What was the stressful experience?	Describe in detail what sensations were present in your body during this experience	What moods/emotions did you notice arising?	What thoughts were present?	What are you thinking as you write about this experience now?
Example. *Waiting for the doctor to call with the results from my scan.*	*My neck and shoulders were all tense, spasms in my back, a sense of tightness in my chest and butterflies in my stomach.*	*Anxious, hopeless.*	*"This is going to show that my spine is crumbling." "It's only a matter of time before I won't be able to walk."*	*Now that I have the results, I hope that having no structural changes since the last scan means I will soon be able to pick up and hold my grandkids.*

Source: Adapted from Segal, Williams, and Teasdale, 2013.

At-Home Daily Practice for Following Session 3

1) Practice with the Seated Meditation, Mindfulness of Breath and Body, and the Body Scan guided meditation audios, alternating each day. The guided Seated Meditation will provide you with the opportunity to practice the meditation we learned today: mindfulness of the breath and body. Continuing to practice the Body Scan is honing your awareness to tune into those messages of the body, those early warning signals that we might be falling into unhelpful habits of mind that we often are not aware of.
2) Engage in at least three short 3-Minute Breathing Spaces every day at set times that you have decided in advance.
3) Complete one entry each day in your Stressful Experiences Diary. This activity hones your awareness of what might trigger the stress response for you, and raise the stress–pain thermometer, and it also trains your mind to become aware of the connection between stress, your thoughts, feelings, and body sensations. It helps to make these entries as close to the experience as you can and record in detail your reactions, noting the precise thoughts and images that may be frequent fliers through your mind, and the exact location of changes in your body.
4) Complete your daily at-home practice record; it helps to fill this in as close to finishing your practice as possible. Make a note in the comment box of anything that comes up in the at-home practice so that we can talk about it at the next meeting.

Therapist Tips, Troubleshooting, and Supervision for Session 3

Mindful Seeing (or Hearing)

At the start of this session clients are guided in a "seeing" or "hearing" meditation, depending on the contextual environment of the therapy space. If a window is available, a "seeing" meditation is recommended; however, if you are in a space with no windows, a "hearing" meditation is the preferred option. The idea is to tune into the experience of these everyday perceptions, letting go of the tendency to think *about* what is seen/heard, and just paying attention to the *experience* of seeing/hearing itself. The instruction is to notice the mind's tendency to label the experience, to categorize, to become attached to particular sights/sounds, and to have aversion to other sights/sounds, and over and over again to simply guide attention back to the experience of the sights/sounds themselves.

Seated Meditation: Mindfulness of Breath and Body

This is the first in a series of Seated Meditations that will be taught in the program. Although this is called a "seated" practice, clients should be encouraged to assume the posture of most comfort so that they can get the most out of the practice (vs. being uncomfortable and unable to focus on anything other than pain). This meditation expands awareness from the body to also include awareness of the breath. In moving from a body-focused meditation (the Body Scan) toward the inclusion of breath-focused awareness, clients train their mind to bring awareness to increasingly ephemeral experiences. It is important to discuss that there is no need to control, deepen, slow, or change the breath in any way—the only thing needed is simply to notice the felt sensation of each breath, focusing on that part of the body where the movement is felt most strongly. Inevitably thoughts will arise, and the instruction is simply to label (using a kind, gentle inner tone of voice) any such thoughts "thinking" and then to return to the object of awareness. In the guided inquiry following the practice, explicitly discuss that "thinking" is no particular failing, and reiterate that becoming aware of the thinking mind is in itself, mindfulness—it is no big deal and, in learning to notice thinking, nonjudgmentally label it, and return to the breath, this is the essence of the mind training that is meditation. It is critical that the clinician emphasize that thinking, noticing thinking, and returning to the object of awareness *is* the process. This practice also emphasizes noticing and mindfully responding to uncomfortable or difficult physical sensations that arise. During this practice, scratching an itch or adjusting posture is not a problem, but this meditation guides clients to have the realization that another option exists: they can choose to mindfully observe the sensation and stay present with it without immediately habitually reacting. It is useful in the guided inquiry to discuss how this way of relating to difficulties is different from how clients typically react to uncomfortable sensations.

The Stressful Experiences Diary

The Stressful Experiences Diary is intended to enhance awareness of the stress–pain–appraisal connection so that clients have the opportunity to experientially learn what effect our judgments have on experience (including but not limited to pain) and how we might learn to relate differently to such judgments. As with the Pleasant Experiences Diary, it is useful to go over the example provided in the handout in session to ensure full understanding of the exercise, giving clients time to ask any questions they might have. It is also helpful to tell clients that they do not have to fill this out "in order" (i.e., left to right)—if their emotion is most prominent in their awareness, they can start there and then backtrack to identify what thought was present. Again, remind clients that this exercise is best completed as soon after the stressful event as possible.

Reference

Segal, Z. V., Williams, J. M. G., & Teasdale, J. D. (2013). *Mindfulness-based cognitive therapy for depression*. New York, NY: Guilford.

8

Session 4: Learning to Stay Present

Therapist Introduction

The first practice taught in this session is a Seated Meditation—mindfulness of sounds and thoughts—which affords the opportunity to learn how to let thoughts pass through awareness just as sounds pass through awareness: arising, lingering for a time, and passing away. Learning to stay present with experience means becoming skillful at disengaging from automatic thinking. Thus, this Seated Meditation practice provides experiential learning in how to relate to thoughts as just events or objects in awareness, not as the Truth, and not as a reflection of one's identity.

The importance of learning how to simply observe thoughts is reinforced with a review of the Stressful Experiences Diary, where clients practiced learning the connection between their judgments of events as "unpleasant" and the associated aversion and changes in body, emotions, thoughts, and pain. This learning is further extended with a discussion of Unhelpful Habits of Mind, with the key idea being to enhance awareness of these unhelpful patterns as a first step. However, staying present with thoughts and emotions can be particularly challenging during times of difficulty. To help with this, the 3-Minute Responsive Breathing Space is introduced.

When thoughts or difficulties seem "too much" and threaten to sweep us away, bringing awareness to the body in movement can bring stability, and provides another place to stand in which to relate to pain, thoughts, and difficulty in whatever form. Mindful Movement and Mindful Walking provide a way to step out of our heads, and into our bodies, tuning into the contrasts between stillness and movement. Both of these techniques are taught in this session.

Mindfulness-Based Cognitive Therapy for Chronic Pain: A Clinical Manual and Guide,
First Edition. Melissa A. Day.

Companion website: www.wiley.com/go/day/mindfulness_based_cognitive_therapy

Therapist Outline

Assessment Measures

Have clients fill out the Assessment Measures. Provide assistance as needed.

Orientation

A central emphasis of this program is that the best way to manage chronic pain is to let go of attempts to fight the pain and push it away. We are learning to respond in a radically different way, by staying present with the pain and what is unpleasant in our experience—mindfully observing it with kindness and a nonjudgmental attitude. Why is this important? Wanting pain to be other than it is takes a great deal of effort; staying present with the pain, as it is already here, allows you to respond wisely to the pain, allowing more effective coping and management strategies the necessary space to arise in the mind.

The practice of applying mindfulness to our experience effectively inserts a "pause" into our habitual reaction, and that pause provides us with the option to *choose* how to respond, rather than have a kneejerk reaction. Moreover, mindfulness strips away judgment, fear, expectation, the layers of thought and emotion that are piled on to our direct experience. Having a certain "lightness of touch" when thoughts, feelings, pain, or other experiences arise gives us more freedom, opening up a potential myriad of possibilities, rather than being closed in by habitual, automatic reactions.

Theme

The mind becomes stirred up like a pond during a storm when it tries to avoid/escape/push away some aspects of experience, and hold on to, and want to keep other experiences. In practicing mindfulness we are cultivating a skill that trains our mind to stay present and observe experience—whether it be considered pleasant, unpleasant, or neutral—and to then wisely respond with equanimity, letting go of attachment and aversion. Awareness of the body in movement is another anchor to the present moment that you can use to manage pain more effectively.

Learning to Stay Present

In this first exercise for today, we are going to further explore how to "stay present" with our experience. In this practice we are about to do, we are training in learning to observe thoughts come and go just as sounds come and go. This presents another place to stand in which we can more wisely respond to thoughts, rather than letting them run us around on autopilot. We can begin to see how thoughts, even particularly worrisome thoughts about our pain, change. In watching thoughts this way, you will begin to notice more clearly the power of the mind in influencing the experience of pain. "Staying present" observing our thoughts is rarely easy. But, if you begin to notice a shift in your experience of pain as you let thoughts come and go, it opens up more options, moving you beyond any typical kneejerk reactions you might have to pain or the anticipation of pain. It is easier to stay in the present moment if you have a sense that the pain flare-up will not last or stay the same forever.

Seated Meditation practice, Mindfulness of Sounds and Thoughts: *lead the group through the Mindfulness of Sounds and Thoughts Seated Meditation; see Appendix B on the website for a script.*

Guided Inquiry

- What did you notice during that practice? *If no one raises any difficulties, explicitly inquire:*
  - What, if any difficulties or challenges did you notice? *Inquiring into how people reacted to these difficulties, i.e., changes in body, mood, and judgments of pleasant/unpleasant/neutral.*
- How was bringing your awareness to sounds and thoughts in this practice different from how you typically relate to sounds and thoughts in your everyday experiences?
- What connections do you see between this practice and living with chronic pain?

To practice being aware of thoughts, even neutral thoughts such as, "What's for supper?," and to practice letting them go is a first step towards being able to free oneself from "hot cognitions" such as rumination about whether one is "damaged goods" or "unlovable." This freedom that comes with staying present or staying grounded is what this practice is all about.

Guided Inquiry of Experience with at-home practice: *Body Scan, Sitting Meditation (Mindfulness of Breath and Body), and 3-Minute Breathing Space, the Stressful Experiences Diary. Review practice logs and make copies if it is part of a research project (i.e., to track dose).*

- Now let's move on to a discussion of your at-home practice. What was that experience like for you?
- How was taking this time for yourself in this way different from the time you would normally take for yourself?
- Having practiced this approach we call mindfulness for 3 weeks now, what thoughts do you now have in relation to how this relates to experiencing persistent pain?

A common theme to emerge from our discussion is the difficulty in dealing with negative thoughts, feelings, and body sensations. *Review the Stressful Experiences Diary.*

- To help us make these distinctions, let's take a look at your Stressful Experiences Diary that you have been working on since last session. What did you notice in engaging in that exercise each day? *Give everyone the chance to reflect with each other on what happened when they tried to record such moments and to record exactly the thoughts, emotions, and body sensations that occurred in the moments they describe. Record responses on the flip chart, differentiating between thoughts, bodily sensations, and emotions by listing them in separate columns.*

A shared experience I am noticing from our discussion is that the situations we find ourselves in, the events of the day that take place, are in and of themselves neither good nor bad. Often it is our state of mind, and our mood entering into those situations that really defines the experience for us and is playing a leading role in raising the stress–pain thermometer.

A number of you have also identified an important discovery in doing this activity: you can see from the changes in your body column that you have identified your own unique warning system that is in place in your body when aversion arises, sending early messages that stress and pain are threatening to take over. Often however, we do not notice these early messages from the body until they reach a screaming volume and we are in the throes of a pain flare-up and they are, at that point, then *demanding* our attention. Even at that point though, remember from Session 1 and the Gate Control Theory that the thought and feeling centers of the brain are also sending signals back toward the body and have the power to influence our perceptions regarding body sensations. It is never too late to catch ourselves.

Mindful awareness is a radically different response from our typical way of relating to experience, which is usually by:

- Numbing ourselves, daydreaming, or spacing out in one form or another: although our bodies may be in a given situation, our minds are off someplace else or in some other time entirely.
- Holding on, craving, and wanting things or experiences to stay the same and last forever: not allowing ourselves to be with experience in the moment and then to let go without resistance as the experience naturally passes, or perhaps wanting some experience other than what is present.
- Fighting our direct experience: resisting, avoiding, or wanting it to go away or be different in some way as we don't like it and do not want it to be here. This is a general theme that it seems many of you encountered with the Stressful Experiences Diary.

What we are learning in this program is how to catch ourselves earlier and earlier when we fall into these ways of relating to experience, and the first step is always awareness. With awareness comes choice. With awareness we have the power to *choose* how to respond, rather than react with these preprogrammed, unhelpful habits.

Unhelpful Habits of Mind: Navigating the Landscape of Chronic Pain

Our minds are typically constantly running story lines, like a running stream of commentary that has become as automatic as breathing. We rarely pay any attention to what it is we are telling ourselves. However, when we experience chronic pain and/or become stressed—as we saw in the Stressful Experiences Diary—oftentimes what we are telling ourselves can become overly harsh, negative, and self-derogating, and because it is all happening automatically, we don't even realize how negative and unhelpful our thoughts have become!

So, as we have been learning and practicing, the first step to lessening the power of negative and unhelpful automatic thoughts is to bring them into awareness, which we have been practicing with during meditation. Another way to bring these thoughts into awareness and to become skillful at catching your automatic thoughts as they arise is to become familiar with the *types* of thoughts that are usually reported by people when they are suffering from chronic pain.

To help with this discussion, utilize the "Unhelpful Habits of Mind" handout. Reading and reflecting on these statements helps people to get some distance from these thoughts and to see them as bundled together with a number of other features of the experience of pain/stress.

In looking at this handout, you can probably already pick your own particular flavor of automatic thinking. The idea here though is to simply bring a sense of humor to this awareness. It can be an amusing exercise to pick out the habits that you seem to have fallen into; the key is to realize that none of these is the Truth. When we are stressed and in pain, though, it is not so easy to be amused! At those times, these thoughts tighten their grip and seem to be 100% true.

When you are having a pain flare-up, perhaps you have the thought, "I can't handle this." What category of unhelpful mind habits would this thought fall under? *Give clients a chance to offer suggestions.* Yes, this could be "Black and White" thinking, or perhaps "Fortune Telling." But that you are sitting here is living proof that some way or another, you *did* handle it, and you did get through the pain flare-up.

It is not our typical approach though to consider the possibility that these thoughts we tell ourselves are not completely true, especially during times when pain has flared up and we are absolutely convinced by them. What effect, though, do you think having the thought "I can't handle this" would have on your emotions, body, and what you do? *Give clients a chance to offer suggestions.* Yes, exactly, we are likely to feel out of control, useless, and to give up, and to not even try any of the pain self-management techniques we are learning in these classes, and pain will likely worsen.

What styles of thinking seem to ring true for you, based on your experience? You might even go back to the thoughts you wrote down on your Stressful Experiences Diary to see if they fit within any of these categories. *Discuss.*

These thoughts have so much power over our pain, how we feel, what we do—feeding into more unhelpful thoughts and more pain—and all this is habitually happening without our awareness. So the key is to catch ourselves; to catch these "hot" cognitions early and see the full landscape of chronic pain—to notice the thoughts and accompanying emotions and behaviors—this full awareness moves us beyond just noticing and being consumed by the pain. In learning to recognize our unique, unhelpful habits of mind that take us away from being in the present moment, we can just observe them over and over again and not get hooked by them, and in this way learn to return more skillfully, and more readily, to the present.

Breathing Space practice: let's practice the 3-Minute Breathing Space to regather ourselves, and again sample "being" mode. *Lead the group through the 3-Minute Breathing Space meditation; see Appendix B on the website for a script.*

Guided Inquiry

- What did you notice with that brief practice? (*Depending on time, you may wish to further this discussion, inquiring into how this was different from how we might typically spend a spare 3 min, and/or how this practice relates to living with chronic pain.*)

This practice allows us to take a brief moment during the day to just step out of automatic pilot mode and step into the present moment, and just be with the breath. Following this session, we will be asking you to expand this practice to times during the day when you become aware that you are experiencing some difficulty in one form or another, whether it be heightened pain, tension, stress, or some other unpleasant experience. This is called a "3-Minute Responsive Breathing Space," and allows you to give the difficult situation some space; to allow it to just be as it is, without piling extra baggage on in the form of negative thoughts or emotions—to just breathe with the difficulty.

Movement Towards Mindfulness

As we learned in the Body Scan meditation, by stepping into awareness of bodily sensations, you can step out of mental chatter and unhelpful habits of mind, giving you a different place to observe what is present, to sample a different mode of *being* with experience. Tuning into the felt sense of a thought or an emotion in the body provides us with insight into our relationship to these thoughts or emotions, and invariably changes the experience of them (remember what happened when we mindfully ate the raisin in Session 1?). Bringing awareness to how we are reacting to something in the body opens up fresh choices for how to respond to present-moment experience. For example, tension in the mind is often expressed as tension in the body; in becoming aware of this tension in the body and then choosing to release it, this will also likely shift the tension in the mind as well. Often people find it easier to notice physical sensations and bring awareness to their body when the body is in motion (rather than when it is still, as in the Body Scan). Moreover, if you find your mind is racing and you have trouble staying still in a Seated Meditation, again, a meditation focused on the body in movement may be more useful in stabilizing the mind at these times. So building on what you have already been practicing, in this next exercise we are going to bring awareness to the body while it is in movement.

Mindful Movement

In movement, we can notice contrast more easily. Just the effort to hold your arm out parallel to the ground for example, and then the release when you let your arm gently fall back to your side is quite noticeable. In this Mindful

Movement meditation you are about to learn, the key practice is to hone in on these contrasts in sensation, and the boundaries of these contrasts, tuning into when and where in the movement you notice them—both the building and release. Physical strengthening or flexibility training is not the goal with this practice. The intention in engaging in these gentle movements is to provide another way for you to get in touch with your body and to step out of unhelpful habits of mind—you will see in your handbook a description of the purpose of this practice. It is particularly important to emphasize moving slowly, gently, paying close attention to the sensations you experience, and honoring the messages from your body. Taking a light touch, rather than pushing or forcing through any resistance or pain. This is not an exercise in self-torture but one of self-kindness!

We are gently working at the edges of any limits or sensations; not holding a posture until it becomes painful, and also not letting our mind impose standards of what we can and can't do. We are gently experimenting with moving into and back out from the point at which a sensation arises and paying close attention to the changes in our bodies. Again, just as you have been practicing in the Body Scan and Seated Meditations, not stopping at a label, and really tuning into the quality of sensation that arises as you do the movements: is it burning? Trembling? Tension? Breathing with the sensations and as best you can, letting any thoughts or emotions that might be attached to the sensations just come and go. Letting the physical sensations be the object of meditation, just as the breath was the object of meditation in your seated practice—just keep bringing your attention back to the physical sensations that arise and pass away as you move.

Mindful Movement meditation practice: *lead the group through the Mindful Movement meditation; see Appendix B on the website for a script for this meditation.*

Guided Inquiry

- What did you notice with that practice? (*Depending on time, you may wish to further this discussion, inquiring into how this was different from how we might typically move, and/or how this practice relates to living with chronic pain.*)

Mindful Walking

We are now going to expand this mindfulness of movement even further, to generalize it to your daily experience. At some time today, you have walked. In this next practice we are going to turn the everyday act of walking into an opportunity to practice mindfulness; to tune into the sensations that are present with each step. Typically we walk to get some place, or to achieve some goal of one form or another. Rarely do we pay attention to the walking itself. Usually, although our body may be walking, we are inhabiting our mind, not our body, and the body is simply doing the mind's bidding. The body mirrors the mind-state; if the mind is rushing, the body will also rush from point "A" to point "B." If the mind is drawn to something that it judges to be pleasant, perhaps the body will pause and look in the direction of this "shiny object" so to speak. Most often, all of this is happening while you are on autopilot, without attention, or intention. Mindful Walking is a way to let go of goals or desires to get someplace else other than where you are, and involves walking while being aware of each step, just intentionally attending to the felt sensations of just the one step you are taking. In paying attention to walking, we do not have to change the way in which we walk, but it does help to slow down the process of walking, to walk at a slow, relaxed pace. You might like to experiment with walking at slightly different speeds, though, to see what pace is suitable for you. It also helps to have a designated path with a start and end point of about 10 paces, although choose what is best for you and what your body needs; each time you reach an end point and turn back around on the path, let this be a reminder to mindfully check in and ask yourself, "Where is my attention? Is it with each step?"

The eyes remain open, and your gaze focused on a point on the ground just slightly in front of you. The idea is to direct most of your attention inwardly to the felt sensations of walking in the body, with just a light attention to your outward experience—enough to keep you on the path so as you don't run into anything. To begin, we first focus on the feet and legs, where the movements of walking can be felt most strongly. As your focus of attention deepens, you can widen your space of awareness to also include the felt sense of walking throughout the body as a whole as you *be* with one step at a time. Included in your handbook is a handout that provides you with instruction on this practice.

Mindful Walking meditation practice: *lead the group through the Mindful Walking meditation practice; see Appendix B on the website for a script for this meditation.*

Guided Inquiry

- What did you notice during that practice? (*Depending on time, you may wish to further this discussion, inquiring into how this was different from how we might typically walk from one location to another, and/or how this practice relates to living with chronic pain.*)

At-Home Daily Practice

During the coming week, your daily practice, as shown in your handouts, will be… *Go over client handout describing at-home practice following Session 4.*

Distribute guided meditation audio files and Session 4 client handouts.

Summary

What we have been working with today is that… *Go over client summary handout: "Learning to Stay Present."*

Client Handbook

Session 4 Summary: Learning to Stay Present

Pain, obstacles, struggles of some form or another, will undoubtedly be faced by all of us at some point in our lives. Awareness is the vehicle for learning how to stay present with these difficulties, for stepping out of autopilot, for switching mental gears from auto mode into mindful mode. With practice in mindfulness, we can eventually choose to let go of the burden of our own particular automatic patterns and unhelpful habits of mind, learning to simply stay present with experience just as it is. The first step in letting go of this extra baggage is awareness.

In the seated practice from today's session, the technique is to invite thoughts *into* the practice, to let thoughts become the object of mindfulness itself, watching them come and go just as sounds come and go. In regularly practicing this meditation during the coming week, we will begin to see more clearly the patterns of the mind, the well-worn pathways of thought that we frequently travel. The meditation technique provides the needed support for noticing when our mind is no longer *observing* the thoughts, but instead has become identified with the thought—seeing it as the Truth—and to then at that point return our awareness, with gentleness and patience, back to being simply the observer.

As we have also practiced today, being mindful of your body in movement is particularly useful for stepping out of mental chatter and for taking a wider perspective. When your mind is racing, using the Mindful Movement or Walking technique is an excellent way to stabilize your mind. These movement-based meditations, or perhaps a breathing space, are ways to bring mindfulness into our day. These portable techniques can slow down the habitual chain of reactions, and bring in space, so that you can wisely respond, rather than react. Just pausing, and allowing this sense of space to emerge, allows you to stay with experience, as opposed to fight against it in some way, and also allows for a sense of nonjudgmental kindness toward yourself to naturally arise.

Again, we do not practice meditation in order to "become good meditators." The training is so that during our day-to-day experience we let go of tendencies to add baggage to the situation, to spin off, and add to our pain—we learn to simply stay present.

Unhelpful Habits of Mind

Extreme Thinking

1) *All or nothing/black and white thinking*: views are split to the extreme, either being all one way *or* the other, with no middle ground, no gray area.
   - For example, "I can't coach my son's football team anymore because of the pain so I am an epic failure of a dad."
2) *Fortune telling*: predicting, usually negative, future outcomes and circumstances.
   - For example, "This tension is going to lead to a full-blown migraine and will knock me out of action for a week!"
3) *Should statements*: doing or expecting others to do what is believed to be the "right" or "moral" thing; or ideas about how the world should be.
   - For example, "The surgeon should have fixed my pain the first time I went under the knife!"

Selective Attention

1) *Overgeneralization*: one experience applies to all situations.
   - For example, "No one would want to hire me, my boss at my last job saw me as damaged goods."
2) *Filtering*: focusing on the negatives of a situation to the exclusion of any positives; not looking at the whole picture.
   - For example, "I am half a person because of this pain."
3) *Disqualifying the positive*: dismissing or discounting positive events or situations.
   - For example, "I vacuumed the whole house today but that is hardly an achievement as it's the first time in months."
4) *Magnification or minimization*: building a negative experience to make it seem worse than it might be, or making positive experiences less than they really are.
   - For example, "This pain is totally unbearable, its killing me!"

Relying on Intuition

1) *Emotional reasoning*: basing your view of a situation, yourself, or others on how you are feeling.
   - For example, "I can feel my spine collapsing. If I exercise like they tell me to I know it will snap."
2) *Mind reading*: inferring someone else's thoughts, thinking you "know" what they are thinking.
   - For example, "My doctor doesn't believe my pain is real."

Blaming

1) *Personalization*: blaming or criticizing yourself when you had limited control over the situation.
   - For example, "It's all my fault my relationship ended when this pain got in the way of me being intimate with my partner in the bedroom."
2) *Labeling and mislabeling*: overgeneralizing and judging yourself or everyone in a group negatively or harshly.
   - For example, "All doctors are just in it for the money, none of them care."

Movement Towards Mindfulness

By stepping into awareness of bodily sensations, you step out of mental chatter, giving you a different place to observe what is present, to sample a different "mode" of being with experience. Often people find it easier to notice physical sensations and bring awareness to their body when the body is in motion. Moreover, if you find your mind is racing and you have trouble staying still in a Seated Meditation, a meditation focused on movement may be more useful in stabilizing the mind at these times.

In practicing Mindful Movement, it is particularly important to emphasize moving slowly, gently, paying close attention to the sensations you are focusing on, and honoring the messages from your body. Taking a light touch, rather than bulldozing through any resistance or pain, paying close attention to the changes in the body and the contrasts between movement and stillness.

The practice in Mindful Movement is to really tune into the quality of the sensation of movement: Is there a sense of tension? Burning? Trembling? Breathing with the sensations and as best you can, letting any thoughts or emotions that might be attached to the sensations just come and go. Letting the physical sensations be the object of meditation, just as the breath was the object of meditation in your seated practice—just keep bringing your attention back to the physical sensations that arise and pass away as you move.

And the good news is, you can do this practice anytime—wherever you go, you always take your body with you! Even something as simple as reaching and picking up a glass of water represents an opportunity to bring more and more mindfulness into your day-to-day life, until it becomes second nature for you to be *in* your body.

Guidance for Practicing Mindful Walking

In the practice of Mindful Walking, we turn the everyday act of walking into an opportunity to practice mindfulness; to tune into the physical sensations that are present with each step. Typically we walk to get some place, or to achieve some goal of one form or another. Rarely, though, do we pay attention to the act of walking itself. Usually, although our body may be walking, we are inhabiting our mind, not our body, and the body is simply doing the mind's bidding. The body mirrors the mind-state; if the mind is rushing, the body will also rush from point "A" to point "B." If the mind is drawn to something that it judges to be pleasant, perhaps the body will pause and look in the direction of this "shiny object" so to speak. Most often, all of this is happening while you are on autopilot, without attention, or intention.

Mindful Walking is a way to let go of goals or desires to get someplace else other than where you are, and involves walking while being aware of each step, just intentionally attending to the felt sensations of just the one step you are taking. In paying attention to walking, we do not have to change the way in which we walk, but it does help to slow down the process of walking, to walk at a slow, relaxed pace. You might like to experiment with walking at slightly different speeds, though, to see what pace is suitable for you. It also helps to have a designated path with a start and end point of about 10 paces, although choose what is best for you and what your body needs; each time you reach an end point and turn back around on the path, let this be a reminder to mindfully check in and ask yourself, "Where is my attention? Is it with each step?"

The eyes remain open, and your gaze focused on a point on the ground just slightly in front of you. The idea is to direct most of your attention inwardly to the felt sensations of walking in the body, with just a light attention to your outward experience—enough to keep you on the path so as you don't run into anything! To keep mindfulness strong, we keep our attention on just one region of the body during the entire Mindful Walking practice (rather than changing the region multiple times). To begin, it helps to first focus on the feet and legs, where the movements of walking can be felt most strongly. As your focus of attention deepens, you can widen your space of awareness to include also the felt sense of walking throughout the body as a whole as you *be* with one step at a time.

At-Home Daily Practice for Following Session 4

1) Practice with the Seated Meditation, Mindfulness of Sounds and Thoughts, and the Mindful Movement guided meditation audios, alternating each day. The guided Seated Meditation will provide you with the opportunity to practice mindfulness of sounds and thoughts. The guided Mindful Movement provides instruction to connect your awareness to the body as you move through gentle movements, noticing perhaps the expression of emotion in the body as you do this. If any of the movements exacerbate your pain problem, you may like to instead practice mindfulness of the breath at those times, and return to the instructions on the guided audio for the other movements. Awareness of the body in movement provides another way to get insight into the mind and to notice our thoughts.
2) Explore using the Mindful Walking practice. You might choose to do this more formally as we did today; or informally by bringing mindfulness to walking as you go about your day. Included in your handouts is further guidance on this practice.
3) Engage in at least three short 3-Minute Breathing Spaces every day at set times that you have decided in advance.
4) Practice the 3-Minute Responsive Breathing Space whenever you notice your stress–pain thermometer rising; for example, when you notice your body becoming tense, or you become emotionally upset, angry, or anxious (or other unpleasant feelings arise), or when you act out or feel like your thoughts are picking up momentum in an unhelpful way.
5) Read over the "Unhelpful Habits of Mind" handout, and consider which of these habits you might engage in, especially during times of stress and pain.
6) Complete your daily at-home practice record; it helps to fill this in as close to finishing your practice as possible. Make note in the comment box of anything that comes up in the at-home practice so that we can talk about it at the next meeting.

Therapist Tips, Troubleshooting, and Supervision for Session 4

Seated Meditation: Mindfulness of Sounds and Thoughts

This practice moves deeper into awareness of the transparency of thoughts, cultivating decentering. The idea here is that just as sounds come and go, if we don't grasp and cling to thoughts, then they too can just come and go. Before this, when thoughts arose in meditation the practice was to label it "thinking," or in other words, to be mindful of the *process* of consciousness. Here, we are bringing mindfulness to the *contents* of consciousness. The ability to observe thoughts without becoming attached or averse to them is the essence of learning to stay. This is an advanced technique: to do this and truly experience it, not just in an intellectual sense. The trap is that we often run story lines in our mind and ruminate; this is qualitatively different from observing thoughts in a meditative sense. Thus, care must be taken that this meditation is not used as a vehicle for promoting maladaptive thinking processes. This meditation also introduces a period of "choiceless awareness," which allows clients to practice open monitoring of their experience, letting go of a specific object to hold attention to, and instead being aware of the entirety of their experience. The idea is that we are "waiting" for the thought or some other experience to arise, like a cat waiting at a mouse hole. And if we find that we get carried along *with* a thought, noticing that, and returning back to being the observer. A core element of this practice is noticing *what happens next* when we judge what arises as "unpleasant"? This is a juicy learning opportunity where we observe first-hand our personal "unhelpful habits of mind," and along with that, what changes in the body arise. Working with difficulties through the body is further introduced with the movement meditations, and will be a central focus of the extended instructions for the Breathing Space as well as the Seated Meditation taught in the next session.

Unhelpful Habits of Mind: Navigating the Landscape of Chronic Pain

This exercise is a more traditional CBT-oriented exercise and the idea is to use the provided client handout to guide a discussion geared toward increasing awareness of clients' automatic patterns of mind. By labeling the patterns that are most relevant to each client, the intention is to enhance earlier recognition of these unhelpful habits of mind, training clients to recognize these thought patterns before they bite the hook and get caught in their powerful grip. Clients may also find it helpful to use these labels within their meditation practice; when they notice their mind has wandered, instead of simply labelling it "thinking," they may like to experiment with, for example, labeling it as "Ahh, here's fortune telling and anxiety"—recognizing the pattern and then using the meditation technique to return back to pure awareness of the object of meditation, thereby training in "not biting the hook."

3-Minute Responsive Breathing Space

This technique generalizes the practice to day-to-day experience, and in particular, experience arising that contains a sense of difficulty. By responding to such difficulties with a 3-Minute "Responsive" Breathing Space, clients learn to experiment with "dipping their toe in" to experience what it is like to stay present with difficulties, which will be built on throughout the rest of the program. It is helpful to communicate that although we practice this technique in session more formally (i.e., in terms of posture, with eyes closed), with practice clients will be able to use this "on the go." The idea is for this to be highly portable in that it may be practiced in an even briefer form, where it entails simply being in touch with one's breath, not necessarily with eyes closed or by oneself, and perhaps even while during a difficult conversation as a means to stay calm, present, and focused. Reflecting this, throughout the remaining sessions, rather than simply delivering the 3-Minute Breathing Space practice at the times suggested in this manual, flexibly implementing it at times where the group may get off track, gets involved in lengthy discussion, or when difficult emotions or experiences arise models for clients how to best use this technique outside of the session to cope with pain, stress and their day-to-day experience.

Mindful Movement and Walking Meditations

As described in Chapter 3 and Chapter 4, given the population is chronic pain, the Mindful Movements included here are modified and simplified. However, even with these adaptations, it is still important to emphasize that clients listen to the messages of their body, respecting (while still gently exploring) any "limits." The idea is for these practices to train clients to "get out of their head" and "into their body." Bringing attention *into* the body is often more readily done when the body is moving, as the interoceptive sensations flowing from that movement are usually more readily apparent than, for example, the sensation in one's big toe during a Body Scan. You might also describe how these practices can be highly effective during those times where the mind is particularly active. For example:

> When you are engaging in a seated meditation and it "just seems impossible" as your mind is racing, experiment with switching to a movement-focused practice. This allows you to *feel* the difference between action and the stillness that was so elusive in your seated practice, and it turns out that this is highly effective in stabilizing the mind. Following that, you might like to return to your seated practice, and to see for yourself what difference there might be in your experience.

Finally, the guidance provided in the script for Mindful Walking suggested clients have their own "path." This is in contrast to delivering this practice where everyone walks behind each other in a circle because this "forces" some people to go at a pace that might be uncomfortable for them (i.e., to walk as fast/slow as the person behind and/or in front of them) and may exacerbate pain.

9

Session 5: Active Acceptance

Therapist Introduction

This session represents the start of the second half of the program, and the emphasis is on transitioning from simply enhancing awareness to also include training in learning how to *wisely respond* to pain, stress, and our moment-to-moment experience. A sitting in silence meditation is the first meditation taught as a means to experientially learn what it is like to "not fill up the space" and to pause, and simply be with experience as it is. This is then followed by a guided inquiry and homework review, and then a 3-Minute Breathing Space to re-anchor back to the present moment after the discussion of the weekly activities.

The process of acceptance is then introduced as a way to actively train in learning to stay with our experience, without needing to rush in and try to immediately change it, push it away, or hold on to it. In discussing steps toward responding with acceptance, an exercise using a tree metaphor is introduced to illustrate the role our automatic thoughts, intermediate beliefs, and core beliefs play in driving habitual responses. This exercise reinforces the notion that first we need to be aware of our patterns of mind that pull us off center, in order to then have the choice, through mindfulness, to be able to wisely respond and return to the present moment. Building on this awareness is a Seated Meditation that trains clients to work with difficulties within the technique of the meditation practice itself, as a means to actively work toward acceptance of pain and life's challenges; this guidance on cultivating active acceptance in meditation is also incorporated into instructions to further clients' use of the 3-Minute Responsive Breathing Space.

Mindfulness-Based Cognitive Therapy for Chronic Pain: A Clinical Manual and Guide,
First Edition. Melissa A. Day.

Companion website: www.wiley.com/go/day/mindfulness_based_cognitive_therapy

Therapist Outline

Assessment Measures

Have clients fill out Assessment Measures. Provide assistance as needed.

Orientation

Over our past 4 weeks together, we have been learning to train the mind to step out of automatic patterns of thought and habituation by intentionally holding the breath or body as our anchor of attention. As we have learned in doing this practice, a central component is noticing when our mind wanders from our anchor—whether it be to thinking, daydreaming, attending to physical sensations, or feelings—and our task up to now has been to notice that, perhaps label it, and then gently but firmly return our attention back to our anchor. Over and over again we practice in this way, with patience and kindness toward ourselves.

Perhaps you have noticed, however, that a pattern has emerged in your practice, that you find your mind being pulled in a similar way or direction each time, whether it be to a memory, sensation, thought, or feeling, or perhaps to ideas about how we ourselves, or others or the world, should be, ought to be, or must be. Oftentimes, and especially when suffering from chronic pain, our thoughts and these standards or rules we have for ourselves become negative, overly strict or harsh, or distorted in some way. And what happens then, when we have this tendency to become hooked on the same thing time after time?

As we learned last week, what typically happens is one of three things: we daydream or numb out in one form or another; or if we like it we hold on, crave it, and want it to last; and if we don't like it, we fight against it and push it away. When we pause however, and don't spin out with our habitual thing, another possibility arises: we have the choice to respond by allowing whatever is present to be present, to simply hold it in our awareness, and respond with nonjudgmental acceptance. This idea of bringing space to difficult thoughts, emotions, and sensations—of opening to them and allowing them to be present—is radically different from our typical, habitual response patterns.

Theme

A small pause can make all the difference, and can open up space to allow things to be, without imposing any standards or judgments of how we feel they *should* or *ought* to be. Acceptance is a cornerstone of self-care, and allows for a fresh perspective to emerge, for your wise mind to see clearly what, if anything at all, needs to shift or change.

Silence

In our first practice today we are going to explore sitting in silence. Silence is a rare experience. We usually fill it. With speech, music, TV, radio… What are we avoiding with these "fillers"? What is left when we just sit with ourselves in stillness, staying with the pause, open to experience? What's there? When we bring silence into our experience, it has the capacity to not only quiet our body, and quiet our mind, but to open us up to a whole world of experience that we don't typically notice (*guide clients to notice the sound of a light flickering, or the hum of an air conditioner in the therapy room*)—all of this is happening in the background, not noticed until we have silence and pay attention, what else is happening "in the background" of our lives?

We are now going to practice simply sitting in silence, with awareness of the breath without any verbal "guidance" from me. During this practice, it helps to bring yourself to a dignified sitting posture; this is a signal to your mind that you are bringing to bear a different quality of attention. Then, gather your awareness to your breath as you breathe in and as you breathe out. Noticing where in the body you sense the breath most prominently—the nostrils, the back of the throat, the chest, the belly. The technique is, as best you can, to follow the rise of the inbreath and the fall of the outbreath as it enters and leaves the body. When you notice thoughts arising, it is no problem—this awareness of the rising of thoughts is mindfulness itself. Simply label the thoughts (regardless of their content) "thinking," and return your awareness back to the breath. As many times as your mind wanders, the technique is to just gently but firmly, move your attention back to the breath.

Sitting in Silence Meditation: *lead the group through the Session 5, Sitting in Silence, with awareness of the breath, Seated Meditation practice; see Appendix B on the website for a script for this meditation.*

Guided Inquiry

- What did you notice during that practice? (*Depending on client responses, you might also further the inquiry into exploring how this practice was different from how clients typically relate to silence, and/or how this practice might relate to living with chronic pain.*)

Guided inquiry of experience with the at-home practice: *Seated Meditation, Mindfulness of Sounds and Thoughts, Mindful Movement, Walking Meditation, 3-Minute Breathing Space, and 3-Minute Responsive Breathing Space. Also inquire into the "Unhelpful Habits of Mind" handout. Review practice logs and make copies if it is part of a research project (i.e., to track dose).*

- Now let's move on to a discussion of your at-home practice. What was that experience like for you?
- How was engaging in the 3-minute Responsive Breathing Space (when you noticed a difficult situation arise) different from the way you would normally react to difficulties?
- What did you notice in terms of your own particular flavor of thinking while looking over the "Unhelpful Habits of Mind" handout?
- Are you noticing any changes in your attitude towards, or experience with, your daily at-home meditation practice?
- In what ways is practice becoming a habit for you?
- What, if any, new challenges or barriers have emerged?

Breathing Space practice: let's practice the 3-Minute Breathing Space to regather ourselves, and again sample "being" mode. *Lead the group through the 3-Minute Breathing Space meditation; see Appendix B on the website for a script.*

Guided Inquiry

- What did you notice with that brief practice? (*Depending on time, you may wish to further this discussion, inquiring into how this was different from how we might typically spend a spare 3 min, and/or how this practice relates to living with chronic pain.*)

Steps Toward Acceptance of Pain: The Root of Our Thought and Beliefs

Acceptance to many of us at first may bring to mind notions of "giving up," "quitting," or "resignation." Truly though, acceptance is an *active*, purposeful process in response to thoughts and feelings—quite the opposite of giving up, which requires no effort at all. Acceptance holds at its core the intention to allow your experience to *be* your experience, whatever it may be, without rushing in to fix or change that experience in any way. As always, awareness is the foundation: to allow difficult thoughts, feelings, and sensations to be present means first registering their existence. We then pause, and hold this awareness in a cradle of kindness, before choosing how to respond. This is very different to an automatic reaction, or passive resignation, as this process of acceptance rests on a *conscious intention* to respond in this way.

Over time, you may notice a running theme throughout your meditation practice of where your mind often trails off to, perhaps (as we learned in Session 4), a theme of "mind reading," "personalization," or some other theme. Like a production that is put on many times over the years, the performers on the stage may change, but the underlying story line or thought stream stays the same. Or perhaps it is the underlying energy that feels the same? Guilt? Anger? Sadness? Or maybe you find your awareness repeatedly pulled to painful sensations? Most typically, our usual reaction is to respond to these thoughts, beliefs, and feelings as the Truth. People who have chronic pain, and for that matter, all people, spend a great deal of effort clinging on to beliefs about how themselves, others, and the world should be, ought to be, or must be. We all have expectations of ourselves, and ideas about the kind of person we need to be to be competent, worthy, lovable ... just to name a few. Keeping up with these ideas of ourselves takes energy and work, and for many people who are experiencing long-term stress (as is the case with chronic pain), these ideas or beliefs may become overly rigid, negative, or unrealistic given that perhaps our context has changed since the time these beliefs were formed, which is often in childhood. But we doggedly hold on to these beliefs, which leads us to resist change, resist pain, and ultimately puts up a barrier to flexibly moving toward acceptance. Oftentimes we are not even aware of our underlying beliefs or the power they hold in driving our thoughts, and how we feel and how we relate to pain. Bringing these beliefs into awareness is the first step toward working with them, and accepting our experience just as it is, letting go of all this extra baggage.

Draw a picture of a tree (see client handout, "Getting Down to the Root of Our Thoughts and Beliefs about Paint") on the flip chart—depicting automatic thoughts, intermediate beliefs, and core beliefs—go through an example linking an automatic thought to a should belief to a core belief, and ask clients what effect this would have on their mood, behavior, pain. See if they can identify their own linkages from their personal experiences, perhaps starting with an automatic thought theme they identified in the "Unhelpful Habits of Mind" handout.

We have positive and helpful core beliefs too, however typically our negative core beliefs come out during stressful times, and these have a negative effect on our thoughts, emotions, body, behavior, and pain. As we have talked about, staying with these negative thoughts, emotions, sensations, even painful sensations, and holding them in awareness with acceptance is radically different from how we typically relate to these experiences. Learning to stay open and accept difficulties is typically a gradual process, and we start where we are; the basic approach to moving in this direction, which we are going to practice next, entails two fundamental steps:

1) As always, the first step is awareness. After settling into the meditation, we rest our attention on what is most predominant in our experience. Whether it is difficult feelings calling for your attention, thoughts, physical sensations—we intentionally move our awareness to whatever is most strongly calling for attention. If you are struggling to pinpoint a difficulty, as a tool to hone your awareness, return back to your handout with the tree, which outlines some "typical" negative beliefs people hold about themselves during times of stress; reviewing this handout may help with becoming aware of beliefs that may be present (or just underneath the surface) for you that may underlie distress or a sense of unease.
2) The second step is to shift your primary focus, so that while the difficulty or whatever your mind is repeatedly drawn to is held in the background, you bring to the foreground of your awareness where in the *body* you are noticing the felt sensation of this difficulty. Just as with the Body Scan, deliberately moving your spotlight of attention to that place, and then breathing with the sensations, opening and softening to them.

We are now going to practice a Seated Meditation that guides you in how to take these two steps to actively work with difficulties in your meditation practice, responding with acceptance.

Sitting Meditation: Mindfulness of Breath, Body, Sounds, Thoughts; and Introducing Working with a Difficulty in the Practice

During this practice, you will be guided to, as best you can, welcome or "invite" a difficulty or problem to mind that you might experience. Perhaps during meditation you have often found your mind wandering to boredom, uncomfortableness, or a relationship of some kind. It is best to start with a "moderate" problem, rather than the biggest concern on your mind—this will give you practice in learning the technique so that later you can apply it to more intense problems. If at any time you find it is too overwhelming during this practice to bring to mind a problem, simply return awareness to the breath, and then perhaps gently going back and forth between your breath, and working with the meditation technique, maintaining a kind, nonjudgmental approach to working with the difficulty. The idea is not to force yourself to have prolonged exposure, rather it is to practice being in touch with difficulties with gentleness, in short moments, again and again: in touch with the difficulty for a short while, pausing and breathing, and then touching in again. And if no problem or difficult experience is paramount on your mind at this point in time, experiment with learning the technique by working with some difficulty you may have experienced during the program, perhaps something you noted in the Stressful Experiences Diary, and intentionally bringing that to mind.

Lead the group through the Session 5, Mindfulness of Breath, Body, Sounds and Thoughts and Seated Meditation, Introducing Working with a Difficulty in the Practice; see Appendix B on the website for a script.

Guided Inquiry

- This practice aims to explore what happens when the habitual tendency of the mind to move away from difficulties is reversed. Without telling us specifically what difficulty you chose to work with or the details about it, I am curious about what that experience was like for you?
- In what ways was this practice different to how you might typically relate to difficulties?
- How do you think working with difficulties beyond pain, such as thoughts, emotional responses, or interpersonal difficulties etc., might affect your day-to-day living with pain?

Physical discomfort is actually a useful way to practice this skill because it can easily be brought into awareness as it is a strong sensation. Obviously this is not a typical response to pain: the natural tendency is to tense, brace, or push away pain or physical discomfort. However, simply being aware of our tendency to push these feelings away and bring an open, friendly, curiosity to that tendency provides a very useful practice. Working with these difficulties in this way, though, may open up more ways of responding. Staying *with* difficulties, and bringing a gentle curiosity to them, is, itself, part of acceptance. With this in mind, we are also going to invite you to extend your use of the 3-Minute Responsive Breathing Space during the coming week, with added instruction for working with difficulties through the body in a similar way to what we just practiced in this seated meditation. *Go over the client handout, "Wisely Responding to Difficulties in the Real World: the 3-Minute 'Responsive' Breathing Space—Staying Open to Difficulties."*

At-Home Daily Practice

During the coming week, your daily practice, as shown in your handouts, will be… *Go over client handout describing at-home practice following Session 5.*

Distribute guided meditation audio files and Session 5 client handouts.

Summary

What we have been learning today is that… *Go over client summary handout: "Active Acceptance."*

Client Handbook

Session 5 Summary: Active Acceptance

When we find our mind repeatedly drawn to a particular difficulty, whether it be to a thought, emotion, or physical sensation, we are learning at that point to shift our focus and bring our awareness to how we are relating to this experience in our body. The practice is to become mindfully aware of those physical sensations that are most prominent when we bring this difficulty to mind, and to intentionally shift our spotlight of attention to the part of the body where those sensations are strongest, and breathe with those sensations, perhaps gently saying to yourself "Whatever arises is okay, let me stay open and feel it, and breathe with it." Learning to work with, make space for, and move toward accepting pain and difficulty in any form takes practice, and it takes a light touch.

At first, you may find you can only stay with the difficulty for a few breaths; this is okay. If this is your experience, practice *gently* touching in with the difficulty, like touching a bubble with a feather: we have a light touch in making contact with the difficulty, touching in, pausing with it and breathing with the sensations, then stepping back and just staying with awareness of the breath for a moment or so as we re-anchor ourselves, and then gently touching back in again, perhaps staying a little longer each time. Just staying with this process, breathing with the sensations, staying open and present with the sensations for as long as they have a pull on your attention.

This practice opens up space so that you can then choose how to respond in a skillful way, rather than react in a habitual, automatic fashion. In this way, acceptance is an *active* process, it is not resignation. We are not pushing away, holding on to, avoiding or changing our experience; rather, we *stay with* our moment-to-moment experience, without needing it to be different from the way it is. We let our experience *be* our experience, noticing it, mindfully observing it, breathing with it, and, little by little, accepting it.

Getting Down to the Root of Our Thoughts and Beliefs about Pain

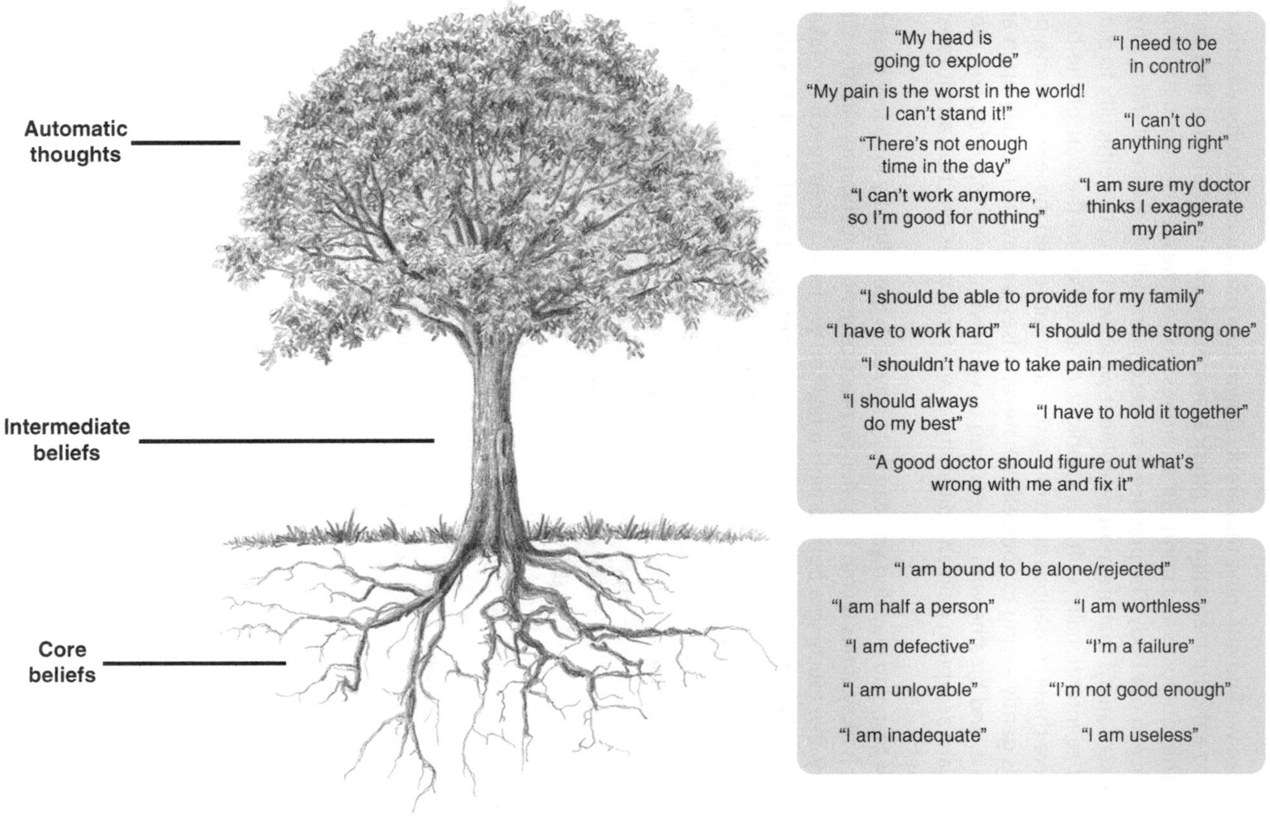
Automatic thoughts
Intermediate beliefs
Core beliefs
"My head is going to explode"
"I need to be in control"
"My pain is the worst in the world! I can't stand it!"
"I can't do anything right"
"There's not enough time in the day"
"I can't work anymore, so I'm good for nothing"
"I am sure my doctor thinks I exaggerate my pain"
"I should be able to provide for my family"
"I have to work hard"
"I should be the strong one"
"I shouldn't have to take pain medication"
"I should always do my best"
"I have to hold it together"
"A good doctor should figure out what's wrong with me and fix it"
"I am bound to be alone/rejected"
"I am half a person"
"I am worthless"
"I am defective"
"I'm a failure"
"I am unlovable"
"I'm not good enough"
"I am inadequate"
"I am useless"

Wisely Responding to Difficulties in the Real World

The 3-Minute "Responsive" Breathing Space—Staying Open to Difficulties[1]

When you experience difficulty in some form or another during your day, whether it be troubling thoughts, emotions, a pain flare-up, the 3-Minute Responsive Breathing Space provides a portable practice that you can use on the go. Just as in the regular Breathing Space you have been practicing, this responsive practice has three basic steps. Here is some further guidance on how you can use this practice to work with difficulties through the body and stay open with acceptance:

1) *Awareness*: as this is a brief practice, you bring yourself into a dignified sitting posture to signal to your mind you are switching into "being" mode. Closing your eyes, bringing awareness to what is happening in this moment, turning toward the sense of difficulty you are experiencing. As you hold this in awareness, tuning into what thoughts are around? What emotions? What sensations are present in the body? Perhaps choosing to gently label what you observe, "Frustration and muscle tension are here" or "Sadness and a sense of loss are here."
2) *Shifting attention*: having acknowledged your experience, shifting your attention, redirecting it to rest firmly on the breath, aware as you breathe in, and aware as you breathe out. If thoughts *about* the difficulty keep arising, when you notice this, return your awareness back to the breath, perhaps more firmly anchoring yourself on the breath by saying to yourself, "Breathing in … breathing out," or if you prefer, counting each breath, "Inhaling, one … exhaling, one; inhaling, two … exhaling, two" etc.
3) *Opening*: having now anchored yourself to your breathing and the present moment, letting your attention expand back outwards to include not only the breath, but also the body as a whole, opening particularly to any sense of unpleasant physical sensations or discomfort in the body that might be present, breathing into it on the inbreath, and back out from it on the outbreath. Continuing to breathe with all that is present, softening and opening to your experience, holding it all—including any sense of tension, holding, or troubling experience—in a cradle of nonjudgmental kindness toward yourself and whatever it is you are experiencing as you go about your day.

At-Home Daily Practice for Following Session 5

1) Alternate each day between practicing with this session's Seated Meditation, Mindfulness of Breath, Body, Sounds, Thoughts and Seated Meditation, Introducing Working with a Difficulty in the Practice, guided meditation audio and sitting in silence for 30 to 45 min without a guided audio. The guided Seated Meditation will provide you with the opportunity to practice working with a difficulty through the body as we did today. Remember to start by picking a "light" difficulty, to give you practice in honing this skill before moving to any "heavier" difficulties you might experience. Sitting in silence will give you the opportunity to observe the mind when we don't do the habitual thing to "fill the silence" or "fill the space." It is helpful to set a timer with a soft, relatively unobtrusive tone to alert you when the 30 to 45 min has elapsed.
2) Engage in at least three short 3-Minute Breathing Spaces every day at set times that you have decided in advance.
3) Practice the 3-Minute Responsive Breathing Space whenever you notice your stress–pain thermometer rising; for example, when you notice your body becoming tense, or you become emotionally upset, angry, or anxious (or other unpleasant feelings arise), or when you act out or feel like your thoughts are picking up momentum in an unhelpful way. Included in your handouts are some tips for practicing this brief meditation "on the go" to stay present and open, practicing working with and accepting difficulties through the body.
4) Read over the examples on your "Getting Down to the Root of our Thoughts and Beliefs about Pain" handout. When you become aware of a negative automatic thought, practice asking yourself, "What does this thought mean to me?" Be on the lookout for any "should," "must be," or "ought to be" types of responses—this is your "Should Belief." Then ask yourself, if this belief is true, "What does that mean about me as a person?" The answer to this question is your core belief, and likely will revolve around your sense of lovability, worth, and/or capability. Remember, the idea is to let this handout be another tool for increasing your awareness of your thinking, and then with this awareness we practice meditation to learn how to respond wisely to our unhelpful habits of mind and to work with difficulties.
5) Complete your daily at-home practice record; it helps to fill this in as close to finishing your practice as possible. Make a note in the comment box of anything that comes up in the at-home practice so that we can talk about it at the next meeting.

Therapist Tips, Troubleshooting, and Supervision for Session 5

Seated Meditation: Sitting in Silence

Throughout the course of the program, clients' at-home practice has included encouragement to practice a 3-Minute Breathing Space meditation without the guided audio and a 10-min breath-focused meditation, practicing in silence. In this session, essentially this same technique is practiced for an extended period, and this is assigned for at-home practice. The intention of this practice is to (1) bring awareness to our own particular flavor of "filling up the space" (i.e., what patterns of automatic thoughts or beliefs might arise), and (2) further facilitate generalization of the skill beyond needing to have a guided audio, so that the experience and practice of mindfulness is always available to clients. They *own* this skill. By engaging in this silent meditation practice, clients learn that whatever benefits they may have come to experience in mindfulness meditation are simply as close to them as the next breath away—all it takes is awareness of the breath as it enters and leaves the body. And even if they have fallen off the bandwagon, so to speak, and haven't been practicing, as soon as they bring their awareness back to the breath, they are right back on board again. So the idea is to briefly introduce the practice, to guide clients to take on a dignified sitting posture, to anchor them on their breath, and then to use minimal instruction—the less said the better.

The Root of Our Thoughts and Beliefs: The Tree Metaphor

Often in meditation, when one has observed the mind for extended periods of time, it becomes apparent that the same or a similar story line is repeated; it has a recurring theme or "energy" (perhaps a sense of urgency, loss, or maybe a background static of elusive unease that is hard to pinpoint or to even describe). The tree metaphor provides a way to introduce a discussion of underlying belief systems that drive what we think, how we feel, what we do, and they operate on a level that is usually below our level of awareness, yet they pose a barrier to moving toward acceptance. In coming to "know" our core beliefs, we can recognize them and work with them in meditation so we are no longer rigidly driven by them, and we can simply allow our experience to be as it is. In presenting this, it helps to draw a schematic of the tree depicted in the handout on the flip chart, and then to provide an example for clients, illustrating Beck's downward arrow technique:

> Let's start with an example situation, "I'm in my armchair, watching my kids go off to school and my wife go off to work." In this situation, you might have the thought, "I hate that I cannot work anymore; I contribute nothing to my family." The question then to ask is: what does that thought mean to you? This will identify the underlying intermediate belief, which might be, "I should be able to provide for my family." If that is true, and right now you are unable to work, what does that mean about you as a

person? This gets at our underlying deep-seated core beliefs about ourselves, which in this example might be, "I am defective" or "I am worthless." This, we can see, is a form of resistance to experience—the opposite of acceptance. Our core beliefs typically revolve around themes of our lovability, worth, and capability. What effect do you think this core belief from this example might have on pain?

It is useful then for clients to identify their own patterns, perhaps by going back to the Stressful Experiences Diary and/or the "Unhelpful Habits of Mind" handout as helpful tools to guide this awareness. Core beliefs are often quite emotionally powerful to bring to awareness, and this awareness is a useful transition to the following Seated Meditation, which provides training in working with difficulties. Again, the idea here is simply to enhance awareness, not to engage in restructuring clients' beliefs in any way. Learning how to respond with acceptance to these beliefs, and to see them as "just thoughts" is further developed throughout the program.

Seated Meditation, Introducing Working with a Difficulty in the Practice

This meditation practice is taught in this session, as well as again in Sessions 6 and 7 as it provides clients with a tangible skill they can use to actively work with difficulties directly and ultimately to move toward responding with acceptance. The idea is to use mindfulness to contact the rawness of the experience with a lightness of touch, like "touching a bubble with a feather." The instruction is to bring the difficulty into awareness, and to check in and see where that difficulty is experienced in the body, and then to breathe with that sensation in the body; this is similarly encouraged in the extended instructions provided in this session for the 3-Minute Responsive Breathing Space. You might describe this seated meditation technique by providing instruction that the skill is to sit with the underlying *energy* of the difficulty. It is important to emphasize to clients that it is best not to start with a highly emotionally charged, on-going, intense difficulty, but rather to pick first a lighter difficulty to build skill with the technique before applying it to increasingly more salient, emotionally charged difficulties. Further, sometimes we do not know how much of a hold a difficulty has on us until we bring awareness to it in a practice such as this, so some clients may find they unexpectedly become "overwhelmed." Thus, it is important to communicate (prior to starting this meditation) that if at any point it feels too much, the practice is to not to "push through" but simply to return to your anchor—your breath—and to stay there until you feel stabilized, and then perhaps experimenting with alternating between gently touching back into the difficulty and returning once more to your anchor. The balance is to learn to stay with the difficulty, while being kind to yourself, and using the breath as an anchor, which is qualitatively different from using the breath as a means to suppress our experience of the difficulty. In this way, kindness and openness are key qualities to emphasize.

Note

1 Adapted from Segal, Williams, and Teasdale, 2013.

Reference

Segal, Z. V., Williams, J. M. G., & Teasdale, J. D. (2013). *Mindfulness-based cognitive therapy for depression*. New York, NY: Guilford.

10

Session 6: Seeing Thoughts as Just Thoughts

Therapist Introduction

This session starts with an exercise from Segal, Williams, and Teasdale's original text that is designed to facilitate direct experience of the ways in which our mind jumps to conclusions ahead of the bare facts, automatically adding to the story line, with perhaps minimal basis in truth. This illustrates the core theme of the session, which is to learn to see thinking as just thinking, with thoughts ultimately being simply secretions of this thinking mind, not facts, and not the Truth. The awareness gained in this opening exercise is built on with: (1) a second in-session practice of the Seated Meditation technique learnt last session, where clients invite a difficult experience in to the practice, and (2) an exercise designed to cultivate awareness of how what we feel, emotionally as well as physically, feeds into what we think.

A further emphasis in Session 6 is introducing the notion of intentionally developing an on-going, personalized daily practice following the program, a "Mindfulness Maintenance Plan." This is introduced in the homework review by explicitly inquiring into clients' experience with the practices since the start of the program. This later transitions into a discussion of keeping the 3-Minute Breathing Space as the first step when "hot" thoughts, pain, and stress threaten to overwhelm and undermine our practice, as well as a discussion of other ways to wisely respond to such thoughts following taking this Breathing Space. To further personalize the pain management skill set following this session, clients are encouraged to practice with their own selection of the meditation practices that have been learned in the program.

Mindfulness-Based Cognitive Therapy for Chronic Pain: A Clinical Manual and Guide,
First Edition. Melissa A. Day.

Companion website: www.wiley.com/go/day/mindfulness_based_cognitive_therapy

Therapist Outline

Assessment Measures

Have clients fill out Assessment Measures. Provide assistance as needed.

Orientation

Write the following sentences one by one (giving them a chance to read as you write) on the flip chart for group members to read:

> John was on his way to school.
> He was worried about the math lesson.
> He was not sure he could control the class again today.
> It was not part of a janitor's duty.
>
> *(Segal, Williams, & Teasdale, 2013, p. 299)*

What did you notice as you read these sentences?

For most people, the interpretation of the story line gets updated with each sentence, moving from a little boy worried about a math lesson, and then most people then think of John as a teacher, and finally the scene in the mind's eye changes to a janitor. We are typically not aware of this "meaning making" function of our minds but we are always adding judgments to our direct experience, so that the reality we do experience is actually a filtered interpretation of the bare facts. We are hardly ever conscious that this is happening, until perhaps some little exercise such as this series of sentences sparks recognition.

This tendency to overlay the bare facts of a situation with our interpretations and ensuing emotional reactions can lead to increased pain. People who have chronic pain, and the associated stress of chronic pain, often have a lot of negative automatic thoughts that are typically directed toward, or about, themselves. Although these thoughts often have a grain of truth to them (which is why they are typically so believable!), usually there is also an element of interpretation or judgment that may make them overly negative or unrealistic, and negative core beliefs such as "I am defective" or "I am a useless" that we learned about last session bubble up to the surface.

Once a negative stream of commentary starts up in our mind, because it is usually running on autopilot, we often don't catch it as it is happening, and so it builds momentum and the stream can quickly turn into a raging river torrent! Spinning off the negative core beliefs are more negative intermediate beliefs and more negative automatic thoughts—and so now even unrelated future events are also interpreted in this destructive, negative torrent of thought. In this program we have been working on stepping out of autopilot and recognizing our thoughts and reactions. Today we will be exploring further ways for you to shift your relationship with your thoughts, to step out of such thought streams, and to see thoughts as just thoughts; not necessarily *the* truth, and not necessarily needing our immediate action.

Theme

Negative thoughts and feelings can put the blinders on us so to speak, narrowing our viewpoint and closing us off from a vast openness of possible ways of responding to experience. It is liberating to realize that our thoughts are just thoughts, not facts, and we can learn to watch them come and go, without getting hooked by them.

Seeing Thoughts as Secretions of the Thinking Mind

In working with difficulties in meditation, we are training our minds to see thinking simply as thinking; to see thoughts as secretions of the mind without necessarily a basis in reality or any great degree of truth. And even if a thought does seem to be true (as thoughts will often claim themselves to be), in this moment, is it bearable? When I tune into my body, in this moment, is it okay to let this experience just be as it is, acknowledging whatever is present with gentle curiosity, patience, and kindness?

We have approached the practice of working with difficulties by bringing to them a light touch, not bulldozing through. Sometimes, thoughts, beliefs, or situations may seem so negative or difficult that to bring awareness to them might seem too unbearable. If this is your experience, rather than fighting with it, we have a number of ways we might respond available to us. One option, as we have been learning, is to bring to awareness how we are relating to the difficulty within the body, whether it be with physical sensations or perhaps emotions. If when you bring to mind the difficulty or the negative thought or belief, you notice a strong sensation in the body arising, we can move our attention to that place, softening, opening, and breathing with the sensations, giving them space and allowing them to be present. And when the sensation no longer has a strong pull on your attention, just resting your awareness with the movements of the breath or to the body as a whole.

Another option for working with difficulties in meditation is that if, rather than a strong physical sensation, you notice a strong emotion bubbling to the surface, we might sit with the emotional charge of that energy, rather than the thought itself: breathing with the emotion, giving it space, opening, just as we are learning to do with physical sensations that arise. In staying with the emotional charge of energy, as opposed to getting lost in thinking, we learn to stay present with experience, without adding further fuel to the fire. We are going to practice this meditation technique of intentionally working with difficulties now.

Sitting Meditation: Mindfulness of Breath, Body, Sounds, Thoughts; and Seated Meditation, Introducing Working with a Difficulty in the Practice

Preface guiding this meditation in the same way as in Session 5, by providing guidance to not select the "biggest," "most emotionally laden" difficulty to work with, but instead inviting a "moderate" problem to the workbench of the mind, and emphasizing to approach this with kindness. Lead the group through the Session 6, Mindfulness of Breath, Body, Sounds and Thoughts Seated Meditation, Introducing Working with a Difficulty in the Practice; see Appendix B on the website for a script.

Guided Inquiry

- Without telling us specifically what difficulty you chose to work with or the details about it, I am curious about what you noticed during that practice?
- How is working with difficulty in this way different (or similar) to how you usually approach challenging circumstances in your life, such as pain?
- In what ways do you see this practice relating to your day-to-day living with chronic pain?

Guided inquiry of experience with at-home practice: *alternating Seated Meditation, Introducing Working with a Difficulty in the Practice, with no guided meditation audio, 3-Minute Breathing Space, 3-Minute Responsive Breathing Space. Also inquire into the "Getting Down to the Root of Our Thoughts and Beliefs about Pain" handout. Review practice logs and make copies if it is part of a research project.*

- Now let's move on to a discussion of your at-home practice. What was that experience like for you?
- What did you notice in bringing difficulties to the "work bench" of the mind during your meditation practice this week?
  - What, if any, challenges did you experience?
- How was practicing without the guided audio different from your usual practice over the past few weeks?
- How was engaging in the 3-Minute Responsive Breathing Space (when you noticed a difficult situation arise) different from the way you would normally react to difficulties?
- What is your relationship to practice now after having been engaging in daily meditation for the past 5 weeks?
  - Are you noticing any changes? (*i.e., attachment or aversion to the practice?*)
- What did you notice in reading over and working with the "Getting Down to the Root of Our Thoughts and Beliefs about Pain" handout?

When Our Viewpoint Gets Trapped by Thoughts and Emotions

We are now going to do an exercise to further explore the connections between thoughts, emotions, and how we feel.

Provide participants with the Version 1 handout (do not *give them Version 2 at this stage), and invite them to write down on the handout what they would think.*

Version 1 says:

- "You woke up feeling down this morning after a bad night's sleep due to pain. You get to the kitchen and see your partner who rushes off, saying he or she couldn't stop and needed to run. What would you think?"

After a few minutes, next provide participants with the Version 2 handout, and invite them to write down what they would think in this situation.

Version 2 says:

- "You woke up feeling happy this morning after a good night's sleep with few interruptions from pain. You get to the kitchen and see your partner who rushes off, saying he or she couldn't stop and needed to run. What would you think?"

Discuss client's responses first to Version 1 and then Version 2, comparing the thoughts and feelings brought up by each scenario. Write their responses on the flip chart.

We have been learning how thoughts effect our emotions and how we feel (i.e., as in the stress–pain connection we discussed in Session 2). Here in this example—where we have objectively the same situation of our partner needing to rush off—we see that the new piece is that the context and our mood going into a situation lead us to make very different interpretations of the same event, which tells us there is no one single truth. So what we perceive as reality is largely determined by what we bring into the situation (i.e., our mood or our frame of mind), as opposed to purely the situation itself.

If the mood we bring to the event is negative, it is likely that the interpretations or conclusions we reach will also be negative/unhelpful and this feeds back to create a vicious cycle leading to worsening mood, more negative thinking, and likely more pain. So a negative mood is a sign that we need to lean in, and pay close attention to our thoughts so that we can catch this chain reaction early on by seeing thoughts as thoughts, not facts. As we have discussed, meditation trains our minds to become skillful at making this distinction, to observe our thoughts, to note when we are getting carried downstream in their content, and to return, over and over again, to our anchor, to awareness of the movements of the breath.

Tools to Shift Your Viewpoint on "Hot" Thoughts

When you are feeling as though the pain is "too much" and you are overwhelmed and caught up in a raging torrent of negative thoughts and feelings, the first step is always the same: take a Breathing Space. The 3-Minute Breathing Space is a portable technique and is something you can do on the spot, in the moment, wherever you find yourself. Bringing your awareness to the breath allows you to step back, bring in space, and allow your wise mind to gently and kindly acknowledge what is happening, without shutting down, without acting out, to just acknowledge. This space removes the blinders, and allows you to see with greater clarity what is happening with you, what is the situation, and what choices there might be in how to respond.

No matter what is happening, the critical point is that there is *always* a choice; even if that is a choice to take no action—no action can sometimes be the best action. But the process of realizing this remains the same, a 3-Minute Breathing Space is always the first step. Following this, there are a number of options for steps to shift your viewpoint and to see the choices that are available to you, which are shown in your handouts... *Go over and discuss the "Tools to Shift your Viewpoint on "Hot" Thoughts" handout.*

As we become more skillful with this practice we may begin to see thinking in the same way as we see breathing; for example, it's just a natural process, a natural activity, and we can observe this activity of the thinking mind without getting lost in the activity, that is to say, lost in the story line of our thoughts. The power of this practice of recognizing thoughts simply as mental events is that it opens up choices in any situation; it shows you what options are present, what other viewpoints there might be, and all of this gives you the opportunity to *choose* how you want to respond. This allows you to see difficulties in a different light; thoughts, emotions, pain—any difficulty—becomes (not a breeze, but…) more manageable, less stressful.

3-Minute Breathing Space: Let's practice taking this first step now. *Lead the group through the 3-Minute Breathing Space meditation; see Appendix B on the website for a script for this meditation.*

Guided Inquiry

- What did you notice with that brief practice? (*Depending on time, you may wish to further this discussion, inquiring into how this was different from how we might typically spend a spare 3 min, and/or how this practice relates to living with chronic pain.*)

Identifying Red Flags for a Rising Stress–Pain Thermometer

An important way to learn how to manage pain is to heighten your awareness of when you might *need* a breathing space or to use one of the other strategies we just discussed to shift your viewpoint. Knowing those red flags that are unique to each of us—which might be changes in emotions, thoughts, or changes in your body such as a sense of tightening, or changes in activity—is important. As we learned in the Gate Control Theory in Session 1, stress and these reactions contribute to worsening pain. It is helpful to learn to catch the early warning signs that you are over- or underdoing activity, overscheduled with depleting activities, or perhaps judging a situation as stressful, or when you are sensing that out of control feeling when pain seems to be creeping up. Awareness of these early signs (without being overly hypervigilant) can then be an impetus for you to apply the skills you have been practicing, and to take wise action—to respond rather than react—so you can better take care of yourself when the stress–pain thermometer is threatening to boil over.

Examine flare-up triggers in pairs or small groups and make a list of the specific warning signals that the stress–pain thermometer might be rising. Follow this with a group discussion, and write some of the red flags on the flip chart; provide the following as examples if clients are having difficulty:

- Completely absorbing yourself with work or avoiding work completely.
- Letting yourself go (i.e., not exercising, eating unhealthily, not taking time for self-care).
- Experiencing your mind "racing" into the future or dwelling on the past.
- Feeling tense/anxious, angry, and/or depressed.
- Sleeping a lot more or a lot less than usual.
- Isolating yourself and not wanting to talk to anyone.
- Pushing through the pain without listening to your body, or resting when needed.

Noticing these red flags provides a useful basis for making the shift toward better self-care, which we will be continuing to work on throughout the remainder of the program. Part of your take-home activities this week is to work with this exercise further and enhance your awareness of these red flags and what might keep you stuck.

Developing a Mindfulness Maintenance Plan

After today, we will have two more classes left. The end of this course though is really the beginning, the beginning of a new way going forward to live a full, meaningful life with pain. In preparing to move toward this, we invite you to really explore how you can personalize the practices you have been learning and make them part of your day-to-day life to develop a Mindfulness Maintenance Plan.

As you have likely discovered, mindfulness is not a "cure" for pain, and it does not "work" like pain medication in that you may not always experience immediate symptom relief. The idea is that mindfulness becomes infused in to your day-to-day life and becomes a way to manage the pain, and becomes a way of life. Keeping up the momentum with your formal meditation practice time each day is the best way to make this happen, and for the changes you have noticed throughout this program to continue.

In the coming week as you go about finding your own way to personalize the practice, be sure also to consider ways to supplement your daily formal practices with the informal mindfulness practices that we have been working with, which "top you up on mindfulness" during the day: bringing mindfulness into routine activities such as eating, washing the dishes, brushing your teeth. The more you can embody these informal practices on a daily level, the more in tune with your experience you will become: noticing perhaps when the stress–pain thermometer may be rising, and also noticing and taking pleasure in the pleasant moments of your experience.

At-Home Daily Practice

During the coming week your daily practice, as shown on your handouts, will be... *Go over client handout describing at-home practice following Session 6.*

Distribute guided meditation audio files and Session 6 client handouts.

Summary

What we have been learning today is that... *Go over client summary handout: "Seeing Thoughts as Just Thoughts."*

In-Session Worksheet: Version 1

You woke up feeling down this morning after a bad night's sleep due to pain. You get to the kitchen and see your partner who rushes off, saying he or she couldn't stop and needed to run. What would you think?

____

____

____

____

____

____

____

____

In-Session Worksheet: Version 2

You woke up feeling happy this morning after a good night's sleep with few interruptions from pain. You get to the kitchen and see your partner who rushes off, saying he or she couldn't stop and needed to run. What would you think?

____

____

____

____

____

____

____

____

Client Handbook

Session 6 Summary: Seeing Thoughts as Just Thoughts

Usually our minds run on automatic pilot, making judgments, interpretations, running story lines—all typically happening without our awareness. However, our thoughts have a powerful effect on how we feel emotionally and physically, and also on what we do (or do not do). Learning to become aware of the patterns of our minds and simply labeling it all as "thinking," and then intentionally letting it go and returning to the breath takes practice.

In knowing and becoming friends with our typical, automatic unhelpful thinking patterns we can become more skillful in catching "hot" thoughts and red flags early, before they pick up momentum and lead to a rising stress–pain thermometer, leaving us with unpleasant emotions and worsening pain. Thoughts that may challenge your practice of mindfulness, such as "This is never going to help my pain" are also critical to catch early as they have the potential to undermine the work you are doing in this program by convincing you not to practice the very tools that you can use to take back control of your life from the pain. Moreover, it is important to see these negative thought patterns for what they are, as just thoughts, and also as extra baggage that over time adds to pain, making it feel overwhelming.

The practices you have been learning in this program translate directly into action, and allow you to choose ways of responding that skillfully manage your pain, thoughts, mood, and well-being. Most importantly, we begin to see that thoughts are not immutable facts, we are not our thinking mind, and we are not our pain. Simply observing our thoughts allows us to step back and gain freedom from the control that thinking and pain hold over us.

Tools to Shift Your Viewpoint on "Hot" Thoughts

When "hot" thoughts are raising the stress–pain thermometer, you might choose to experiment with relating to the thoughts with one (or more!) of these approaches:

1) Step 1 is always to take a 3-Minute Breathing Space. Then…
2) You may choose to simply watch your thoughts, as if they are projected on to a screen, and you watch them as an observer, waiting and watching, without getting taken along with any of them, as they flash across the screen.
3) To label all thoughts, whether they are positive, neutral or negative, as just "thinking." In this way, all thoughts, even particularly juicy ones, are seen simply as mental events, without necessarily any substance or truth. And even if you believe there is at least a grain of truth to a thought, it is up to you to see it for what it is, and then to choose how to respond.
4) Perhaps you might choose to return to your "Unhelpful Habits of Mind" handout, and to ask yourself if you are engaging in any of those habits? Perhaps labeling it, "Ah, fortune telling," and then bringing awareness to your breath.
5) To express your thoughts by writing them down on paper. This also gives you a degree of distance from your thoughts so that you can see them for what they are. There is something about getting thoughts down on paper, and the pause between having the thought and getting it written, that opens up a fresh perspective and allows you to process the thought and emotion and to reflect without getting carried away by the thought or emotion.
6) You might wish to ask yourself: "Where did this thought come from?" "What mood state might be accompanying this thought?" "How am I relating to this thought or mood in my body?" "Am I adding more baggage to the bare facts, and is there something I can acknowledge with kindness, and let go?" Perhaps gently saying to yourself that there may be another way to view this situation.
7) When working with particularly challenging thoughts, or if the same difficult thought keeps coming up, it might be helpful to bring these thoughts to the work bench of the mind in meditation—using the Seated Meditation practice we did together earlier today and that you have been practicing during the week—so you can mindfully observe them in a balanced, intentional, accepting way and to see what might come up for you in such an open context.

At-Home Daily Practice for Following Session 6

1) Practice with your own selection from the guided meditation audios for a minimum of 45 min a day (e.g., guided Seated Meditations, Body Scan, Mindful Movement). The idea is to begin settling into your own personal practice that is just right for you.
2) Engage in at least three short (regular) 3-Minute Breathing Spaces every day at set times that you have decided in advance.
3) Practice the 3-Minute Responsive Breathing Space whenever you notice your stress–pain thermometer rising.
4) If you notice your stress–pain thermometer is still raised following the 3-Minute Responsive Breathing Space, take a moment to read over your "Tools to Shift your Viewpoint on 'Hot' Thoughts" handout and experiment with one of the options suggested.
5) Identify your unique warning signs that your stress–pain thermometer is rising—what keeps you "stuck"? And what you can do to lower it? Carry a small notepad around with you during the day to jot down, as close to the moment as possible, those changes in mind (going back to the "Unhelpful Habits of Mind" and "Getting Down to the Root of Our Thoughts and Beliefs about Pain" handouts for tips), emotion, body, and activity (returning to your Stressful Experiences Diary for ideas) that may be triggers for increased pain and stress that would be helpful to be aware of (without becoming overly vigilant). If it feels comfortable, you might even ask people close to you if they have noticed any signals that a pain flare-up is on the way.
6) Complete your daily at-home practice record; it helps to fill this in as close to finishing your practice as possible. Make a note in the comment box of anything that comes up in the at-home practice so that we can talk about it at the next meeting.

Therapist Tips, Troubleshooting, and Supervision for Session 6

Session Opening Exercise ("John")

The opening exercise is best delivered with minimal introduction, simply by saying something along the lines of, "We are going to start today's session with a brief exercise. I am going to write some sentences up on the flip chart, and I invite you to read them one by one as I write them." And then proceed to write the sentences, stepping away from the flip chart and pausing at the end of writing each sentence to give clients a chance to read it. This exercise, cleverly developed by Segal, Williams, and Teasdale, clearly illustrates, through direct experience, the meaning-making function of our minds and how we get carried along and *believe* our thoughts. The power of automatic thoughts and their connection to pain and stress has been a recurring theme throughout the program. This exercise sets the stage for the focus of this session, which is to begin to further our capacity to relate differently to our thoughts and beliefs: to see thoughts as just thoughts, not as the truth, and not as something that we need to "obey."

When Viewpoints Get Trapped

The alternative viewpoints exercise introduces a new piece to the puzzle. In this exercise, clients observe via their own and the group's shared responses to the two example scenarios that (1) not only do automatic thoughts influence how we behave and feel, but that (2) context and how we feel also loop around and influence how we think. When fatigue, stress, pain, and negative mood are present, these are likely to trigger unhelpful thinking habits that put us in a negative frame of mind, which further clouds how we see our outer (and inner) circumstances. Thus, both the opening exercise and this viewpoint exercise illustrate how we are constantly adding meaning and interpretations to scenarios and situations, and this awareness opens up freedom to choose how to respond. Included in the client handouts is a description of some of the ways clients may choose to shift their viewpoint on "hot" thoughts once they are aware that they are getting swept away in unhelpful thinking patterns, stress, and/or negative mood, and within this, the 3-Minute Responsive Breathing space is taught as the first step. The handout describes a number of options for next steps following this Breathing Space; steps to take skillful action rather than run off pre-programmed habitual, unhelpful patterns of reacting.

Identifying Red Flags for a Rising Stress–Pain Thermometer

The intention of this interactive exercise is to enhance clients' awareness of those changes in mind, body, emotion, and behavior that might be red flags or warning signals that stress and pain are rising. This activity is also assigned for clients' at-home practice so that they can build on it during the coming week as they make direct observations of their experiences. Clients are the experts on what makes their pain better or worse; this interactive group exercise is helpful to cue awareness on what other factors might be influencing pain and stress that have been operating "below the surface" of awareness which they might not yet have recognized. Some clients might not be aware of *any* triggers for their pain (i.e., the pain seems to "come out of the blue"), and so it can be helpful to connect this exercise back to the Gate Control Theory from Session 1—instead of asking about "red flags" or triggers, inquiring into what things they have noticed "open the gates." Often this different way of explaining the exercise can reach different people. If clients are really stuck, starting by writing up on the flip chart some of the example responses from the therapist outline can be a helpful way to stimulate thoughts and facilitate the discussion.

Mindfulness Maintenance Plan

Following this session, there are only two remaining classes, so it is important that the notion of finding ways to keep up momentum and maintain a personalized, daily formal mindfulness practice following the program be introduced. As the therapist, you should elicit, reflect, and reinforce motivational statements about practice, and encourage clients to explore their own ways of integrating the meditation techniques taught into their day-to-day lives. Building on this, the at-home activities following Session 6 are mostly self-directed in that clients are encouraged to practice with their own selection of the techniques that have been taught. This notion is reinforced in Session 7, where clients are further encouraged to continue to develop routines for practicing on their own, and again in Session 8, where clients are guided to identify a personalized reason for maintaining the practice.

Reference

Segal, Z. V., Williams, J. M. G., & Teasdale, J. D. (2013). *Mindfulness-based cognitive therapy for depression*. New York, NY: Guilford.

11

Session 7: Taking Care of Myself

Therapist Introduction

A core emphasis of this session is development of a Mindfulness Maintenance Plan for on-going self-care following the conclusion of the program. The session starts with once more practicing the Seated Meditation practice where a difficulty is intentionally introduced into the practice, and clients harness the meditation technique to stay open to the difficulty, training in responding with nonjudgmental acceptance. This practice is followed by a guided inquiry, that transitions into a discussion of client's at-home practice.

For self-care to be effective, at base, we need to notice our warning signs and then have a plan in place for taking proactive steps to lower the stress–pain thermometer. Therefore, in the second half of this session, to heighten awareness of daily activity routines and how these may contribute to stress and pain, clients are invited to participate in an activity where they make note of the details of what they do in a typical day, and then to break these activities down into those that are nourishing, and those that are depleting—highlighting the link between activity and mood/energy. Clients then work toward identifying ways to build in more nourishing activities (perhaps returning to their Pleasant Experiences Diary from Session 2 for ideas). This then transitions into a discussion of clients' unique red flags for stress and pain flare-up, and how activity may be effectively used as a means to defuse these destructive patterns and foster better self-care and effective pain management.

Mindfulness-Based Cognitive Therapy for Chronic Pain: A Clinical Manual and Guide,
First Edition. Melissa A. Day.

Companion website: www.wiley.com/go/day/mindfulness_based_cognitive_therapy

Therapist Outline

Assessment Measures

Have clients fill out Assessment Measures. Provide assistance as needed.

Orientation

During this program, a recurring theme has been to tune in and bring mindful awareness to our mind, emotions, body, and also our pain. Learning to step out of automatic pilot, and to check in with what thoughts are present, what emotions are present, what sensations, including painful sensations are present (and going beyond just the label of "pain"). This opens up a new way of relating to experience and allows you to notice when you might be getting carried away with thoughts, and when pain is beginning to take over your mind space.

At times, especially when pain or emotions may be spiraling out of control, exploring how activity may help manage chronic pain represents another way to respond wisely to the needs of any given moment. In exploring this option of activity, it may become apparent that perhaps the type of activity you are engaging in may need to shift, or perhaps the amount, intensity, or quality might need to change in order for you to best take care of yourself.

Theme

In learning to tune in, you will likely become aware of your own unique warning signs or red flags that pain or an emotional flare-up are imminent. If you can catch it at that early stage, there are more options in terms of action to take to respond to these signs before they threaten to take over. The important message is that there are things *you can do* to better manage pain, and precisely what that is will be unique for each of you.

Sitting Meditation: Mindfulness of Breath, Body, Sounds, Thoughts; and Seated Meditation, Introducing Working with a Difficulty in the Practice

Part of taking care of ourselves is learning how to work with pain and difficult situations so as they are less overwhelming. We are now going to practice the specific meditation technique we have been working with the past two sessions, which is an ideal vehicle for gently building our ability to stay present with difficult situations. During this meditation you will be guided to bring a difficulty or problem to mind, working with staying in touch with the difficulty with openness and kindness, as best you can.

Lead the group through the Session 7, Mindfulness of Breath, Body, Sounds and Thoughts and Seated Meditation, Introducing Working with a Difficulty in the Practice; see Appendix B on the website for a script.

Guided Inquiry

- Without telling us specifically what difficulty you chose to work with or the details about it, what did you notice with that practice? (*Depending on client responses, you might also further the inquiry into exploring how this practice was different from how clients typically relate to challenging circumstances, and how this practice might relate to living with pain.)*

Guided inquiry of experience with at-home practice: *Practice with your own selection from the guided audio files; 3-Minute Breathing Space (Regular and Responsive). Also inquire into the "Tools to Shift your Viewpoint on 'Hot' Thoughts" handout, and noticing red flags that the stress–pain thermometer is rising. Review practice logs and make copies if it is part of a research project.*

- What was the experience of your at-home practice, working with your own selection of the guided meditations like this past week?
- Of the practices you have learned, what are you finding yourself settling on?
- What have you found is helpful in keeping up your daily practice?
- What challenges, if any, have you noticed?
  - How might you overcome these barriers?

Part of your take-home activities was also to explore those changes in your thinking, emotions, behavior, and physical sensations which are red flags or triggers that your stress–pain thermometer is rising. What red flags did you notice that might be your own unique warning signals? What seems to keep you "stuck" when these red flags arise? *Discuss clients' experiences.* We are going to continue to work with identifying ways to respond wisely when you notice these red flags, so that you can move towards better self-care. This next exercise is going to drill down even further to bring deeper awareness to how what we do in the moments of our days might be a further red flag, or on the other hand, might be rejuvenating.

The Relationship Between Activity and Pain

When you are having a pain flare-up, you may not "feel up to it" when it comes to engaging in activity to take care of yourself; or perhaps you are having a good day, and so you overdo it and want to squeeze in everything you can as you are feeling so good, right? Or perhaps there is a certain anxiety in not knowing how you are going to feel from one day to the next, and so it becomes harder to plan and commit to doing something you might enjoy "just in case" you might experience a pain flare-up. Living with pain, stress, and the whole spectrum of emotion that comes along with the territory of chronic pain—anxiety, anger, sadness—can also lead to a sense of not *wanting* to do anything. Perhaps because all of this takes away your motivation or perhaps because you can't do things "like you used to" so you might think "what's the point?" We each have our own tendencies in the face of pain; if you are aware of those tendencies as they are happening however, you can see if in this moment it is helpful, or not, to go along with those tendencies. Self-care is not selfish. And sometimes you need to put yourself first, and sometimes you need to continue to do things you enjoy instead of letting pain be the dictator.

We are going to do an exercise now to heighten our awareness of our tendencies and what precisely it is that we do day to day. So I invite you to bring to mind how you spend a typical day and write those things you do down on this piece of paper (*hand out paper*). Starting from the moment you wake up, and examining the activities in fine detail—perhaps washing your face, making coffee, breakfast, talking to family—all the way to the evening and when you lay your head down to go to bed. *Allow time for clients to write down their daily activities.*

And now, I would like for you to see if you can divide your list into:

1) Nourishing activities: put an "N" next to those things you do in your day-to-day life that you value, that energize you, nourish you, rejuvenate you.
2) Depleting activities: put a "D" next to those activities you do in your day-to-day life that zap your energy, leave you feeling emotionally drained, take you out of the moment, or that place a strain on your well-being in some way.

For now, you can just leave those activities that may be "neutral." *Allow time for clients to divide their list in this way.*

What did you notice in doing this activity? Did you discover you had more Ns than Ds or vice versa, or was it reasonably balanced? *Discuss clients' experiences.*

To build in more nourishing, valued activities during our day and to decrease the amount of time spent in depleting activities takes planning and intention. So I invite you to look back over your list and consider: of those activities in your daily life that are depleting, "What little shifts in my day, or in my approach to my day, might allow me to do these less frequently and/or differently so as they don't drag me down?" And, of those activities you value and find nourishing, "What little shifts in my day, or in my approach to my day, might bring more of these into my daily experiences, and/or help me to be more fully present with them when they are happening?" *Allow time for clients to write down their ideas and discuss, writing responses on the flip chart.*

A number of you have commented that you have competing demands on your schedule, and that you feel you "should be doing x, y, z for others" before taking care of you. Another emerging theme is that you feel locked into the various patterns of your life and you feel it's beyond your control for your days to look different, to include more nourishing activities and less depleting activities. Self-care seems like a luxury, an optional extra "if there is time."

So it's a bit of a bind, if we want our days to look and feel different, to be doing more of what we value and what energizes us, and yet our thoughts tell us, "Well, that would be nice, but it's just not possible," then things won't shift or change in the direction we want them to and we are stuck. But just in noticing that thought stream, in bringing awareness to how you are spending your day, to pay attention even in the midst of feeling rushed as you move from one activity to another, you might find that there are gaps or spaces of time, or shifts that can be made in your approach where self-care can become the priority. Bringing awareness to those gaps opens up space for you to *choose* how you spend those spaces of time, allowing you to make a mindful decision about what you really need—perhaps by taking a moment to slow down and have a cup of tea out in the garden—rather than just running on autopilot and checking emails or Facebook, for example, or however you might habitually fill up those precious spaces of time. At base, the message here is to mindfully check in with yourself (multiple times a day), asking yourself "What do I need to do in this moment to best take care of myself?"

Tips for Better Self-Care

Sometimes in the moment we may not know what it is we need to take care of ourselves, perhaps the pain feels overwhelming or we just don't know what might give us a sense of pleasure or mastery. It helps to have a "go to" list, which will be unique for all of us, of activities (or nonactivities) that are nourishing to you or that give you a sense of mastery, so that when you notice perhaps your pain building, your mind falling into unhelpful habits, or your mood sinking, you can go to this list (which you might keep on the fridge or somewhere visible), and no matter how "good" or "bad" you feel, you can proactively choose to do something that will nurture you. So let's take a few moments to start making this list now, jotting down some things that are nourishing or that give you a sense of mastery—making sure to include some things that are big and small, require effort and require little effort, so that no matter how we feel, there is always something on this list we can do that will uplift our mood and take care of ourselves in some way. And if you are stuck for ideas, perhaps return to your Pleasant Experiences Diary from Session 2 to see what you found uplifting. *Allow time for clients to write down activities.*

It is best to have a variety of options in self-care activities on your list, to keep things fresh and interesting. If the option comes up though, be open to spontaneously experimenting with something new that you haven't done before or that isn't on the list. An approach of curiosity and inquisitiveness often overrides a sense of withdrawal, retreat, or fear-based reactions, and how you feel afterwards might surprise you! Now, looking back at your list of daily activities, what "gaps" or windows of time might be present, and where you can schedule in those activities that give you a sense of pleasure or mastery? *Allow time for clients to look at their list, and schedule in nourishing activities.*

Part of your take-home activities will be to continue developing these plans to increase the moments in your days that are nourishing, and to add to this list of self-care activities. In learning to take better care of yourself in this way, it is likely that thoughts such as "This isn't going to change anything," or even the thought "I am going to feel a thousand times better after this" will come up. As best you can, simply note those as just thoughts, and lay them aside, choose one activity from your list to engage in, and bring an open mind to the activity without prejudging how you are going to feel afterwards, and also not waiting until you "feel like" doing it to do it.

A key message is not to expect miracles straight away. The idea is to think of it like steering a ship: initially you slightly turn the wheel of the ship, steering it in a different direction only by perhaps a change in a few degrees, but over time, that slight change in direction sends the ship on an entirely different course. By building more nourishing activities into your day, and limiting or removing those activities that drain you, this builds your sense of control in the face of pain and pain flare-up—you are not just at the mercy of how your pain feels on a given day, there are things *you can do* to manage the pain. As always, it is helpful to use the 3-Minute Breathing Space as a first step to tune in, and to mindfully observe what it is that would be most nourishing for you in this moment—taking this brief pause allows your wise mind to see more clearly what action, if any, is then needed to best take care of yourself.

3-Minute Breathing Space: let's practice taking this first step now. *Lead the group through the 3-Minute Breathing Space meditation; see Appendix B on the website for a script for this meditation.*

Guided Inquiry

What did you notice? (*Depending on time, you may wish to further this discussion.*)

Steps Towards Self-Care in the Face of a Rising Stress–Pain Thermometer

When your stress–pain thermometer is rising, knowing your red flags and knowing in advance what is nourishing for you are key elements of a good self-care plan. What we are learning today is that to move toward better self-care in the face of pain and stress, at base involves two steps:

Step 1 is always to take a 3-Minute Breathing Space.

Step 2 is to then respond, to make a wise choice as to what would be the kindest, most nourishing thing you could do to best take care of yourself in this moment. This might be something that gives you a sense of pleasure, mastery, or sense of achievement and control. It could be practicing a longer meditation, going back and reading over a handout that you connected with from this program, or engaging in some other activity you have identified as nourishing for you in your list that we started making earlier.

When pain is intense it is often the case that we are also taken over by a running stream of negative thoughts about the pain ("This is terrible"), its effects ("It's ruined my whole day and put me further behind"), and about our own self-worth ("I am worthless; who is going to want to keep me on the job?"). In taking a Breathing Space as a first step, this puts us in a better position to see these thoughts clearly for what they are, as just thoughts. Following this, you might choose to return to your handout from Session 6, "Tools to Shift Your Viewpoint on 'Hot' Thoughts" to refresh your mind on the tools you have available to you.

You may also become aware of how pain is affecting your emotions and the rest of your body. For example, you may find that a pain flare-up results in anger as well as increased muscle tension throughout your body. As in the

Seated Meditation we practiced earlier today, it may be helpful to bring these difficulties to the workbench of your mind and to intentionally "soften" and "open" to them, rather than continue to resist and fight against them. This approach can help clear your mind, so you are in a better "mental space" to choose the best course of action.

Many people report that the most difficult times are when they haven't seen any red flags or signs that their pain is about to intensify, and the flare-up seems to come out of the blue and takes them by surprise. Without knowing how long the pain will last, if even still during these times you start by taking a Breathing Space and then bring an open, inquiring mind to the situation, this allows your mind to settle (to whatever degree it does) and to see what could be the most nourishing thing you could do to take care of yourself, as best you can, until the pain flare-up shifts. The task is to stay in the moment as best you can, without piling extra baggage on top of the pain, to stay with experience just as it is, with kindness and openness. Included in your handouts this week are some tips for better self-care, and for what action you might take when your stress–pain thermometer is rising.

At-Home Daily Practice

This will be your last "assigned" daily at-home practice in the program, so the key point is to settle into a meditation practice routine that allows you to best take care of yourself. During the coming week, your daily practice, as shown in your handouts, will be… *Go over client handout describing at-home practice following Session 7.*

Distribute guided meditation audio files and Session 7 client handouts.

Summary

What we are training in observing, and that was a focus of today's session is that… *Go over client summary handout: "Taking Care of Myself."*

Client Handbook

Session 7 Summary: Taking Care of Myself

How we spend the moments of our lives is essentially how we spend our minutes, hours, days, weeks, years … essentially our entire life. Each moment is really all we have and how we choose to respond to each moment and what we decide to do in each moment accumulates to have a powerful influence on our thoughts, emotions, our pain, and our general overall sense of self-worth and lovability. To live a meaningful life in line with our values, it is helpful to (following a Breathing Space) routinely check in and ask ourselves:

- In my daily life, what am I doing that is nourishing me, making me feel alive, energized, connected, and grounded?
- In my daily life, what am I doing that drains me, throws me off course, and makes me feel I am just going through the motions with no meaning and no purpose?
- Some things cannot be changed, accepting that, am I mindfully choosing to bring in to my life more nourishing moments, and less depleting moments?

When we bring awareness to what we are doing in the moments of our lives, this brings with it the choice of whether we want to continue what we are doing, or to make a shift. By becoming skillful at regularly checking in with ourselves and bringing awareness to the quality of the activity we are engaging in from one moment to the next, we learn to make more mindful decisions about what it is we really need to move toward more effectively managing pain. In doing this, we can use our daily activities to work *for us* rather than *against us*: we can cultivate our own personal balance of activities to not only manage the routine daily pattern of our lives to become more energizing, but also to help cope through times of pain flare-up, and the negative mood and unhelpful thinking that is so often a part of the chronic pain landscape.

Practicing building in more nourishing activities, and lessening our time spent on draining activities is something we need to learn to do even when we are feeling good. Practicing in this way also means that the skill of self-care (yes, it is a skill as for most of us it doesn't come naturally!) is well honed and ready for difficult times such as when pain threatens to take over.

Tips for Better Self-Care

When your stress–pain thermometer is rising, knowing your red flags and knowing in advance what is nourishing for you are key elements of any good self-care plan. With this awareness, no matter how good or bad we feel or what our minds are telling us, we then need to choose to take some form of wise action—to take steps toward better self-care. By building more nourishing activities into your day (by actually scheduling them in!), and limiting or removing those activities that drain you, this builds your sense of control in the face of pain and pain flare-up—you are not just at the mercy of how your pain feels on a given day, there are things *you can do* to manage the pain.

It is best to have a variety of options in self-care activities included on your personalized list of activities that give you a sense of pleasure, mastery, or accomplishment (which we started working on in today's session) that you can go to which will keep things fresh and interesting. If the option comes up though, be open to spontaneously experimenting with something new that you haven't done before or that is not on the list. An approach of curiosity and inquisitiveness often overrides a sense of withdrawal, retreat, or fear-based reactions, and how you feel afterwards might surprise you!

A key message is not to expect miracles straight away. The idea is to think of it like steering a ship: initially you slightly turn the wheel of the ship, steering it in a different direction only by perhaps a change in a few degrees, but over time, that slight change in direction sends the ship on an entirely different course.

Steps Towards Better Self-Care in the Face of a Rising Stress–Pain Thermometer

Many people report that the most difficult times are when they haven't seen any red flags or signs that their pain is about to intensify, and the flare-up seems to come out of the blue and takes them by surprise. Without knowing how long the pain will last, even during these times, to move towards better self-care in the face of a pain and stress flare-up involves two basic steps:

Step 1 is always to take a 3-Minute Breathing Space.

Step 2 is to then respond, to make a wise choice as to what would be the kindest, most nourishing thing you could do to best take care of yourself in this moment. This might be something that gives you a sense of pleasure, mastery, or sense of achievement and control. It could be practicing a longer meditation, going back and reading over a handout that you connected with from this program, or engaging in some other activity that you have identified as nourishing for you in your list that we started making during this session.

When pain is intense it is often the case that we are also taken over by a running stream of negative thoughts about the pain ("This is terrible"), its effects ("It's ruined my whole day and put me further behind"), and about our own self-worth ("I am worthless; who is going to want to keep me on the job?"). In taking a Breathing Space as a first step, this puts us in a better position to see these thoughts clearly for what they are, as just thoughts. Following this, you might choose to return to your handout from Session 6 "Tools to Shift Your Viewpoint on 'Hot' Thoughts," to refresh your mind on the tools that you have available to you.

You might also become aware of how pain is affecting your emotions and the rest of your body. For example, you may find that a pain flare-up results in anger as well as increased muscle tension throughout your body. As in the Seated Meditation we practiced in this session, it may be helpful to bring these difficulties to the workbench of your mind and to intentionally "soften" and "open" to them, rather than continue to resist and fight against them. This approach can help clear your mind, so you are in a better "mental space" to choose the best course of action.

At-Home Daily Practice for Following Session 7

1) Develop your own personalized practice that you intend to engage in following this program. Settle on your own form of practice that is just right for you by selecting from the meditation techniques you have learned during this program to practice each day for a minimum of 45 min a day (e.g., guided Sitting Meditation, Body Scan, Mindful Movement).
2) Engage in at least three short (regular) 3-Minute Breathing Spaces every day at set times.
3) Practice the 3-Minute Responsive Breathing Space whenever you notice your stress–pain thermometer rising, and follow that by engaging in one nourishing activity. This nourishing activity can even be a nonactivity, and can be just a small thing you do for yourself that makes you feel energized, perhaps even something as simple as making a nice hot cup of tea.
4) To develop your own personalized action plan, continue to add to your list that we started making today of nourishing activities (or nonactivities) that you can engage in not only once you notice a red flag, but that you can schedule in and proactively use for your own self-care so that you are triggered less often. It helps to have options of nourishing activities that entail varying degrees of planning, time and "effort." For example, higher on effort might be going for a picnic by the lake, and lower down the scale might be listening to a guided Body Scan, or having a relaxing hot bath or even listening to a guided Body Scan practice *while* having a hot bath! This way, there is something you *can* do, even during times when your mind might be telling you "There is nothing I can do to manage this pain."
5) Complete your daily at-home practice record; it helps to fill this in as close to finishing your practice as possible. Make a note in the comment box of anything that comes up in the at-home practice so that we can talk about it at the next meeting.

Therapist Tips, Troubleshooting, and Supervision for Session 7

The Relationship Between Activity and Pain

We are typically not aware of precisely what we do in each moment of each day; we usually go through habitual routines and, without our knowing it, these automatic routines may be imbalanced in that the amount of depleting activities we engage in may outweigh the amount of nourishing, valued activities included in our day. In inviting clients to do this exercise, be sure to let them know that what they write down is just for them only, they do not have to "turn it in"—this gives clients permission to let go of any reservations about fully engaging in the activity. As how we spend our moments is how we spend our lives, seeing it written on paper in front of us can be quite illuminating. Often it will come up that on a given day the same activity could be either nourishing or depleting (depending on pain, fatigue, time, or any number of other factors), and this is perfectly okay—clients can write "N/D" next to those activities. Also, some activities may not be particularly nourishing or depleting and are relatively neutral, and you can tell clients to just leave those ones for now.

In the discussion that follows, the idea is not that all depleting activities be eliminated (as this is not realistic); rather, it is to explore ways to possibly cut back these activities. Or if a depleting activity *needs* to be done (i.e., not just because it is expected by others or clients feel they "should," but actually it does just literally need to be done, e.g., preparing something to eat), exploring how it could be done with a different quality, so it is less draining. In terms of building in more nourishing activities, a key message to convey, as one of my clients put it is: "self-care is not selfish." In other words, self-care is not an optional extra if there is time "left over" after taking care of everyone else, but rather self-care is an essential component of effective pain management that needs to be scheduled in and prioritized.

It is important to discuss how nourishing activities can be both those that bring a sense of pleasure (as in, for example, those experiences noted in the Pleasant Experiences Diary) as well as those that bring a sense of mastery or a sense of having accomplished something meaningful—both of these are uplifting. Having a readily available sense of what *is* nourishing and expanding the repertoire of activities that provide a sense of pleasure, mastery, or accomplishment is particularly helpful in overcoming inertia barriers often experienced with chronic pain, as is beginning to actually schedule these activities into a client's day in-session. In making their list of self-care activities, it is helpful to remind clients to include activities that entail varying degrees of effort, planning, and time, so there is always *something* that clients can do to take care of themselves in essentially any circumstance. A final "new" component in this session is encouraging clients to use the 3-Minute Breathing Space as the entry point to opening up their mind to allow them to then wisely choose what self-care activity from their list they need to engage in to best take care of themselves in any given moment.

12

Session 8: Harnessing the Power of the Mind for Chronic Pain Management

Therapist Introduction

In this last session we return to the Body Scan as the first meditation delivered to give a sense of having come full circle. Returning to the Body Scan is a metaphor for illustrating that this journey of practicing mindfulness meditation is at just the beginning; as Jon Kabat-Zinn points out, the real practice is for the rest of our lives. This practice is then followed by a review of client's experiences during the week, and a discussion of the take-home activity targeted toward identifying red flags for stress and pain flare-ups as well as identifying options of nourishing activities, and using these as a way to prevent relapse following the program. Following this, the program as a whole is reviewed, and clients are given the opportunity to reflect on their experiences over the course of the program. The "Mindfulness Knapsack" handout is used to facilitate discussion of all the portable pain coping techniques clients have learned in the program that they can carry forward with them.

A crucial component of this session is working with clients on their Mindfulness Maintenance Plans for keeping up regular practice going forward. The practices clients have chosen to settle on following the program are discussed, and clients are guided to identify a meaningful reason for continuing to practice and take care of themselves. The class concludes with a meditation in which the object of attention is a shell, stone, or bead (or some other object), and this is a tangible reminder for clients of all they have put into, and gotten out of, the program.

Mindfulness-Based Cognitive Therapy for Chronic Pain: A Clinical Manual and Guide, First Edition. Melissa A. Day.

Companion website: www.wiley.com/go/day/mindfulness_based_cognitive_therapy

Therapist Outline

Assessment Measures

Have clients fill out Assessment Measures. Provide assistance as needed.

Orientation

Today is our last meeting together as a group; however, your practice does not stop just because these classes stop. From this program, you have been practicing, building momentum, training your mind, and developing skills you can use to manage chronic pain and to live a meaningful life with the pain; by this point, you are firmly in the driver's seat. This eighth session is much more a beginning than an ending as this is the start of the rest of your lives.

Although your own felt experience of this program will be unique for each of you, if there were a way to condense it all down in to just a few words to describe the central theme of the course, the closest thing may be this:

- With awareness, we see our automatic ways of reacting to pain, of thinking and feeling, and in being mindful of this, we see that there are skillful ways of responding available to us, that there is a choice.

This doesn't change the fact that you have pain, sadness, or some other "problem" that you are facing, but it does open up the freedom to choose to take wise action, to face the pain in a radically different way rather than being driven by and controlled by pain and unexamined, automatic thinking patterns – there is another way. The instruction has been to bring a friendly curiosity to our thoughts, feelings, and sensations, and to hold them in a cradle of mindfulness. The task is to stay with our direct experience, using the breath as an anchor.

Theme

The intention to keep up the practices you have settled on can be strengthened by linking this intention to positive reasons for taking care of yourself. Just as food needs to be eaten for it to nourish you, mindfulness needs to be regularly practiced for it to continue to be a tool to manage your pain and to maintain a balance in life.

Returning Full Circle: The Body Scan Practice

We are going to start today's session by coming full circle—ending at the beginning, beginning at the ending—by practicing the Body Scan together.

Lead the group through the Body Scan meditation; see Appendix B on the website for a script.

Guided Inquiry

Followed by only a brief review.

- What did you notice in returning to the Body Scan practice?

Guided inquiry of experience with at-home practice: *Practicing with own selection from the guided audios, 3-Minute Breathing Space (Regular and Responsive and Nourishing activity), Steps Towards Better Self-Care. Review practice logs and make copies if it is part of a research project.*

- What was the experience of practicing with your own selection of the guided practices like for you?
- What schedule do you find yourself settling into?

During this past week, part of your take-home activities was to develop a list of activities (or non-activities) that are nourishing, that give you a sense of pleasure, mastery, or accomplishment, and to identify ways to schedule these into your day-to-day lives. The reason for doing this was to heighten your awareness of all the self-care options that are available to you, so that you can draw on these when pain and stress might be starting to take over and also to schedule them in as a prevention strategy. *Discuss clients' experiences, and write their examples of nourishing activities up on the flip chart. Nourishing activities might include:*

- Call or visit a friend or family member you like to spend time with.
- Have a nice, long, hot soak in the bathtub.
- Read an enjoyable book or do some other enjoyable hobby.
- Make yourself a cup of tea or your favorite hot drink.
- Go for a walk outside.
- Cook a meal for yourself.
- Listen to your favorite music album.
- Do some gardening, housework, or some other household task.

It is helpful to write down your own unique go-to nourishing activities on a small notepad or list that you might carry with you in your wallet or purse, or maybe that you put up on the fridge. Make sure that you include on the list some activities that do not take a lot of planning or energy, so that even during difficult times, there is some activity you can still do to take care of yourself. You might start the list with a brief, gentle, encouraging statement such as "self-care is not selfish; do something today to look after you." With heightened awareness—without being overly vigilant!—you can use this list to nip in the bud early warning signs of pain flare-up or stress overload. The earlier on you catch the warning signs, the less momentum will be behind the flare-up, and the more likely you will be able to better manage and engage in one of these self-care activities and prevent relapse.

Review Whole Course (As a Whole Group, with Flip Chart)

As this is our last session together, arising naturally from this is perhaps a variety of thoughts and feelings about the program ending. So we are going to spend some time to reflect on our experiences during the course of the program. *Reflect on the following questions:*

- When you first learned of this program, what was it that made you decide to join the group? What did you hope to get out of the program?

- Did you get what you had wanted from these groups? Were there any surprises?
- What were the most important or useful things you learned during the program?
- What obstacles do you see that might get in the way of your continuing to practice what you have learned in this program?
- What might help you to overcome any obstacles you see for yourself?

Allow time for clients to share responses to the above questions, writing responses on the flip chart. In addition to this exercise, clients should spend a few moments writing down (just for themselves) their own personal reflections about their experiences over the past 7 weeks.

Your Mindfulness Knapsack

Your "Mindfulness Knapsack" handout is a go-to for reminding you how you can continue to practice daily the skills you have learned, as part of your Mindfulness Maintenance Plan. Throughout the past 7 weeks you have been packing this knapsack with a variety of both formal and informal mindfulness practices, and these are portable skills you can keep in your knapsack to carry forward and bring out regularly during the day to manage chronic pain and stress. (*Go over handout and give clients the opportunity to discuss.*)

The Path Forward

In the absence of the structure of our regular weekly meetings, it can be challenging to develop and maintain your own regular, personalized mindfulness practice. There are a number of options and combinations of options, so likely the practices you each settle on will be unique to you. For the past couple of weeks, part of your take-home activities has been to experiment with which practices work best for you so you can develop your own way forward. What form of practice(s) have you settled on? *It may be helpful to list clients' responses on the flip chart.*

Deciding on a regular practice and sticking with it helps to make meditation simply a part of your daily routine, which helps to keep you on the path going forward, and to maintain the momentum to keep up the practice. Remember though, at the core of mindfulness is kindness to yourself, and keeping a flexible mind. Circumstances change, barriers to practice may arise … keep your practice fresh and be open to modifying your practice to match your circumstances. Having close at hand a favorite guided mindfulness practice or book, or a meaningful quote, can be a strong support for connecting back and keeping up your daily practice of mindfulness.

It helps to develop a plan for going forward on the path of regular daily mindfulness practice and to keep your Mindfulness Knapsack close at hand (as opposed to stuffed in the cupboard waiting to start the journey!), ready and available to you at any time, and especially at times of a pain or stress flare-up. Like learning any new skill, mindfulness takes practice and a key way to keep yourself motivated to do that is to keep your practice regular and to keep your practice fresh. Pain and stress can often times be unpredictable; if we practice mindfulness each day, it becomes a skill that is available to us when we need it most.

Answering the Question: Why am I Doing This?

No matter how good or strong our "resolutions" may be, it seems it is often human nature to "fall off the wagon" so to speak. Research has shown that what helps to keep you on track with your intention to practice mindfulness daily is to link it to a deeply meaningful reason, so that your intention is clearly linked to an answer to the question: "Why am I doing this?" Finding at least one meaningful or positive reason to practice is a powerful motivator and helps to keep up the momentum to maintain your mindfulness practice, and to have pain and stress flare-up prevention and management strategies in place.

For example, one client completing a past program described that having meaningful conversations with loved ones and friends was one of her most valued activities. Prior to starting the program though, she had been feeling sad and frustrated as she was finding that because the pain was demanding so much of her attention and energy, she had started having a great deal of difficulty keeping up with conversations and found she was isolating herself more and more. She was afraid that as a result she was losing "closeness" in her most valued relationships. As the program progressed though, she found that practicing mindfulness made her better able to focus and shift her attention, so that she was no longer "captive" to the pain, realizing that even with the pain, she could still enjoy talking with her loved ones. And when she was having a meaningful conversation, she noticed the pain, but was no longer absorbed by it, and she was able to really *be* with the loved one she was talking with, staying with that experience, despite the pain still being there.

Take a few moments now to quieten your mind, and think about what is it that you value the most in life that you have noticed is fostered, strengthened, or helped in some way by training in regular mindfulness? And when you are ready, when an answer to this question rises to the surface, write what comes to mind down on paper. *Give clients time to think and to write ideas down on paper; this reason for continuing the practice is just for clients, however, if anyone would like to share their experience of this exercise with the group, invite them to do so.*

What you have written down is you own personalized reason for maintaining the practice going forward. You may find that your reasons for practice evolve over time and also that your motivation may flux and change from one day to the next. It is important to watch for decreases in motivation to engage in self-care, and to explore different ways of relating to this experience. Bringing a gentle curiosity so that even in these times, you can find a reason to practice, perhaps even if that is just by seeing that maintaining your practice gives you something within your control that can ground you until the storm passes.

The effort we are talking about in keeping up this practice is not the typical *striving* type of effort you might automatically think of. Instead, this is about holding a deep-seated intention to take care of yourself by being aware of where you are from one moment to the next, keeping some of your attention placed inwards, keeping you in "human being" mode, and allowing you to step out of the more typical "human doing" mode we often find ourselves in when we lose touch with the present moment. Keeping up the mindfulness practice daily keeps you on the path going forward.

The Final Meditation of the Program

Give each client a small object, such as a shell, stone, or bead, and guide clients through a short meditation with the object as the focus of attention in much the same way as they examined the raisin in the first session. Instruct clients to mindfully examine the object, tuning into details such as its shape, weight, texture, how the light reflects off its surface etc. and to intentionally link their reason for keeping up the practice to this object.

At the conclusion of the meditation: the object is a reminder of your experience in having undertaken this program, symbolizing perhaps the hard work you have put in, the time and effort, the insights you have gained, perhaps a shift in your relationship to your pain, and a reminder of all the people you have shared this experience with. Some people have kept this object in their car so that each time they "go somewhere" they are reminded of their time in this program, others have kept it in their purse or desk—perhaps you might choose to keep it somewhere where you see it often and are reminded to continue the process that you have started, to continue to explore learning to live a meaningful life with the pain, and to tune in and listen to your body with kindness and acceptance, to take care of yourself.

Summary

So to once more pull together what we have been learning… *Go over the client summary handout: "Harnessing the Power of the Mind for Chronic Pain Management."*

The Beginning Always Exists in the Present Moment

Each moment is a new beginning. Hold your intention, from this point forward, to stick to your practice as best you can; it's not so much about the form or length of the practice you decide on, as it is about the everydayness of the practice. It is better to fit in only short practices every day during the week, than to only engage in a long meditation practice on a weekend—everyday consistency in your practice is the most important thing, not the duration.

The 3-Minute Breathing Space is an ideal short practice to engage in each day. This technique provides a portable way of tuning in, to see what your experience is, what thoughts, emotions, and feelings in your body are present, and to anchor yourself in awareness a few times a day. Let this practice be your first step in responding during times of increased pain, stress, and difficulty.

Even if you find a period of time has elapsed and you haven't practiced, the moment you pause, tune into your breath, return to the present as if you had invited it—in that moment, you are right back on the path. Each moment is the first moment of the rest of your life. "Now" is all we ever have, and is truly the only time we have to live.

Completion Certificates: present Certificates (*see Appendix D on the website for a template*).

Client Handbook

Session 8 Summary: Harnessing the Power of the Mind for Chronic Pain Management

Over the course of this program, a major theme has been learning that there is another place to stand, another place to view our pain, feelings, thoughts, and circumstances. In being the mindful observer, bringing acceptance to what is (as it *already is*), we see that we can *choose to respond* with wise action, rather than *react* in preprogrammed, habitual, kneejerk ways. In harnessing the healing power of our own mind by bringing mindfulness and acceptance to the situation, we may see that there are other options for skillful action available to us—even if sometimes that means taking no action, this can sometimes be the best action. We let things be as they are, without adding something extra.

Some things cannot be changed, for many of you here chronic pain is and will continue to be a part of your daily experience. Other feelings and situations may also be difficult, if not near impossible to change. Refusing to accept this, we may spend a lot of time resisting this reality, fighting against it, expending fruitless effort to get things to be different in some way from how they actually are—all of which adds baggage and only serves to increase our pain. Even when faced with a situation you desire to change but cannot, you can still respond to this with a sense of dignity and a sense of control. As you have learned in this program, the option to intentionally face all that life brings with an approach of mindfulness and acceptance always exists—is always available to you.

There exists always the possibility to return, to return to the present moment and be anchored, grounded with awareness of your breath. This possibility is as close as the next breath.

The Beginning Always Exists in the Present Moment

Each moment is a new beginning. Hold your intention, from this point forward, to patiently persist with your practice as best you can. It's not so much about the form or length of the practice you decide on, as it is about the everydayness of the practice. It is better to fit in only short practices every day during the week, than to only engage in a long meditation practice on a weekend—everyday consistency in your practice is the most important thing, not the duration.

The 3-Minute Breathing Space is an ideal short practice to engage in each day. This technique provides a portable way of tuning in, to see what your experience is, what thoughts, emotions, and feelings in your body are present, and to anchor yourself in awareness a few times a day. Let this practice be your first step in responding during times of increased pain, stress, and difficulty.

Even if you find a period of time has elapsed and you haven't practiced, the moment you pause, tune into your breath, return to the present as if you had invited it—in that moment, you are right back on the path. Each moment is the first moment of the rest of your life. "Now" is all we ever have, and is truly the only time we have to live.

Your Mindfulness Knapsack: Packed with Portable Pain Coping Skills to Carry Forward

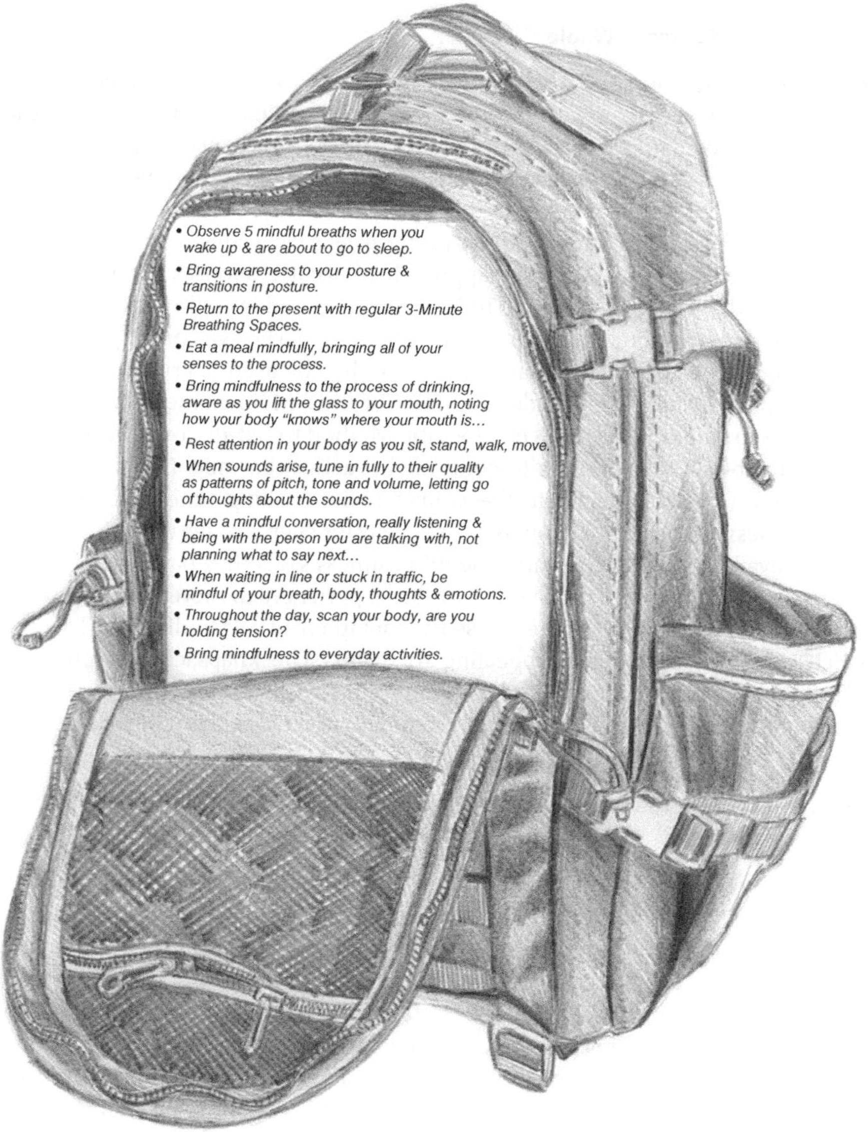
• Observe 5 mindful breaths when you wake up & are about to go to sleep.
• Bring awareness to your posture & transitions in posture.
• Return to the present with regular 3-Minute Breathing Spaces.
• Eat a meal mindfully, bringing all of your senses to the process.
• Bring mindfulness to the process of drinking, aware as you lift the glass to your mouth, noting how your body "knows" where your mouth is…
• Rest attention in your body as you sit, stand, walk, move.
• When sounds arise, tune in fully to their quality as patterns of pitch, tone and volume, letting go of thoughts about the sounds.
• Have a mindful conversation, really listening & being with the person you are talking with, not planning what to say next…
• When waiting in line or stuck in traffic, be mindful of your breath, body, thoughts & emotions.
• Throughout the day, scan your body, are you holding tension?
• Bring mindfulness to everyday activities.

Therapist Tips, Troubleshooting, and Supervision for Session 8

Reviewing the Course as Whole

In reviewing the course as a whole, it is helpful to focus the discussion on the clients' direct experiences with the program, and what insights and learning they have accomplished for themselves through this direct experience. So the idea is not to provide a session-by-session review of what technique was taught when and what themes were covered, but rather to provide a loosely structured way for clients to explore and to reflect on the past 7 weeks via asking open-ended questions, and using a guided inquiry approach to what responses clients provide. During this discussion, it is helpful to be especially cued in to listening for client's reasons and motivation for keeping up the practice, maybe even putting a star next to these responses on the flip chart, as this can then be used as grist for the mill in the later part of the session in development of their Maintenance Plan. It is also important to guide clients using the Socratic Method to self-discover ways to overcome any obstacles or barriers to continued practice that might come up in the discussion. To further facilitate the course review, taking time to go over the "Mindfulness Knapsack" handout is a useful way for clients to see the many options that are available to them, to carry the mindfulness skills they have been learning and practicing forward in to their day-to-day experiences to more effectively manage pain. You might also choose to use the metaphor of a "Mindfulness Toolbox," which might be particularly appealing to males. The knapsack metaphor was selected here to be gender neutral and to highlight the notion of portability and carrying these skills with you during the day, and practicing them "on the go."

Mindfulness Maintenance Plan and Linking to a Meaningful Reason to Practice

Many clients report feeling worried they will "fall off the bandwagon" once the structure of the program is no longer there to support them each week. Thus, an important part of this session is discussing client's Mindfulness Maintenance Plans that they have been working on, and what daily practices they have selected to settle on. There are lots of potential options for practices clients can choose, and emphasizing the "everydayness" of the practice is what is most important, more so than how long one practices. Keeping the practice fresh is also key; so if clients find their motivation wavering, encouraging changing it up by perhaps practicing a Mindful Walking meditation outside is a useful way to reignite the best intentions. Although as the therapist you certainly want to be supportive of clients' goals, it is important to ensure that the plans clients propose are realistic, setting them up for success rather than failure. It is particularly helpful to work with clients to come up with a personalized answer to the question, "Why am I doing this?" Undoubtedly this question will come up in meditation, when we are just sitting there, essentially "doing nothing" ... and so linking the practice to a meaningful reason that clients feel deeply about allows them to reconnect to their motivation, linking the practice back to what it is that clients value in engaging in this daily practice. If clients are stuck and are struggling to articulate a reason, again returning back to the flip chart from the earlier discussion—where clients identified what was helpful to them in the program, and why they stuck with it—can be helpful. It is important that clients know that their reason(s) for maintaining the practice is entirely personal—it is for their benefit—and they do not have to share their reason with the group; however, usually at least one group member values the opportunity to share their experience with this exercise and that is also completely fine.

Concluding the Program: Final Meditation and Completion Certificates

The final meditation of the program entails providing clients with a stone, shell, bead, or some other object to which they anchor their attention. In this meditation, you as the therapist guide clients to explore the object in much the same way as you did with the raisin in Session 1, guiding their attention to qualities such as weight, texture, hardness or softness, light reflections etc. and to intentionally link their reason for keeping up the practice to this object. Many clients really value this object to hold on to going forward as a concrete, tangible reminder of their experiences with the program. I have had clients contact me years after a program ended and on multiple occasions part of their message was to communicate how much they have valued this object, keeping it with them in the car as they travel around; one client even described being crouched over by the pain and still holding this object in her hand as a connection to the present moment and as a reminder that "this too shall pass." You might also consider other ways to conclude the program that perhaps better fit with your client population and within your practice setting; for example, you might choose to provide clients with a copy of Jon Kabat-Zinn's *Full Catastrophe Living*. In our programs we have also always provided a Certificate of Completion (see Appendix D on the website for a template) on a piece of quality thick paper, and while these can serve as documentation, many clients even frame these certificates and feel pride for seeing the program through, completing it, and advancing their pain coping skill set.

Reference

Kabat-Zinn, J. (2013). *Full catastrophe living (revised edition): Using the wisdom of your body and mind to face stress, pain, and illness*. New York, NY: Bantam Books.

13

Integrating MBCT for Chronic Pain with Existing Treatments

The MBCT for chronic pain protocol is designed to provide clients with skills they themselves can use to train their mind and reprogram neurological patterns of pain processing in the brain so that these patterns work *for* them rather than against them in managing pain. For some individuals with chronic pain this approach may function as an effective *alternative* treatment, for most however it will likely be *complementary* to their standard medical care, including pharmacological, physical therapy (PT), and occupational therapy (OT). This brief eight-session program is extremely accessible for clinicians as a standalone alternative or complementary approach that is well suited for incorporation into intensive individual or group-delivered interdisciplinary pain rehabilitation programs.

There are, however, some considerations to contemplate before adapting this treatment to best meet the various contextual factors you may be working with in your own particular clinical practice and/or research setting, to optimize fluidity of integration. In this chapter I will describe some of the ways you can adapt and include the concepts of this approach within existing programs while still maintaining the essence of the MBCT model and treatment framework. This includes specific MBCT exercises that can be delivered in "isolation," how to adapt the approach to fit a transdiagnostic frame, and also brief and long-term therapy delivery options. Inevitably though, you will also come up with other creative ideas not covered here, and I will include mention of a "cognitive blueprint" that you can use as a guide if you are considering making further adaptations.

Delivering MBCT for Pain in Various Treatment Contexts

Including MBCT as Part of an Interdisciplinary Pain Management Program

Most chronic pain management programs (if not all) that describe themselves as interdisciplinary (or multidisciplinary) in nature include a psychological component, even if that component is not delivered by a psychologist (e.g., psychoeducation is often delivered by occupational therapists). Given the breadth and depth of the CBT for pain literature, as well as that CBT is usually included in mental

Mindfulness-Based Cognitive Therapy for Chronic Pain: A Clinical Manual and Guide, First Edition. Melissa A. Day.

Companion website: www.wiley.com/go/day/mindfulness_based_cognitive_therapy

healthcare professional training curricula, I would take an educated guess to say that it is CBT-oriented techniques that are the usual source for the psychological content included in these interdisciplinary programs. Techniques such as guided relaxation, activity pacing, scheduling of pleasant events, assertive communication, and a host of others work particularly well alongside an interdisciplinary approach of titrating analgesic/anxiolytic/sedative medications and increasing physical strength and other critical physical function domains with PT/OT. CBT in this context has been shown to work particularly well and I am not advocating for CBT to be discontinued. My view is though, that if you are practicing in such a clinical context, many of the MBCT techniques have the capacity to be flexibly incorporated into CBT-oriented interdisciplinary programs (as well as programs with an ACT-oriented emphasis) to perhaps make engagement in these psychological programs appeal to an even wider net of clients.

In terms of integrating some of the mindfulness aspects of MBCT into a CBT-oriented interdisciplinary approach: most CBT programs include a guided relaxation module; this could be replaced or interchanged with a Body Scan meditation. Teaching the Body Scan as part of a clinical session is a useful technique that has many benefits beyond a relaxation response (as discussed earlier) and once this technique is mastered, it may be followed by some of the more advanced Seated Meditation techniques if desired. The Mindful Walking and/or Mindful Movement techniques might be integrated during rest/break periods within longer therapy sessions to provide a more structured way to get clients out of their chairs, to stretch, and to refresh their minds at the halfway point of a session. The 3-Minute Breathing Space meditation is another excellent, portable technique that is extremely appealing to clients and may be integrated into any therapist's toolkit. Moreover, the informal mindfulness practices are also another excellent, easily integrated aspect of the MBCT program that can be seamlessly incorporated. The "Mindfulness Knapsack" client handout may be a useful tool to foster discussion of ways to informally integrate mindfulness and to support clients in learning this basic approach to everyday living.

Integrating some of the more CBT-oriented MBCT exercises into interdisciplinary programs is also encouraged, and as they are CBT-oriented anyway they have an inherent capacity to "blend in" and may be used to enhance awareness of automatic, reflexive thinking patterns. This enhanced awareness could then potentially be built upon with CBT-oriented cognitive restructuring, which is theoretically opposed to the mindfulness approach of accepting thoughts without needing to change them, but nonetheless, if delivering CBT and cognitive restructuring specifically, awareness of automatic thoughts is the first step to changing them. The "Stressful Experiences Diary" might be useful for this purpose, along with the "Unhelpful Habits of Mind" and the "Getting Down to the Root of Our Thoughts and Beliefs about Pain" handouts. Some of the other less formal in-session cognitive-therapy oriented activities included in the MBCT program, such as the Session 6 exercises of writing the sentences up on the board starting with "John was on his way to school" and the Alternative Viewpoints exercise (When Our Viewpoints Get Trapped by Thoughts and Emotions) may also be useful for experientially demonstrating the power of automatic thinking habits, and then linking this back to chronic pain. Of course, the Gate Control

Theory from Session 1 and introducing the stress–pain thermometer and ABC cognitive model in Session 2 are textbook CBT-oriented exercises, and the handouts provided along with these exercises in this manual may be a useful addition to your practice to provide a fresh way of explaining these concepts.

Finally, the focus on wellness and "positive psychology" in MBCT might be particularly useful to integrate into a CBT-oriented interdisciplinary treatment where historically the main emphasis has been focusing on changing "negative" thoughts, emotions, and behaviors. It is increasingly recognized how important "positive" thoughts, emotions, and behaviors are in pain coping, and many of the MBCT exercises and techniques provide tools to directly target this "well" focused approach. For example, the "Pleasant Experiences Diary" brings a client's awareness to pleasant experiences in their day and this awareness is built upon in the development of self-care and relapse prevention plans. The Session 7 exercise of identifying "The Relationship between Activity and Pain"—which invites clients to list out how they are spending their days and then to identify ways to integrate into their day more nourishing experiences (including those experiences that bring a sense of pleasure and mastery) and to decrease depleting experiences—represents another way that a "positive psychology" approach might be built into existing pain treatments to enhance client self-care.

As one caveat however, given this program is a skills *building* approach with associated advancing complexity, I do not consider the full treatment package to be a "modularized intervention" with complete sessions being able to be delivered in any random order. The treatment is presented in a planned, intentional sequence in the preceding chapters, where techniques build in complexity to engender graduated enhancement of skill in training the mind through meditation in such a way as to better manage pain. Initially, the focus of meditation is the body and learning to move attention around each body part in turn (i.e., the Body Scan meditation); the body is a tangible object of meditation and holding this as an initial focus, along with the breath, functions to stabilize the mind. As treatment progresses, the object of meditation becomes increasingly less tangible (i.e., transitions to sounds, and then eventually thoughts and difficulties) as skill in using the technique and being able to observe the mind without getting swept away by thoughts advances. Thus, while the first half of treatment is based on enhancing awareness and stabilizing the mind, the second half of the treatment trains in how to *respond* once awareness is enhanced, which is interdependent upon first requiring a stable mind. The CBT components also build on each other and advance in increasing complexity; for example, an initial focus is automatic thoughts, and later in treatment the concept of intermediate and core beliefs is addressed. As in traditional CBT, it would be clinically unwise to approach working with core beliefs prior to a client first establishing skill in working with automatic thoughts.

Caveats for attempting to use this approach in a modularized fashion aside, there is still a great deal of flexibility in terms of the application of the MBCT techniques and exercises. As can be seen from the brief examples in this section, there are *many* ways MBCT can be integrated into existing interdisciplinary pain management programs when it is not possible to deliver the full protocol. Some of my suggested ways for integration (and others that you might identify) may be more or less suitable to your context, timeframe, population characteristics, infrastructure etc. You might like to start just by experimenting with including some of these suggestions and if it fits/works well, perhaps eventually considering implementing the full program. As I will discuss later in this chapter, I have also developed and pilot tested a brief, four-session version of the MBCT for chronic pain manual, and this provides a further option for integration of the approach into an interdisciplinary pain program.

MBCT as a Transdiagnostic Intervention to Target Pain and Comorbidities

In community clinical practice (i.e., practice settings not necessarily a part of a pain clinic service), many adult clients presenting with depression, anxiety, sleep problems, or perhaps relationship difficulties are also likely to have chronic pain (given the widespread prevalence of chronic pain conditions), and vice versa if the presenting complaint is chronic pain (i.e., comorbid emotional problems are the norm, not the exception in chronic pain). Historically, this problem of clients presenting with complex comorbid profiles has been faced via assessment to diagnose what is the client's "primary" problem (or what is impacting functioning the most). The answer to this question has informed the sequence of targeted treatment first to treat the identified primary problem, and then later to tackle secondary complaints. One of the challenges with this approach, however, is that when treating pain, and when other common comorbid conditions such as depression and other emotional problems go untreated (i.e., in cases where they are the identified "secondary" complaint to pain), research has shown that there is an increased likelihood of pain treatment failure and relapse (Bair, Robinson, Katon, & Kroenke, 2003; Linton & Bergbom, 2011).

A more recent emphasis has been on the development of a transdiagnostic approach to treating chronic pain and comorbid emotional problems. A transdiagnostic approach focuses on the mechanism overlap between co-occurring problems, and identifies targeted interventions designed to influence shared mechanisms that cut across diagnostic boundaries (Garland & Howard, 2014; Linton, 2013). In the broader field of mental health, the Research Domain Criteria framework has integrated a range of transdiagnostic, shared mechanisms into a matrix that was updated in 2016 (see: http://www.nimh.nih.gov/research-priorities/rdoc/constructs/rdoc-matrix.shtml) and comprehensively conceptualizes symptom constellations across multiple units of analysis (i.e., genes, molecules, cells, circuits, physiology, behavior, self-report, and paradigms). Notably, both chronic pain and emotion share many underlying neurophysiological pathways, as well as cognitive mechanisms that function to amplify both pain and unhelpful emotions, including avoidance, suppression, attentional bias, memory bias, and negative automatic thinking patterns such as catastrophizing (Garland & Howard, 2014; Linton, 2013). Given this shared neurological and cognitive territory between pain and emotion, the empirical findings that treating just the pain does not always concurrently improve the emotional problem and may actually negatively impact treatment outcomes, might seem rather counterintuitive. However, what this shared territory does suggest from a transdiagnostic perspective is that for pain treatment to be optimally effective in concurrently targeting emotional problems, the specific *shared* mechanisms of both problems must be simultaneously targeted.

From this viewpoint, although yet to be empirically established, the MBCT for pain manual presented here appears to have the capacity to be readily adapted as a transdiagnostic approach to concurrently target both pain and emotional problems simultaneously. Theoretically, the MBCT for pain approach, as described in Chapter 3, is designed to specifically target the shared pain–emotion mechanisms identified by Linton (2013) of avoidance (indeed, meditation in some respects might be considered an exposure-based intervention), open nonjudgmental acceptance (as opposed to suppression), as well as unhelpful automatic thinking patterns, and the memory and attentional biases described by Garland and Howard (2014). Moreover, mindfulness meditation is at the heart of the MBCT program and has been shown to ramp down neurophysiological pathways associated with negative thinking, emotion, and pain, and to engender a decoupling of cognitive–evaluative and sensory–discriminative brain networks (Grant et al., 2011; Jensen et al., 2014).

Based on this, the basic structure of the MBCT for pain protocol may be adapted to be helpful for working with patients reporting a variety of other disorders for which there is an evidence base showing that MBCT is of benefit (such as depression, anxiety, and potentially sleep difficulties and a number of other conditions) (Fjorback et al., 2011). This is an important point as in clinical practice it is rare to treat a patient with *just* chronic pain (or *just* depression for that matter); as noted earlier, the archetypal presentation includes a number of comorbid conditions, most often depression and anxiety co-occurring with chronic pain (Gatchel et al., 2007). In this context, the manual described herein provides a highly structured, yet flexible protocol that can be adapted to suit the specific individual needs of clients with a complex comorbid symptom profile, as well as to address the function of those symptoms within the unique context of the presenting client. Although the preliminary evidence suggests that even without transdiagnostic adaptations the MBCT for chronic pain approach does improve mood, there may be specific clients you work with who require more specific emphasis on comorbid emotional symptoms.

To illustrate how you might go about adapting the MBCT approach to transdiagnostically target comorbid conditions, let's take the example of working with a client who is presenting with major depression and disabling low back pain (which will be the most common comorbid presentation based on the epidemiological data). For this client, you might choose to incorporate into the earlier MBCT for pain sessions some examples and psychoeducational content also pertaining to depression. Of course, the mindfulness meditation techniques taught in MBCT have been shown to improve not only pain, but also emotional regulation, so these techniques may be readily incorporated. Moreover, you might choose to use the guided inquiry to connect the in-session and take-home exercises back, not just to pain, but also to symptoms of depression as another way to easily enhance the transdiagnostic capacity of the manual. Importantly, the manual covers how both thinking and emotions entering into a situation influence our viewpoints, as well as how activity may be useful, and indeed *most* of the exercises have a connection to both emotion and pain—hence these are well suited for a transdiagnostic approach. However, given that, to the best of my knowledge, no research has investigated the utility of MBCT delivered specifically as a transdiagnostic approach, careful, frequent tracking of patient outcomes throughout treatment is critical when delivering this approach in this fashion. Chapter 4 provides detailed suggestions on potential psychometrically sound measures that you might consider using for this purpose.

Alternative Treatment Format and Delivery Mode Options

As described earlier in Chapter 4, the standard delivery of MBCT for chronic pain entails eight, 2-hr sessions, once per week for 8 weeks, within a group-delivered format. This mirrors the format described in the original MBCT for depression relapse protocol (Segal, Williams, & Teasdale, 2002), which in turn followed the format of the MBSR protocol developed by Kabat-Zinn at the University of Massachusetts Medical School (Kabat-Zinn, 1990). Lacking however, is a replicated empirical demonstration that this is the *best* or most efficacious format for delivering MBCT (or MBSR for that matter). Moreover, when considered alongside the building evidence that the time commitment to participate in a traditional MBCT (or MBSR) program is a common barrier for treatment engagement (Day, Thorn, et al., 2014), as well as the mixed findings regarding dose–response relationships, there is reason to seriously consider flexibly applying briefer versions of the treatment approach, which would likely be more feasible and acceptable for many people (Carmody & Baer, 2009; Day, Jensen, et al., 2014). Moreover, for any number of other reasons, the standard delivery format may not fit within your particular setting, client population, or reimbursement procedures.

In one of our unpublished pilot trials that I conducted with Dr. Dawn Ehde and Dr. Mark Jensen (funded by the National Multiple Sclerosis Society; NMSS), we developed and implemented a four-session version of the MBCT for chronic pain manual, included in Appendix F on the website. We implemented the four-session protocol within a multiple sclerosis (MS) population because as part of the pilot process, client feedback was that they were not willing to commit to traveling to the clinic for eight sessions.[1] However, uniformly clients were open to attending four sessions, suggesting this brief therapy was a much more feasible alternative in this setting. Thus, we delivered the four-session version to four individuals with MS-related pain. We obtained (currently unpublished) patient global impressions of change (PGIC) at post-treatment, and found: (1) 50% of clients reported pain interference was "Very Much Improved" and another 25% said it was "Much Improved"; (2) 50% reported pain intensity was at least "Minimally Improved"; (3) pain unpleasantness was rated "Much Improved" by 75% of the sample; (4) 75% reported fatigue was at least "Minimally Improved"; (5) Mood was reported "Very Much Improved" by 50% of clients, and the other 50% reported mood was "Much Improved"; (6) mindfulness was "Very Much Improved" in 75% of clients, and for the other 25% it was "Much Improved"; (7) 50% reported pain acceptance was "Very Much Improved"; and (8) negative pain-related thoughts were reported "Very Much Improved" by 50% of the sample. Moreover, across no PGIC outcome domain did anyone report worsening function; the most negative outcome occasionally reported by one person was that no change occurred. Although this is in essence a case study and these results are preliminary, these results suggest that this four-session version of the

MBCT manual is feasible, tolerable to clients, and holds the capacity to engender clinically meaningful improvement. As mentioned earlier, you might find that this four-session version of the manual is more practical for integration into an interdisciplinary pain management program given that inpatient versions of such programs tend to run over a very compressed, brief period of time.

Within the current healthcare system, reimbursement is typically only available for a small number of sessions; hence brief, action-oriented treatment (as opposed to insight-oriented therapies [i.e., talk therapies] which are long term and suitable for a smaller subgroup of patients) seems most appropriate to meet these constraints. However, despite the commonly experienced reimbursement pressures to engender clinical improvements over the shortest period of time possible, you might be operating within a clinical practice setting where the option for delivering long-term therapy for clients who may be requiring it is available to you. In such circumstances, although MBCT is an action-oriented therapy and it is typically delivered as a brief treatment, it is possible to deliver this approach over a longer period of time. It is most likely that in delivering MBCT for chronic pain as a long-term therapeutic approach that it would best be done within an individual therapy setting. In my own practice, although I find group delivery of MBCT optimal (for the reasons discussed earlier, i.e., group support, social learning etc.), the program can be easily adapted and I have found that it lends itself well to individual therapy. This longer-term, 1:1 approach may be particularly useful for individuals who have severe comorbid psychological conditions thereby justifying a longer-term care plan. However, given it is *chronic* pain we are working with here (i.e., the condition itself is inherently long term), longer programs might be beneficial for many clients, not just those with comorbid conditions.

Core factors to consider when deciding whether to undertake an individual therapy and/or long-term approach to MBCT delivery for a given client would be: (1) the complexity of the case conceptualization, and if the extended intake assessment battery did identify multiple, entrenched maladaptive maintaining factors, to ask yourself, *does MBCT theoretically map onto these maintaining mechanisms?*; (2) if MBCT does map onto identified maintaining mechanisms, *what is the capacity to integrate the above transdiagnostic suggestions into treatment delivery in your practice setting?*; (3) whether shortening the standard 2-hr sessions (which is a long session for individual therapy work) down to 1 hr would be beneficial as 2 hr might be too fatiguing/carry too heavy a cognitive load, and if this is the case, considering if it is possible to extend the treatment out to 16 sessions; (4) whether the option exists of spending more time upfront practicing the earlier meditations that are designed to stabilize the mind before transitioning to meditations where the object of meditation is increasingly less tangible; and (5) if booster sessions following treatment completion may be helpful, which really can be added as a component of both brief and long-term therapy, across both individual and group-delivered formats—indeed, collaborative care models speak to the beneficial nature of step-wise care, and regular, brief therapist contact in monitoring progress and maintaining improvement (Ehde et al., 2014). Again, tracking outcomes and progress is critical for guiding clinical decisions regarding the length of treatment, and if considering a brief or longer-term approach it is essential that regular review of client progress as a function of the length of treatment be routinely incorporated into therapy sessions. If progress plateaus, this should be a red flag suggesting considered thought is needed about whether therapy should progress on the same path, or whether perhaps an alternative therapeutic approach might be warranted and/or more beneficial.

It should also be said that there are a number of "middle ground" options for continued on-going care, booster sessions and follow-up. I described earlier in Chapter 4 that many clinicians delivering MBSR and MBCT include in the program an all-day mindfulness retreat (between Sessions 6 and 7) and I mentioned that if your practice context is well suited to this and you would like to include this as part of your program, Segal, Williams, and Teasdale (2013) provide an excellent description of the possible content to include. Offering this all-day retreat has the added benefit that typically past program participants are also invited to take part both to share their experiences, and to continue a sense of community and shared practice, thereby providing them with a "booster" session of sorts. To meet this same purpose, another option would be to hold bi-monthly or bi-quarterly MBCT sessions that past graduates can attend. Alternatively, a regular open-invitation mindfulness meditation practice session held at your clinic once every week (or less frequently if desired), which could be as brief as 1 hr and could even possibly be managed by past graduates themselves, would provide another option for longer-term continuity of care.

Finally, a promising alternative to traditional in-person MBCT treatment delivery modalities is to harness technology as a means to increase access, feasibility, and/or tolerability. For many individuals with disabling chronic pain traveling for extended periods of time is exceptionally uncomfortable, and for others who live in rural areas, even if they could tolerate traveling moderate-long distances, just the time (and resources, i.e., petrol/gas) spent getting into the clinic may not be practical. Thus, the use of technology such as internet-based, telephone, or Therapeutic Interactive Voice Response approaches may offer a viable alternative to overcome access barriers (Dowd et al., 2015; Naylor, 2008). Based on Dowd and colleagues' (2015) recent research, internet-delivered MBCT for pain has a preliminary evidence base to show that it may be a feasible and efficacious alternative. Additionally, utilizing technology platforms (such as Qualtrics, SurveyMonkey, or other programs) for conducting frequent assessment—whether implementing the treatment online or face to face—is a useful means to track client outcomes (as suggested in Chapter 4) as well as client engagement (i.e., including an online meditation practice record, for example), without the frequent assessment impinging on the time available for the actual session.

Retaining MBCT for Chronic Pain Treatment Integrity

Replication vs. Adaptation: The Question of Too Much Fidelity or Not Enough?

In this chapter I have talked about various ways you might go about adapting the manual described in this text to better meet your unique client needs, service system goals and objectives, and perhaps your own personal needs as a therapist.

You might also be considering further creative ways to adapt the manual even further. However, is there a point at which the approach may have been adapted so far that truly it is almost unrecognizable as MBCT? At what point in the adaptation process does MBCT become something *other* than MBCT? Fidelity is an issue of utmost importance in randomized controlled trials. However, as discussed in Chapter 4 it is also of critical importance clinically. The question of replication vs. adaptation underlies a hot topic within the dissemination and implementation literature; some schools of thought argue that community-based programs should implement exact replications of evidence-based therapy models, and others advocate for recognition of the need to adapt models to population, cultural, system/organizational service systems, budget, and community resource needs (just to name a few) (Mowbray et al., 2003).

While there are arguments to be made on either side, on the research side is the data I described earlier in Chapter 4 that indicate clinically implemented programs with higher fidelity have been found to lead to improvement in client outcomes (Paulson et al., 2002), change in key theoretically specific mediator (i.e., mechanism) variables (Ellis et al., 2007; Hansen et al., 1991), and greater client satisfaction (Day et al., 2016). Other research has also shown that interventions that more closely adhere to the theoretical model of the treatment being delivered exert stronger therapeutic effects (Resnick et al., 2005). Some other studies have not replicated these effects (Perepletchikova & Kazdin, 2005; Perepletchikova et al., 2007); however, even if future research does confirm *beyond a doubt* that fidelity is critical for improved outcomes in the real world, from a clinical practical perspective this would likely not be enough in and of itself to gain local buy-in.

The community-based participatory approach[2] has shown that what is needed for local buy-in is inclusion of community members (e.g., clients and care givers), practitioners, and other key community stakeholders early in the process. Incorporation of their knowledge and expertise into the program (i.e., by adapting the program accordingly) is considered essential to optimize the chance of real-world implementation success. This is consistent with the evidence that has found that as clinicians ourselves, we are more engaged and motivated when we feel that we are exercising our own judgment and expertise in the therapy process (Henry, Butler, Strupp, & Schacht, 1993), so it is only natural that when this happens, implementation success is more likely to occur. Thus, it would seem a reasonable, effective approach to future program implementation of MBCT for chronic pain to find a balance between the two—optimizing both fidelity and buy-in/clinician flexibility—the challenge, though, is to identify an effective way to strike this balance. If you are considering making further adaptations in order to strike this balance, it is worth considering: what elements and order of elements are critical? What might be adapted, omitted, or added to meet community needs and to allow therapists to optimally make use of clinical acumen?

Finding the Right Balance

Mowbray and colleagues (2003) reviewed several different potential approaches to answering these questions and to strike a balance between fidelity and the desirability (or in some cases necessity) to adapt treatments. They describe that at one end of the spectrum is a purely practical approach, where adapting a program is acceptable "up to a zone of drastic mutation" (p. 335). However, as Mowbray and colleagues point out, this guideline entails subjective judgment vis à vis what constitutes "drastic" change. Alternatively, at the other end of the spectrum is an empirically driven approach where dismantling designs are implemented to systematically investigate the role of key program elements, with the idea then that those elements identified as nonessential may be adapted, and those elements found to be essential may *not* be adapted. However, in the non-modularized MBCT approach where skills are integrated and build upon each other, such a dismantling approach would be particularly difficult as it is not only identification of the (non)essential elements that is important, but also identifying whether the sequence of those elements is synergistically important.

Mowbray and colleagues (2003) suggest that a powerful alternative to both the practical and purely empirically driven approaches is to implement a theoretically driven approach where the theory of the model provides a "cognitive blueprint" for guiding what adaptations are viable, while maintaining the integrity of the program (p. 335). In this sense, the implemented program is manual-*guided*, where therapists follow the program's theoretical framework, but not manual-*driven*, where therapy is delivered in a cookbook fashion, thereby preserving the art of skillful therapy delivery (that includes but is not limited to, common therapeutic factors such as warmth, congruence, accurate empathy, Socratic dialogue etc.). Although in efficacy research trials more stringent fidelity procedures are required, in clinical practice a manual-*guided* approach scaffolded by in-depth knowledge of the MBCT theoretical model is likely to be most appealing.

The suggested areas for adapting the protocol that I have described in this chapter follow primarily the theoretically driven approach described by Mowbray and colleagues (2003), while also integrating the (albeit limited) empirical knowledge base available on MBCT for chronic pain. This approach yielded multiple adaptation options, showing that there is a great deal of clinical flexibility in terms of changes and adaptations that can be made with an informed, intentional, organized approach. In thinking about making further adaptations of your own beyond those that I have suggested in this chapter to tailor the approach to your unique setting, client characteristics, and organizational factors, the key emphasis is to stay true to the underlying MBCT for chronic pain theoretical model. Thus, a wise first step would be to return to the description of the MBCT for pain theoretical model in Chapter 3, and to then ask yourself whether the adaptation you are thinking of stays true to the essence of this model. In this way, your decisions are guided by a theoretically sound "cognitive blueprint" for adaptation action.

Summary

There are many potential settings in which MBCT for chronic pain can be incorporated to address the unique needs of a wide range of population types and organizational systems. My collaborators and I have run this program in the

Black Belt region of rural Alabama (with a low-literacy, minority population with heterogeneous chronic pain), in the small urban town of Tuscaloosa, Alabama (with a headache pain population), within a bustling busy hospital in the large urban city of Seattle, Washington (in an MS pain population), and currently I am running the program within a university setting in Brisbane, Australia (with a low back pain population)—and each time the basic MBCT approach has been feasible, acceptable to clients, and of benefit. Researchers have also successfully delivered MBCT online, and I would expect increasingly wider implementation of this mode of delivery. Although in my general clinical work I have found limited need to adapt the program, the four-session brief MBCT manual may be a particularly appealing option when access and time constraints or other barriers are present. Further, both the theory on shared mechanisms and the current evidence suggest that MBCT may be a suitable transdiagnostic approach not only for pain, but also for overlapping symptoms of common comorbidities such as depression, anxiety, and sleep problems. I have discussed multiple other ways in which you can tailor the manual to your particular circumstances, and have described that while the flexibility of this approach is appealing, within that, there are also some basic theoretical and therapeutic principles that should be considered prior to further adaptations, in order to optimize outcome. Ideally future research and clinical experiences will advance the MBCT for chronic pain theoretical model and manual, and will guide more precise decisions on what level of adaptation is possible, or indeed recommended to best integrate the approach into your clinical practice setting.

Notes

1 This treatment was delivered in a hospital setting in downtown Seattle, Washington, USA, and so traffic and access issues are a common barrier for individuals with highly disabling medical conditions at this location.
2 This approach has garnered emerging popularity in the US, with the Patient Centered Outcomes Research Institute (PCORI, 2016) funding initiative.

References

Bair, M. J., Robinson, R. L., Katon, W., & Kroenke, K. (2003). Depression and pain comorbidity. *Archives of Internal Medicine, 163*, 2433–2445.

Carmody, J., & Baer, R. A. (2009). How long does a mindfulness-based stress reduction program need to be? A review of class contact hours and effect sizes for psychological distress. *Journal of Clinical Psychology, 65*(6), 627–638.

Day, M. A., Halpin, J., & Thorn, B. E. (2016). An empirical examination of the role of common factors of therapy during a mindfulness-based cognitive therapy intervention for headache pain. *Clinical Journal of Pain, 32*(5), 420–427.

Day, M. A., Jensen, M. P., Ehde, D. M., & Thorn, B. E. (2014). Towards a theoretical model for mindfulness-based pain management. *Journal of Pain, 15*(7), 691–703.

Day, M. A., Thorn, B. E., Ward, L. C., Rubin, N., Hickman, S. D., Scogin, F., & Kilgo, G. R. (2014). Mindfulness-based cognitive therapy for the treatment of headache pain: A pilot study. *Clinical Journal of Pain, 22*(2), 278–285.

Dowd, H., Hogan, M. J., McGuire, B. E., Davis, M. C., Sarma, K. M., Fish, R. A., & Zautra, A. J. (2015). Comparison of an online mindfulness-based cognitive therapy intervention with online pain management psychoeducation: A randomized controlled study. *Clinical Journal of Pain, 31*(6), 517–527.

Ehde, D. M., Dillworth, T. M., & Turner, J. A. (2014). Cognitive behavioural therapy for indiviudals with chronic pain: Efficacy, innovations and directions for research. *American Psychologist, 69*(2), 153–166.

Ellis, D. A., Naar-King, S., Templin, T., Frey, M. A., & Cunningham, P. B. (2007). Improving health outcomes among youth with poorly controlled type I diabetes: The role of treatment fidelity in a randomized clinical trial of multisystemic therapy. *Journal of Family Psychology, 21*(3), 363–371.

Fjorback, L. O., Arendt, M., Ornbol, E., Fink, P., & Walach, H. (2011). Mindfulness-based stress reduction and mindfulness-based cognitive therapy: A systematic review of randomized controlled trials. *Acta Psychiatry Scandinavia, 124*(2), 102–119.

Garland, E. L., & Howard, M. O. (2014). A transdiagnostic perspective on cognitive, affective and neurobiological processes underlying human suffering. *Research on Social Work Practice, 24*(1), 142–151.

Gatchel, R. J., Peng, Y. B., Peters, M. L., Fuchs, P. N., & Turk, D. C. (2007). The biopsychosocial approach to chronic pain: Scientific advances and future directions. *Psychological Bulletin, 133*(4), 581–624.

Grant, J. A., Courtemanche, J., & Rainville, P. (2011). A non-elaborative mental stance and decoupling of executive and pain-related cortices predicts low pain sensitivity in Zen meditators. *Pain, 152*(1), 150–156.

Hansen, W. B., Graham, J. W., Wolkenstein, B. H., & Rohrbach, L. A. (1991). Program integrity as a moderator of prevention program effectiveness: Results for fifth-grade students in the adolescent alcohol prevention trial. *Journal of Studies on Alcohol, 52*(6), 568–579.

Henry, W. P., Butler, S. F., Strupp, H. H., & Schacht, T. E. (1993). Effects of training in time-limited dynamic psychotherapy: Changes in therapist behavior. *Journal of Consulting and Clinical Psychology, 61*, 434–440.

Jensen, M. P., Day, M. A., & Miró, J. (2014). Neuromodulatory treatments for chronic pain: Efficacy and mechanisms. *Nature Reviews Neurology, 10*, 167–168.

Kabat-Zinn, J. (1990). *Full catastrophe living: Using the wisdom of your body and mind to face stress, pain and illness*. New York, NY: Delacourt.

Linton, S. J. (2013). A transdiagnostic approach to pain and emotion. *Journal of Applied Biobehavioral Research, 18*(2), 82–103.

Linton, S. J., & Bergbom, S. (2011). Understanding the link between depression and pain. *Scandinavian Journal of Pain, 2*, 47–54.

Mowbray, C. T., Holter, M. C., Teague, G. B., & Bybee, D. (2003). Fidelity criteria: Development, measurement and validation. *American Journal of Evaluation, 24*(3), 315–340.

Naylor, M. R., Keefe, F. J., Brigidi, B., Naud, S., & Helzer, J. E. (2008). Therapeutic Interactive Voice Response for chronic pain reduction and relapse prevention. *Pain, 134*(3), 335–345.

Paulson, R. I., Post, R. L., Herinckx, H. A., & Risser, P. (2002). Beyond components: Using fidelity scales to measure and assure choice in program implementation and quality assurance. *Community Mental Health Journal, 38*, 119–128.

PCORI. (2016). Patient Centered Outcomes Research Institute, about us. Retrieved from http://www.pcori.org/about-us

Perepletchikova, F., & Kazdin, A. E. (2005). Treatment integrity and therapeutic change: Issues and recommendations. *Clinical Psychology Science and Practice, 12*, 365–383.

Perepletchikova, F., Treat, T. A., & Kazdin, A. E. (2007). Treatment integrity in psychotherapy research: Analysis of the studies and examination of the associated factors. *Journal of Consulting and Clinical Psychology, 75*(6), 829–841.

Resnick, B., Bellg, A. J., Borrelli, B., Defrancesco, C., Breger, R., Hecht, J., … Czajkowski, S. (2005). Examples of implementation and evaluation of treatment fidelity in the BCC studies: Where we are and where we need to go. *Annals of Behavioral Medicine, 29*, 46–54.

Segal, Z., Williams, J. M., & Teasdale, J. (2002). *Mindfulness-based cognitive therapy for depression: A new approach to preventing relapse*. New York, NY: Guilford Press.

Segal, Z. V., Williams, J. M. G., & Teasdale, J. D. (2013). *Mindfulness-based cognitive therapy for depression*. New York, NY: Guilford.

Conclusion

As with the last session of the MBCT for chronic pain program, this "conclusion" is much more a beginning than an ending. We are still in the infancy of discovering the possibilities of MBCT as a therapeutic framework for pain, which is an exciting time indeed. There is much to learn, identify, and potentially refine to streamline MBCT for chronic pain and to identify the ways in which this approach can be best harnessed to optimize benefit. In this last section I will describe some of the future directions that I consider most critical, although there are certainly other needed future directions beyond those which I describe. More RCTs investigating the efficacy of MBCT for chronic pain are unquestionably definitely needed, however my discussion here will focus on more nuanced research questions pertaining to advancing our understanding of not just whether MBCT for chronic pain is effective, but how is it of benefit and for whom?

We also have much work to do in improving access to psychosocial approaches for chronic pain, and to integrate them into mainstream healthcare. Chronic pain is an isolating condition, and many clients feel alone with their pain and many go undiagnosed and untreated, without the opportunity to learn pain coping skills. I consider that central to dissemination efforts is merging input from both scientists and practitioners alike—what is needed is not just empirical evidence guiding practice, but a complete circle in which practice guides research and future needed evidence. Finally, I will provide some recommendations on resources to further your learning, experience, and knowledge base of psychosocial treatments for chronic pain, with an emphasis on suggestions for extending and deepening your experience in mindfulness-based approaches in particular.

Future Directions

Dose–Response: How Much Meditation is Enough?

Meditation is a popular topic that piques the curiosity of people from all walks of life, and along with that comes any number of more or less educated and informed opinions on the practice. If you take a moment to google the question,

Mindfulness-Based Cognitive Therapy for Chronic Pain: A Clinical Manual and Guide,
First Edition. Melissa A. Day.

Companion website: www.wiley.com/go/day/mindfulness_based_cognitive_therapy

"How much meditation is enough?" as I just did, you will be returned with well over 12 *million* hits. Articles or blogs or other media releases will relatedly tell you about "How much is too much meditation?" "Is too much meditation bad for you?" "How long does it take for meditation to work?" "How long should I meditate to see results?" "What is the best time to meditate for greatest benefits?"... The list goes on. Inevitably you, and/or your clients, will ask one or more versions of these questions. Unfortunately, all of these millions of hits and articles on the matter are proffered in the face of exceptionally very little empirical evidence. However, given the practice of mindfulness meditation has been shown to correspond directly with neurological changes in the brain contributing to observed improvements in pain and coping, a critical question is: what is the optimal "dose" of meditation needed to trigger this beneficial neurological cascade for a given individual?

The current standard in the field is to recommend a blanket 45-min daily formal mindfulness meditation practice for everyone. As I have described throughout the text though, the limited available evidence is inconsistent when it comes to dose–response analyses (i.e., the amount of practice needed for a beneficial response) and to the best of my knowledge, there is little evidence to suggest 45 min is the magical number for everyone. Given that the time commitment entailed in participating in a mindfulness-based program is the most common reason clients decline participation, and that for those who do participate time is commonly described as a barrier to continued engagement, future efforts uncovering precise dose recommendations for a given client with a unique set of circumstances and characteristics (i.e., it is not likely that one dose size fits all) is needed.

Related to these mixed, and limited, dose–response findings for clients, a scarcity of research has examined how long should therapists who are delivering mindfulness-based interventions meditate for? Clinical experience and theory suggest that therapists with a regular practice will be in a better position to embody the qualities of mindfulness and a nonjudgmental attitude, to more skillfully initiate the guided inquiry into clients' moment-to-moment experience, and to build therapeutic rapport (Day, Jensen, et al., 2014). However, the moderating role of therapists' personal practice has not been determined so there are no guidelines for how much past therapist experience in meditation practice is needed *before* starting a program, and how much practice is ideal *during* delivering a mindfulness program. Uncovering the influence of this hypothesized effect and again, identifying at least a ballpark figure of how much meditation is enough would likely be useful for many time-poor and incredibly busy clinicians. The good news, however, is that despite a lack of empirical knowledge regarding how your practice may benefit your clients, what we do know is that in all likelihood it will help prevent burnout and optimize well-being for *you*!

Mechanisms: How and for Whom?

The growing enormity of the problem of chronic pain speaks to the critical need to prioritize optimizing psychosocial pain treatments—including but not limited to MBCT—so that we can reduce the incalculable human, financial, and social costs that living a life with chronic pain entails. To meet this challenge, experts in pain and psychotherapy more broadly agree that a critical next step is to streamline our treatments to efficiently target critical mechanisms and to match clients to the treatment most likely to efficiently maximize benefit (Jensen, 2011; Kazdin, 2009; Thorn & Burns, 2011). Identifying treatment mediators will elucidate *how* MBCT for pain is beneficial, and examination of treatment moderators will inform decisions regarding for *whom* MBCT is most appropriate.

In terms of treatment mediators, Burns and colleagues proposed two overarching frameworks applicable to essentially all various treatment theoretical models that might explain their effects: (1) the *Specific Mechanism Model*, in which treatments work primarily via the mediators/reasons specified by theory (e.g., change in mindful attention during MBCT; see Chapter 3 for a detailed description of the theory-specific mechanisms of MBCT for pain); or (2) the *General Mechanism Model*, where treatments work via a widespread network of shared, not necessarily theoretically specific, mechanisms (e.g., change in mindful attention during CBT) (Burns et al., 2015). Although neither of these models has yet been tested in the context of MBCT for chronic pain, the evidence when applied to other treatments has been mixed. Some findings support the Specific Mechanisms Model, where it has been shown that CBT engenders benefit as theorized (i.e., via change in pain catastrophizing) (Thorn et al., 2007; Turner et al., 2007), whereas other research has found CBT works via change in both pain catastrophizing *and* pain acceptance (a theorized mechanism of ACT), supporting a General Mechanism Model (Baranoff et al., 2013; Vowles, McCracken, & Eccleston, 2007). Future research is needed to clearly elucidate how MBCT may engender benefit, and whether this is a function of whether the individual was well suited to MBCT to begin with (i.e., was "well matched" to MBCT); this would inform streamlining efforts such that only active treatment components are retained for given individuals.

Similarly, we also need to learn when sudden gains are likely to occur, as this has important clinical implications. For example, if change in key mediators is *not* occurring early on in treatment, and if associated sudden gains have not occurred via an identified time point, this provides critical decisional-tree information on whether treatment should proceed or if a change in approach might be needed. Following on from this, we also need to know when sudden *losses* might occur following treatment. Currently we have a very limited understanding of the mechanisms of post-treatment maintenance, continued gain, and relapse; hence, we have less than ideal post-treatment maintenance models informing our relapse prevention strategies.

As touched on above, equally important is to determine *who* is most likely to benefit from the MBCT for chronic pain approach. Turk and colleagues were among the first to formally identify the need to move beyond the "patient uniformity myth" in pain management, recognizing that clients may be more or less suited to one treatment vs. another (Turk, 2005). In Chapter 4, I described some of the most important considerations that have been identified when deciding if MBCT is well suited to a given individual, including pre-treatment preferences, motivation, and expectations (among others). To refine these recommendations further however, uncovering the key moderators of MBCT is needed. In our recent review of the moderation research within the area of pain (Day et al., 2015), we identified that to date, most of this moderation research has focused on patient weaknesses as moderating factors, and has been conducted in an exploratory, post hoc manner. As such, past research has not led to an a priori theoretical framework upon which to build patient–treatment matching principles.

To address this gap, my collaborators and I proposed the "Limit, Activate and Enhance Model of Moderating Effects in Psychosocial Pain Management" (Day et al., 2015). This model makes specific predictions about which patients are expected to respond to which treatments, and accounts for both patient weaknesses (i.e., responses that are either maladaptive and need to be "Limited," or deficits in the use of an adaptive coping strategy that needs to be "Activated") as well as strengths (i.e., skills and resources that could facilitate the efficacy of treatment, and therefore are factors that need to be recognized, utilized, and "Enhanced"). To date, no research has investigated the utility of this model in matching clients to MBCT vs. CBT, for example. However, in proposing the model our intention was that it would spark much-needed investigation into treatment moderators, and move us toward clearly articulated treatment plans for a given client operating in a unique context. This then has the capacity to limit the burden that therapy may place on the client, while also maximizing the use of limited healthcare resources.

Common Factors: More than Just MBCT Techniques and Tools

Common factors of therapy refer to those elements that the majority of psychotherapies have in common and that have long been purported to importantly influence the process and outcome of treatment (e.g., therapeutic working alliance). Although these factors might fall within Burns' and colleagues (2015) *General Mechanisms Model* understanding, they are worth particular mention here as, within the broad psychotherapy outcome literature, Lambert (1992) found in his review that specific factors only accounted for an estimated 15% of the benefits of therapy. This relatively small contribution is likely one critical reason why, when two active treatments are compared, they typically show similar effects on outcome (Day et al., 2012).

Although I discussed in Chapter 3 what we currently know about the role of common factors in MBCT (which is limited), there is one powerful common factor I only alluded to: the so called "placebo effect." The placebo effect is uniformly found across treatments, including biomedical treatments. Verum and sham acupuncture have been reported to produce nearly identical effects on chronic pain intensity (Madsen, Gøtzsche, & Hróbjartsson, 2009). If that is not enough to convince you of the power of placebo, though, a double-blinded RCT found that placebo knee surgery for osteoarthritis (i.e., where patients randomized to this condition received skin incisions and underwent a simulated debridement without insertion of the arthroscope) was just as effective as arthroscopic debridement or arthroscopic lavage in improving pain and function, even at 1- and 2-year follow-up (Moseley et al., 2002). Unfortunately, too few studies have systematically evaluated both specific and common factors (including those variously described as placebo effects) to determine their unique and potentially synergistic effects in psychosocial treatments for chronic pain. Carefully constructed research and clinically informed examinations of these factors are needed before we can conclude how MBCT and other treatments for pain are exerting effects.

Reaching Clients

Improving Access

I wrote recently that chronic pain is an "invisible killer" (Day, 2016). Arthritis, headaches, bulging discs—none of this can be *seen* from the outside, and indeed there is no blood test to measure the amount of pain one is experiencing. Thus, many individuals with chronic pain report feeling alone, isolated, misunderstood, and many become hopeless and see no way forward through the pain and, sadly, many do end their life. Compounding the "invisibility" of the problem even further is that chronic pain tends to go underdiagnosed and undertreated even by primary care doctors and other trained healthcare professionals (IOM, 2011; Tait & Chibnall, 2005). Moreover, when surgeries, medication, imaging, and other biomedical approaches "fail," many of my clients report to me that they have been given the spoken or unspoken message to "just deal with it." And they are left wondering, "but how?"

There is a general lack of awareness in both stakeholders and the general public alike of just how effective psychosocial treatments are in teaching clients a valuable skill set to effectively (and nonpharmacologically) self-manage pain (Darnall et al., 2016). Further, although barriers to receiving skills management training and adequate chronic pain treatment more generally are well documented, we have not established effective means to overcome the barriers underlying these circumstances and we are failing to reach clients. Access and treatment barriers exist in the form of geographical isolation (i.e., large areas of Australia and the US, for example, are rurally located and therefore access to services is limited), socioeconomic constraints, cultural factors (i.e., most treatments have been developed in the context of White, relatively highly educated clients, and have not been appropriately adapted for minorities and low-literacy individuals), and barriers within the healthcare system (i.e., not only reimbursement issues but also barriers in the form of providers who are frequently not familiar with the role of a psychologist in pain management and therefore don't refer for services such as MBCT; Darnall et al., 2016; Day, in press).

Current efforts are underway to identify effective means to begin to reduce these barriers. A core theme of Dr. Beverly Thorn's program of research over the past 10 years has focused on adapting CBT for pain to reduce the associated cognitive demands, and to be culturally sensitive and accessible for low-literacy, minority individuals, and research investigating this approach is promising (Eyer & Thorn, 2015; Thorn, 2015; Thorn et al., 2011). Additionally, Dr. Dawn Ehde and colleagues recently reviewed the literature and reported that internet-delivered, interactive voice response technology, video conferencing, and web-based programs may all be effective in overcoming barriers to treatment access and improving pain outcomes (Ehde et al., 2014). Of course, there is continued debate regarding reimbursement procedures for technology-enhanced treatment delivery in some contexts, likely a function of technology advancing faster than the systems of the institutions affiliated with, and housing the systems. What is still urgently needed, to make chronic pain "visible" and to address systemic healthcare barriers, is continued sustained efforts to educate other healthcare providers and to advocate for government and industry support for psychological approaches to become mainstream treatments for pain within the medical system.

Dissemination and Implementation

Historically there has been a gap between research evidence and clinical practice, and the evidence-based practice (EBP) movement was an attempt to bridge that gap. Sackett and colleagues (Sackett, Rosenberg, Gray, Haynes, & Richardson, 1996) conceptualized the key components of EBP in their "three-legged stool" metaphor, which describes how clinical decisions are optimally informed through: (1) an integration of the best available evidence,[1] with (2) clinical expertise in the context of (3) client characteristics, values, culture, and preferences. This conceptualization has been adopted as the definition of EBP by leading organizations in psychology (APA, 2005). However, just the term "evidence-based practice" is a "loaded" one for many individuals, eliciting strong emotional reactions and viewpoints. Researchers typically express concern that the process of EBP gives permission to clinicians to rely on their clinical experience and ignore the evidence. Whereas clinicians view the evidence as biased (i.e., the strict inclusion and exclusion criteria of RCTs have been described to exclude one-third to two-thirds of presenting clients, and those excluded are described as more representative of what is experienced in clinical practice) and express concerns that the EBP movement will mean others can dictate what treatment they must deliver for a given client in order to be reimbursed (Westen, Novotny, & Thompson-Brenner, 2004).

Personally, as I described in Chapter 13, I think there is a middle ground where both scientists and practitioners can meet, where clinical practice is *guided* (but not driven by) manuals that are supported by evidence and that are adapted for unique client and contextual needs, and where clinicians weave in their in-depth knowledge of the MBCT theoretical model and experience. To me, this is the true spirit of EBP. However, what has been lacking in the field is a systematic effort to complete the circle via intentional integration of clinical experiences to guide research questions. As I mentioned earlier, community-based participatory research is the perfect vehicle to bring together the knowledge and expertise of scientists, clinicians, and key community stakeholders to inform an on-going circle of research-guided practice and practice-guided research. Harnessing an approach such as this has the capacity to more effectively disseminate and sustain the long-term implementation of MBCT and other psychosocial treatments for chronic pain so that they are accessible, feasible, and applicable to clients where they are needed the most: in the real world.

Suggested Resources for Continued Learning

In whatever way(s) you might choose to explore including and/or adapting MBCT for chronic pain, I hope that this text will be a helpful guide and that it may be of benefit. There are also a number of other excellent resources to support and further your learning about MBCT, mindfulness, and psychosocial approaches for chronic pain, and below I provide some suggestions for resources that you might like to consider reading and perhaps recommending to your clients. Given that cognitive and behavioral therapy is so well integrated into most training programs for mental health professionals, most of the resources suggested are intended to deepen your exploration of mindfulness. Although not exhaustive, the suggested mindfulness resources offer further guidance and support on the pathway toward shifting how you or your clients relate to experience (including but not limited to pain), and to move toward an increased sense of wholeness, well-being, balance, and deeper levels of self-discovery in the only moment you ever have: this moment.

Books: Mindfulness (Secular) and Psychosocial Approaches (Alphabetically)

Collard, P. (2013). *Mindfulness-based cognitive therapy for dummies*. Chichester: John Wiley & Sons.

Kabat-Zinn, J. (1994). *Wherever you go, there you are: Mindfulness meditation in everyday life*. New York, NY: Hyperion.

Kabat-Zinn, J. (2009). Mindfulness meditation for pain relief: Guided practices for reclaiming your body and your life (Audio CD series). Louisville, CO: Sounds True.

Kabat-Zinn, J. (2013). *Full catastrophe living (revised edition): Using the wisdom of your body and mind to face stress, pain, and illness*. New York, NY: Bantam Books.

Sears, R. W. (2015). *Building competence in mindfulness-based cognitive therapy*. New York, NY: Routledge.

Segal, Z. V., Williams, J. M. G., & Teasdale, J. D. (2013). *Mindfulness-based cognitive therapy for depression* (2nd ed.). New York, NY: Guilford Press.

Shapiro, S. L., & Carlson, L. E. (2009). *The art and science of mindfulness: Integrating mindfulness into psychology and the helping professions*. Washington, DC: American Psychological Association.

Thorn, B. E. (2004). *Cognitive therapy for chronic pain: A step-by-step guide*. New York, NY: Guilford Press.

Web-Links, Blogs, and Listservs (Alphabetically)

Most of these webpages, include embedded links to a range of resources including links to therapist training and certification programs, free downloadable guided video and audio meditation and yoga practices, drop-in and online classes, reading materials, blogs and more:

MBCT listserv: https://groups.yahoo.com/neo/groups/MBCT/info Oxford Mindfulness Centre: http://www.oxfordmindfulness.org/

University of California San Diego, Centre for Mindfulness website: http://health.ucsd.edu/specialties/mindfulness/Pages/default.aspxl and blog: https://ucsdcfm.wordpress.com/

University of California Los Angeles, Mindful Awareness Research: http://marc.ucla.edu/

University of Exeter, Mindfulness: http://cedar.exeter.ac.uk/mindfulness/

University of Geneva, Mindfulness-Based Interventions: http://www.unige.ch/formcont/caspleineconscience/

University of Massachusetts, Center for Mindfulness: http://www.umassmed.edu/cfm/

University of Wales Bangor, The Centre for Mindfulness: https://www.bangor.ac.uk/mindfulness/

Non-Secular Texts, Websites, and Magazines

Pema Chödrön is a wonderful teacher who seamlessly translates Eastern concepts to reach Western audiences with humor, gentleness, kindness, and clear seeing. As a start, consider reading: *Living beautifully: With uncertainty and change*, or *When things fall apart: Heart Advice for difficult times*. Boulder, CO: Shambhala Publications. A number of her books are also available in the form of audio recordings.

Sharon Salzberg's *The force of kindness: Change your life with love and compassion*. Boulder, CO: Sounds True, provides excellent teaching and instruction that is particularly helpful for learning to work with a harsh, overly critical mind.

If you are a therapist practicing within the context of palliative care or another setting where your clients are experiencing persistent pain associated with terminal illness and/or end of life pain, a wonderful resource for you is a book by Stephen and Ondrea Levine, *Who dies? An investigation of conscious living and conscious dying*. New York, NY: Anchor Books.

Insight Meditation—meditation retreats, classes, and other resources:

- USA: http://www.dharma.org/or www.spiritrock.org
- Australia: http://www.dharma.org.au
- UK: www.gaiahouse.co.uk

Lion's Roar (previously Shambhala Sun) website and magazine: http://www.lionsroar.com/

Mindful, Taking Time for What Matters: brief mindfulness articles applied to a range or various topics: http://www.mindful.org/#'

Mind and Life Institute, mindfulness events and resources: https://www.mindandlife.org/

Note

1 The "best available evidence" is considered practice guidelines or summaries. See the National Institute for Health and Clinical Excellence (NICE) guidelines for examples: https://www.nice.org.uk/

References

American Psychological Association (APA). (2005). *Policy statement on evidence-based practice in psychology*. Retrieved from http://www.apa.org/practice/ebpstatement.pdf

Baranoff, J. H. S., Kapur, D., & Conner, J. P. (2013). Acceptance as a process variable in relation to catastrophizing in multidisciplinary pain treatment. *European Journal of Pain, 17*, 101–110.

Burns, J., Nielson, W. R., Jensen, M. P., Heapy, A., Czlapinski, R., & Kerns, R. D. (2015). Does change occur for the reasons we think it does? A test of specific therapeutic operations during cognitive-behavioral treatment of chronic pain. *Clinical Journal of Pain, 31*, 603–611.

Darnall, B. D., Scheman, J., Davin, S., Burns, J. W., Murphy, J. L., Wilson, A. C., ... Mackey, S. C. (2016). Pain psychology: A global needs assessment and national call to action. *Pain Medicine, 17*, 250–263.

Day, M. A. (2016). Chronic pain: The invisible killer. *InPsych, 38*(2), 26.

Day, M. A. (2017). Pain and its optimal management. In J. Dorrian, E. Thorsteinsson, M. Di Benedetto, K. Lane-Krebs, M. Day, A. Hutchinson, K. Sherman., *Health Psychology in Australia* (pp. 261–281). Port Melbourne: Cambridge University Press.

Day, M. A., Ehde, D. M., & Jensen, M. P. (2015). Psychosocial pain management moderation: The limit, activate and enhance model. *The Journal of Pain, 16*(10), 947–960.

Day, M. A., Jensen, M. P., Ehde, D. M., & Thorn, B. E. (2014). Towards a theoretical model for mindfulness-based pain management. *Journal of Pain, 15*(7), 691–703.

Day, M. A., Thorn, B. E., & Burns, J. (2012). The continuing evolution of biopsychosocial interventions for chronic pain. *Journal of Cognitive Psychotherapy: An International Quarterly, 26*(2), 114–129.

Ehde, D. M., Dillworth, T. M., & Turner, J. A. (2014). Cognitive behavioural therapy for indiviudals with chronic pain: Efficacy, innovations and directions for research. *American Psychologist, 69*(2), 153–166.

Eyer, J. C., & Thorn, B. E. (2015). The Learning About My Pain study protocol: Reducing disparaties with literacy-adapted psychosocial treatments for chronic pain, a comparative behavioral trial. *Journal of Health Psychology*, 1–12.

IOM. (2011). *Relieving pain in America: A blueprint for transforming prevention, care, education, and research*. Washington, DC: The National Academics Press.

Jensen, M. P. (2011). Psychosocial approaches to pain management: An organizational framework. *Pain, 152*(4), 717–725.

Kazdin, A. E. (2009). Understanding how and why psychotherapy leads to change. *Psychotherapy Research, 19*(4–5), 418–428.

Lambert, M. J. (1992). Implications of outcome research for psychotherapy integration. In N. J. C. & M. R. Goldstein (Eds.), *Handbook of psychotherapy integration* (pp. 94–129). New York, NY: Basic Books.

Madsen, M. V., Gøtzsche, P. C., & Hróbjartsson, A. (2009). Acupuncture treatment for pain: Systematic review of randomised clinical trials with acupuncture,

placebo acupuncture, and no acupuncture groups. *British Medical Journal, 338*(a3115), 1–8.
Moseley, J. B., O'Malley, K., Petersen, N. J., Menke, T. J., Brody, B. A., Kuykendall, D. H., ... Wray, N. P. (2002). A controlled trial of arthroscopic surgery for osteoarthritis of the knee. *New England Journal of Medicine, 347*(2), 81–88.
Sackett, D. L., Rosenberg, W. M., Gray, J. A., Haynes, R. B., & Richardson, W. S. (1996). Evidence based medicine: What it is and what it isn't. *British Medical Journal, 312*(7023), 71–72.
Tait, R. C., & Chibnall, J. T. (2005). Racial and ethnic disparities in the evaluation and treatment of pain: Psychological perspectives. *Professional Psychology: Research and Practice, 36*(6), 595–601.
Thorn, B. E. (2015). Reducing the cognitive demands of psychosocial treatments for chronic pain: Clinical research. *The California Psychologist, 48*(3), 11–16.
Thorn, B. E., & Burns, J. W. (2011). Common and specific treatment mechanisms in psychosocial pain interventions: The need for a new research agenda. *Pain, 152*(4), 705–706.
Thorn, B. E., Day, M. A., Burns, J., Kuhajda, M. C., Gaskins, S. W., Sweeney, K., ... Cabbil, C. (2011). Randomized trial of group cognitive behavioral therapy compared with a pain education control for low-literacy rural people with chronic pain. *Pain, 152*(12), 2710–2720.
Thorn, B. E., Pence, L. B., Ward, L. C., Kilgo, G., Clements, K. L., Cross, T. H., ... Tsui, P. W. (2007). A randomized clinical trial of targeted cognitive behavioral treatments to reduce catastrophizing in chronic headache sufferers. *The Journal of Pain, 8*(12), 938–949.
Turk, D. C. (2005). The potential of treatment matching for subgroups of patients with chronic pain: lumping versus splitting. *Clinical Journal of Pain, 21*(1), 44–55.
Turner, J. A., Holtzman, S., & Mancl, L. (2007). Mediators, moderators, and predictors of therapeutic change in cognitive-behavioral therapy for chronic pain. *Pain, 127*, 276–286.
Vowles, K. E., McCracken, L. M., & Eccleston, C. (2007). Processes of change in treatment for chronic pain: The contributions of pain, acceptance, and catastrophizing. *European Journal of Pain, 11*, 779–787.
Westen, D., Novotny, C. M., & Thompson-Brenner, H. (2004). The empirical status of empirically supported psychotherapies: Assumptions, findings and reporting in controlled clinical trials. *Psychological Bulletin, 130*(4), 631–663.

Index

Page references to non-textual material such as worksheets will be in *italics*, while references to Notes will be followed by the letter "n"

Mindfulness-Based Cognitive Therapy for Chronic Pain: A Clinical Manual and Guide, First Edition. Melissa A. Day.

Companion website: www.wiley.com/go/day/mindfulness_based_cognitive_therapy

b

i

o

p

t

u

v

w

y